Serono Symposia Publications from Raven Press
Volume 45

THE STATUS OF DIFFERENTIATION
THERAPY OF CANCER

Serono Symposia Publications from Raven Press

Serono Symposia Publications from Raven Press
Volume 45

The Status of Differentiation Therapy of Cancer

Editors

S. Waxman, M.D.
*Clinical Professor of Medicine
Head, Cancer Chemotherapy
Foundation Laboratory
The Mt. Sinai Medical Center
1, Gustave L. Levy Place
New York, N.Y. 10029*

G.B. Rossi, M.D.
*Chairman, Laboratory of Virology
Istituto Superiore di Sanità
Viale Regina Elena, 299
00161 Rome, Italy*

F. Takaku, M.D.
*Chairman,
The Third Department of
Internal Medicine Faculty of Medicine
University of Tokyo,
Hongo, Tokyo, Japan*

RC 270.8
S73
1988

Raven Press ■ New York

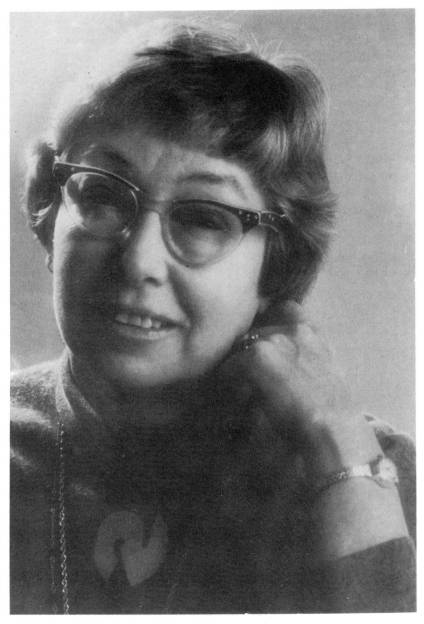

Charlotte Friend, Ph.D

Dedication to Charlotte Friend

On January 13, 1987 Charlotte Friend died of a disease similar to that which she studied throughout her professional life. Her struggle lasted long, always endowed with dignity, relentless work, and lack of self-pity. If psychological defiance of neoplasia could bear a lively fruit, she would have been spared death.

Her illness prevented her from attending the First Conference on Differentiation Therapy, something we both deeply regretted. The organization of a Conference of this nature, first envisaged by Sam Waxman, and quickly joined by Dr. Takaku and myself, sounded as a melody to her ears. In the 60's, when I had the privilege of meeting and working with Charlotte for three wonderful and fundamental years, she was a lonely pioneer. Together with Drs. Pierce, Ichikawa, Sachs and few others, she observed that neoplastic cells did indeed differentiate. Under appropriate conditions, e.g., exposure to dimethly-sulfoxide (DMSO), it appeared, in 1971, that events related to *differentiation* of murine erythroid leukemic (MEL) cells into orthochromatic erythroblasts would override the mechanism(s) leading leukemic cells into indefinite self-renewal. A 2-log difference was observed when DMSO-treated MEL cells were assayed for tumorigenicity in susceptible syngeneic mice. That experiment, though a bit naive, was one of the earliest to test differentiation-related inhibition of tumorigenicity.

It was heartening to Charlotte to know that a group of her distinguished colleagues were going to meet for the purpose of discussing basic and clinical research focused on "differentiation therapy of cancer". Indeed, it showed that her pioneering vision of fighting leukemic cells by reestablishing the physiological control mechanisms of their growth was perhaps getting close to success.

I deeply miss Charlotte's presence and her guidance. Her advice, both professionally and personally, was always astute and on target. This notwithstanding, I am indebted to Sam Waxman for this generous offer to dedicate this Conference, and the Proceedings thereof, to Charlotte. I am certain that the recognization of her contribution to the field of choice of this Conference will undoubtedly harden our resolve to see it through.

GIOVANNI ROSSI

Raven Press, 1185 Avenue of the Americas, New York, New York 10036

© 1988 by Raven Press Book, Ltd. All rights reserved. This book is protected by copyright. No part of it may be reproduced, stored in a retrieval system or transmitted, in any form or by any means, electronic, mechanical, photo-copying, recording, or otherwise, without the prior written permission of the publisher.

THE STATUS OF DIFFERENTIATION THERAPY OF CANCER
(Serono Symposia Publications from Raven Press; v. 45)

International Standard Book Number 0-88167-325-0
Library of Congress Catalog Number 87-043067

Papers or parts thereof have been used as camera-ready copy as submitted by the authors whenever possible; when retyped, they have been edited by the editorial staff only to extent considered necessary for the assistance of an inter-national readership. The views expressed and the general style adopted re-main, however, the responsibility of the named authors. Great care has been taken to maintain the accuracy of the information contained in the volume. However, neither Raven Press, Serono Symposia, nor the editors can be held responsible for errors or any consequences arising from the use of information contained herein.

The use in this book of particular designations of countries or territories does not imply any judgment by the publisher or editors as to the legal status of such countries or territories, of their authorities or institutions or of the delimi-tation of their boundaries.

Some of the names of products referred to in this book may be registered trade marks or proprietary names, although specific references to this fact may not be made; however, the use of a name with designation is not to be con-strued as a representation by the publisher or editors that it is in the public do-main. In addition, the mention of specific companies or of their products or proprietary names does not imply any endorsement or recommendation on the part of the publisher or editors.

Authors were themselves responsible for obtaining the necessary permission to reproduce copyright material from other sources. With respect to the pub-lisher's copyright, material appearing in this book prepared by individuals as part of their official duties as government employees is only covered by this copyright to the extent permitted by the appropriate national regulations.

Printed in Rome, Italy
by Christengraf

Preface

In the last decade research on the mechanisms which control normal and neoplastic cell growth and differentiation has received a tremendous impetus. The discovery of biological response modifiers, oncogenes, specific genetic regions encoding for growth factors and their receptors and messengers, combined with the understanding of complex regulatory processes at the molecular level, has shed new light on the possibility of utilizing differentiation therapy as a practical treatment.

The Conference on Differentiation Therapy, which had its first meeting in Sardinia in 1986, and its second in Bermuda in 1987, was established with this purpose in mind. The goals of this three-year workshop are to bring together scientists, all of whom are working on different aspects of this multifaceted problem, to establish collaborations, share data and materials, and discuss the efficacy of differentiation therapy of cancer. The organization is comprised of ten working sub-groups, has nearly 150 participants, and covers virtually every aspect of the field from its molecular biology through its use in clinical trials.

These Proceedings, published a few months after the Second Conference, are aimed at providing the reader with an up-to-date overview of the status of differentiation therapy, with emphasis on the progress made by the entire group in the last year. The reports of the various co-chairman and several of the plenary speakers are presented in this volume.

We are indebted to Ares-Serono Symposia for sponsoring and organizing the Second Conference, and want to acknowledge the following organizations for their sponsorship of the First Conference: Industria Farmaceutica Serono, Prodotti Roche Itàlia, Boehringer Ingelheim, Wellcome Italia, the National Institutes of Health, Eizai Co. Ltd Japan, Samuel Waxman Cancer Research Foundation, Schering Plough Inc., Beckman Analytical, Gruppo Flow, Merck Sharp and Dohme, Pfizer Italiana, Chemotherapy Foundation, E.I. Du Pont de Nemours and Co., Bristol Myers Co., Farmitalia Carlo Erba, Pfizer Inc., Sclavo, Upjohn Co., Cetus Corp.

Plans for the Third Conference, which will be held in Sardinia in September, 1988, are underway.

Finally, we would like to thank Francine Zuckerman for her efforts and invaluable service in compiling this volume.

November, 1987   SAMUEL WAXMAN, M.D.

Contents

Future Strategies

Contributors

J.P. Abita
Institute de Recherches sur les Maladies du Sang
Hopital St. Louis - Place du Dr. Fornier
Paris, France

P. Alexander
CRC Medical Oncology Unit
Southampton General Hospital
Southampton SO9 4X9, England

T.L. Breitman
Laboratory of Biological Chemistry
Division of Cancer Treatment
National Cancer Institute
National Institutes of Health
Bethesda, MD 20892
USA

P. Calabresi
Dept. of Medicine
Roger Williams Avenue
Providence, RI 02908
USA

E.H. Chang
Dept. of Pathology
Uniformed Services University of Health Sciences
F. Edward Hebert School of Medicine
4301 Jones Bridge Road
Bethesda, MD 20814
USA

K. Christman
Molecular Biology Division
Michigan Cancer Center
110 East Warren St.
Detroit, MI 48201
USA

L. Degos
Institute de Recherches sur les Maladie du Sang
Hopital St. Louis - Place du Dr. Fournier
Paris, France

T.M. Dexter
Paterson Laboratories
Christie Hospital
Wimslow Road
Withington, Manchester M209 BX, England

J. Egorin
Department of Developmental Therapeutics
University of Maryland Cancer Center
655 West Baltimore Street
Baltimore, MD 21201
USA

J. Fingert
Department of Surgery
The Cox Building
Massachusetts General Hospital
Boston, MA 02114
USA

G.E. Francis
Dept. of Hematology
The Royal Free Hospital
Pond Street
Hampstead, London NW3, 3QG, England

R.M. Friedman
Dept. of Pathology
Uniformed Services University of Health Sciences
F. Edward Hebert School of Medicine
4301 Jones Bridge Road
Bethesda, MD 20814
USA

F. Gavosto
1 Clinica Medica
University of Turin
Via Genova, 3
10126 Turin, Italy

J.A. Hickman
Cancer Research Campaign
Experimental Cancer
Chemotherapy Research Group
University of Aston at Birmingham
Gosta Green
Birmingham, England

M. Hozumi
Dept. of Chemotherapy
Saitama Cancer Center Research
Institute
Saitama-Ken 362, Japan

E. Huberman
Division of Biological and Medical
Research
The University of Chicago
Argonne National Laboratories
9700 South Cass Avenue
Argonne, IL 60439
USA

D.E. Ingber
Dept. of Surgery
The Children's Hospital
300 Longwood Avenue
Boston, MA 02115
USA

Y.S. Kim
Dept. of Medicine
University of California School of
Medicine
4150 Clement Street
San Francisco, CA 94143
USA

R. Lotan
Biology Section
The University of Texas
M.D. Anderson Hospital and Tumor
Institute
5723 Bertner Avenue
Houston, TX 77030
USA

P.A. Marks
Memorial Sloan Kettering Cancer
Center
1275 York Avenue
New York, NY 10021
USA

D. Medina
Dept. of Cell Biology
Baylor College of Medicine
Houston, TX
USA

F.L. Meyskens, Jr.
Arizona Cancer Center
Section of Hematology and Oncology
The University of Arizona
Tucson, AZ
USA

M.A.S. Moore
Laboratory of Developmental
Hematopoiesis
Memorial Sloan Kettering Cancer
Center
1275 York Avenue
New York, NY 10021
USA

M. Oishi
Institute of Applied Microbiology
University of Tokyo
Bunkyo-ku, Japan

J. Paul
Beatson Institute for Cancer Research
Garscube Estate
Switchback Road
Glasgow, Scotland

C.M. Pinsky
Biological Resources Branch
Frederick Cancer Research Facility
NCI, DHHS
Frederick, MD 21701
USA

H.D. Preisler
Roswell Park Memorial Institute
666 Elm Street
Buffalo, NY 14263
USA

A. Raza
Roswell Park Memorial Institute
666 Elm Street
Buffalo, NY 14263
USA

R.A. Rifkind
Sloan Kettering Institute
Memorial Sloan Kettering Cancer
Center
1275 York Avenue
New York, NY 10021
USA

D. Roop
Laboratory of Cellular Carcinogenesis
DCE, NCI, NIH
Bethesda, MD 20892
USA

G. Rossi
Laboratory of Virology
Ist. Superiore di Sanità
Viale Regina Elena, 299
00161 Rome, Italy

P. Rowley
Division of Medical Genetics
University of Rochester School of
Medicine and Dentistry
Rochester, NY 14642
USA

R.E. Scott
Section of Experimental Pathology
Mayo Medical School
Mayo Clinic/Foundation
Rochester, MN 55905
USA

M. Sherman
Director of Oncology
Hoffman-La Roche, Inc.
Nutley, NJ 07110
USA

F. Sigaux
Institut National de la Santé et de la
Recherche Medical
Hôpital St. Louis
Paris, France

F. Takaku
The Third Departments of Internal
Medicine
Faculty of Medicine
University of Tokyo
Hongo, Tokyo, Japan

T. Watanabe
Institute of Applied Microbiology
University of Tokyo
Bunkyo-ku, Japan

S. Waxman
Division of Medical Oncology
Mt. Sinai School of Medicine
1 Gustave L. Levy Place
New York, NY 10029
USA

M. Weimann
Dept. of Medicine
Brown University
Roger Williams Hospital
825 Chalkstone Avenue
Providence, RI 02908
USA

S.H. Yuspa
Laboratory of Cellular Carcinogenesis
DCE, NCI, NIH
Bethesda, MD 20892
USA

DIFFERENTIATION CONTROL IN NORMAL AND NONTRANSFORMED CELLS

Cellular Differentiation and the Prevention and Treatment of Cancer

R.E. Scott, M. Edens, D.N. Estervig, M. Filipak, B.J. Hoerl,
B.M. Hsu, P.B. Maercklein, P. Minoo, C.-Y. Tzen,
M.R. Wilke and M.A. Zschunke

Section of Experimental Pathology
Mayo Clinic/Foundation
Rochester, MN 55905

INTRODUCTION

Numerous approaches have been developed to treat cancer and
new approaches are currently being sought to prevent cancer. The
traditional approach to treat cancer employs the use of cytotoxic
agents that attempt to selectively kill the cancer cells. Cytotoxic chemotherapy has provided valuable treatments for many
types of cancers in the past 20 years but it has significant
limitations and side effects.

Another approach for cancer chemotherapy is to inhibit cancer
cell growth without cytotoxicity. This new concept specifically
attempts to induce terminal differentiation in cancer cells so
that they remain viable but irreversibly lose their proliferative
potential. In this regard, the goal of many current studies is
to identify pharmacological and/or physiological agents that
effectively induce the selective loss of proliferative potential
in cancer cells without affecting normal stem cells. Notwithstanding the attractiveness of this approach to cancer therapy,
the mechanisms that mediate the irreversible loss of a cell's
proliferative potential are very poorly defined.

The final new concept for cancer therapy involves the attempt
to induce cancer cells to revert to a nontransformed and essentially normal physiological state in which they retain their
viability and their ability to reproduce. From this perspective
the ideal cancer remedy would be to identify approaches to make
cells resistant to neoplastic transformation and thereby prevent
the process of carcinogenesis. For the sake of discussion in
this paper, we define the process by which cells are made
resistant to neoplastic transformation as "anticancer activity"

and the process by which cancer cells are induced to revert to
a nontransformed state as "cancer suppressor activity."

Figure 1 specifically illustrates the concepts described
above for cancer prevention and therapy and suggests that anticancer and cancer suppressor activity can be induced by nonterminal differentiation whereas the induction of the loss of
proliferative potential is mediated by the process of terminal
differentiation.

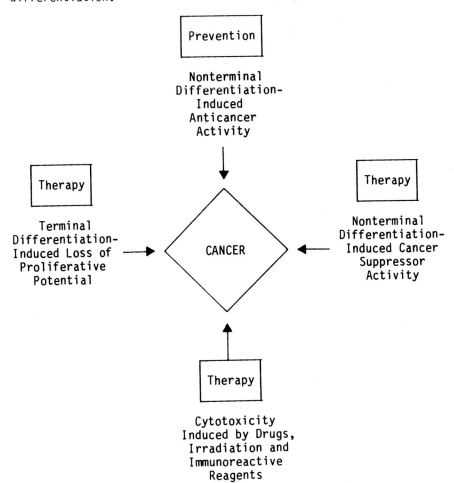

FIG. 1. Biological concepts for cancer prevention and therapy.

The current paper specifically summarizes the results of our
studies on murine mesenchymal stem cells and human keratinocyte
progenitor cells with respect to mechanisms which induce the
irreversible loss of proliferative potential associated with

cellular differentiation. In addition, this paper reviews
evidence that nonterminal differentiation can specifically induce
anticancer activity and cancer suppressor activity in cells that
retain their stem cell characteristics.

Mechanisms that Mediate the Irreversible Loss of Proliferative Potential

A. Murine mesenchymal stem cells.

Experiments performed during the past decade have established
that the controls of proliferation and differentiation are integrally regulated processes (18,23). In this regard, Figure 2
illustrates the results of our studies on cultured 3T3 T mesenchymal stem cells in diagrammatic form. First, it shows that
rapidly growing cells can undergo growth arrest if the culture
medium is deprived of essential growth factors. This type of
state can also be induced by the process termed contact
inhibition and it has been referred to as the G_0 restriction
point (14). Although mesenchymal stem cells can arrest proliferation at this state, the available evidence suggests that
such cells are not able to differentiate (18). However, we
established that prior to adipocyte differentiation, 3T3 T
mesenchymal stem cells must arrest their growth at a distinct
predifferentiation state (18) that has been functionally and
biochemically characterized (2,5,25,26,38,40). Recent preliminary studies also suggest that a specific protein factor(s)

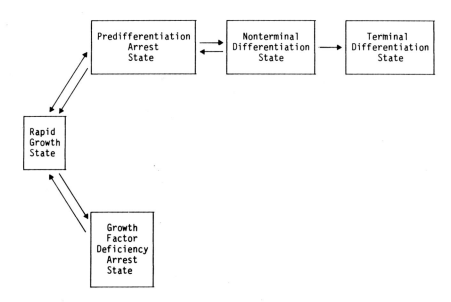

FIG. 2. Model for the integrated control of proliferation and
differentiation in mesenchymal stem cells.

that is present in human plasma and serum acts to induce growth arrest at this specific state. Once cells arrest their growth at this predifferentiation state, they acquire the potential to differentiate if they are not first induced to reinitiate pro-liferation by the addition of mitogenic factors. In this regard, it should be stressed that the predifferentiation arrest state is pivotal because such cells can make decisions to either differentiate or to reinitiate proliferation depending on the availability of growth factors or differentiation factors in the medium.

If the culture conditions are appropriate to support differentiation, at least two steps are involved. First, the growth arrested cells undergo nonterminal differentiation wherein they develop an adipocyte morphology yet retain their prolifera-tive potential (11). This process of nonterminal differentiation can be induced by a variety of factors including plasma/serum factors, insulin, dexamethasone, methyl isobutyl xanthine, and certain prostaglandins. It is also inhibited by TGF-ß (27) and TPA (40). Nonterminally differentiated cells can also be induced to dedifferentiate if treated with retinoic acid, TPA, or other reagents (34).

During the process of nonterminal differentiation cells not only acquire a completely differentiated phenotype but they also down regulate their response to growth factors even though this does not prevent the nonterminally differentiated cells from growing if exposed to a high concentration of appropriate growth factors. For example, whereas predifferentiation growth arrested cells can be induced to proliferate with 5% FCS, nonterminally differentiated adipocytes require 30% FCS + 50 µg/ml insulin to express a maximum response (Hoerl and Scott, manuscript in preparation).

The final step in the differentiation process in mesenchymal stem cells is the actual irreversible loss of proliferative potential. To define as carefully as possible the mechanisms that mediate the irreversible loss of proliferative potential, we have performed a series of biological, biochemical, and molecular studies. First, we have purified 20,000-fold a human plasma protein that induces the terminal event in differentiation, i.e., the irreversible loss of proliferative potential. This protein, designated aproliferin, can convert nonterminal cells to terminal cells within 12 hours of exposure (33). The mechanism by which aproliferin mediates this effect is still under investigation. Experiments are also in progress to prepare an anti-aproliferin monoclonal antibody. We have in addition clearly demonstrated that protein synthesis is required for the terminal event in differentiation (33), that the expression of less than 10 pro-teins occurs during the process of terminal differentiation (35), and that cell clones can be isolated that are defective in their ability to undergo the terminal event in differentiation (32). The most interesting of these proteins is a 36 kd basic nuclear protein (BNP-36) that is lost during the process of terminal

differentiation. The use of monoclonal antibodies to BNP-36
shows cross reaction with heat shock protein 90 and shows that
BNP-36 is conserved throughout evolution (Minoo and Scott,
manuscript in preparation). Additional studies are currently in
progress to further characterize the structure and function of
this potentially highly significant protein as are experiments to
clone and characterize the gene for BNP-36.

   In summary, at the present time it is our hypothesis that
the terminal event in mesenchymal stem cell differentiation is
mediated by specific extracellular aproliferin-like factors that
modulate important biochemical and molecular events that irreversibly change the expression of proteins required for cellular
proliferation. Since it clearly has been established that
neoplastic or preneoplastic cell clones can specifically lose the
ability to undergo the terminal event in differentiation, we
suggest that a major advance in cancer therapy could result if
specific approaches/drugs could be found that selectively induce
the terminal event in differentiation in such aberrant cells.
Several recent studies have in fact suggested that terminal
differentiation-inducing agents exist that act on hematopoietic
neoplasms especially erythroid/myeloid leukemias (19).

   The most frequent cancers in humans, however, are epithelial
malignancies. Therefore, it is important not only to study the
mechanisms for the control of proliferation and differentiation
in mesenchymal cells but also such control mechanisms in normal
and transformed human epithelial cells.

   B. Human skin epithelial cells.

   The development of serum free and defined medium for the
culture of normal human skin epithelial cells (31)•has made it
possible to accurately study the biological mechanisms that
regulate their proliferation and differentiation (16,37).
Figure 3 summarizes the results of our studies and demonstrates
that proliferation and differentiation are also integrally
regulated in these cells. More specifically, during the
differentiation process cells first undergo reversible growth
arrest, then irreversibly lose their proliferative potential, and
finally express a terminally differentiated phenotype (Wilke and
Scott, manuscript in preparation).

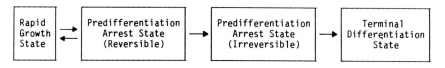

FIG. 3. Model for the integrated control of proliferation and
differentiation in normal human skin epithelial cells.

   Comparison of Figures 2 and 3 demonstrates that mesenchymal
stem cells and normal human skin epithelial cells show certain
similarities and certain differences. Both cell types, for

example, undergo reversible growth arrest prior to differentiation and in both cell types the process of differentiation
involves multiple steps. However, in 3T3 T stem cells, reversible predifferentiation growth arrest occurs at a distinct G_1
cell cycle state whereas in normal human skin epithelial cells
predifferentiation growth arrest can occur either in G_1 or G_2
(Table 1). Other differences also exist. In mesenchymal stem
cells following reversible predifferentiation growth arrest,
nonterminal differentiation occurs prior to loss of proliferative
potential, i.e., terminal differentiation. In contrast, in human
skin epithelial cells the irreversible loss of proliferative
potential occurs before the final step in overt keratinocyte
differentiation.

TABLE 1. Growth arrest and differentiation characteristics of
cultured normal human skin epithelial cells

Initial type growth arrest state[a]	Growth arrest inducing agent/process	Predominant cell cycle arrest state	Potential to express the terminally differentiated phenotype without cell cycle Progression
Reversible	TGF-β	G_1	+
	Ethionine	G_1	+
	Isoleucine deficiency	G_1	+
	Growth factor deficiency[b]	G_1	+
Irreversible	Razoxane	G_2	+
	Senescence	G_1	+
	TPA	G_1/G_2	+

[a]If cells are maintained at a reversible growth arrest state for
an extended interval, some cells progress or decay into an
irreversible growth arrest state.
[b]The growth arrest state induced by growth factor deficiency is
complex and can rapidly progress to a state of terminal
differentiation.

The differences between these two cell types could result from
numerous factors. 3T3 T murine cells of mesenchymal origin are
immortalized and aneuploid whereas the human cells are normal,
mortal, diploid, and of epithelial origin. In our opinion, the
most important difference is that 3T3 T cells exhibit stem cell
characteristics of being able to differentiate into multiple
cell types whereas cultured normal human skin epithelial cells

actually represent unipotential keratinocyte progenitor cells. Evidence for this latter conclusion is that the normal human keratinocytes that grow in culture are primarily derived from suprabasal skin cells and therefore cannot by definition represent stem cells (Wilke and Scott, manuscript in preparation). Furthermore, when cultured skin cells are transplanted onto patients, no evidence of differentiation into nonkeratinocytes can be detected (15).

With respect to this review, the most important aspect of these observations concerns the mechanisms by which normal human keratinocyte progenitor cells can be induced to irreversibly lose their proliferative potential. Although these studies are still in progress, the available data strongly suggest that 1) the irreversible loss of proliferative potential occurs prior to the expression of overt terminal differentiation, 2) the irreversible loss of proliferative potential can occur as a sequential event following reversible predifferentiation growth arrest, and 3) that exposure of growth arrested cells to high calcium concentration accelerates the process of terminal differentiation. Most interesting, the terminal differentiation of normal human keratinocyte progenitor cells also appears to be associated with a marked reduction in the expression of the same unique 36 kd basic nuclear protein that is associated with the irreversible loss of proliferative potential during mesenchymal stem cell terminal differentiation (Minoo and Scott, manuscript in preparation). We therefore speculate that similar mechanisms may mediate the irreversible loss of proliferative potential in many cell types.

C. Preneoplastic and neoplastic human and murine cells.

Numerous clones of preneoplastic and neoplastic human and murine cells have been developed in our laboratory during the past 10 years and essentially all of these cell clones show significant defects in their ability to respond to signals that induce terminal differentiation and/or the irreversible loss of proliferative potential (24,36,39). Although such defects need not be absolute, they are expressed in the vast majority of these cell populations. For example, we recently established that a line of human squamous carcinoma cells (SCC-25) is clearly defective in its ability to irreversibly lose its proliferative potential/terminally differentiate even under the most stringent differentiation-promoting conditions (Scott et al., manuscript in preparation).

If all preneoplastic and neoplastic cells express significant defects in their ability to irreversibly lose their proliferative potential either at a predifferentiation state or in association with terminal differentiation, how will it be possible to develop therapeutic approaches that induce such aberrant cells to become terminal? Another significant question concerns whether it is reasonable to strive to develop new cancer therapies that are designed to selectively induce the irreversible loss of proliferative potential in cancer cells without affecting normal stem/progenitor cell populations. What advantage does this approach have over traditional cytotoxic chemotherapy which also must be specifically targeted to affect cancer cells while sparing normal stem/progenitor cells?

The best answer to these questions, in our opinion, is more research. Before we can answer these questions, we must first understand in much greater detail the biological, biochemical, and molecular mechanisms that make cells irreversibly lose their proliferative potential. Hopefully, the results of future studies will clearly define an approach by which cancer cells selectively can be induced to irreversibly lose their proliferative potential by specific pharmacological reagents and thereby to be removed from the malignant cell pool.

Since a major focus of our research is to discover the mechanisms that mediate regulation of the irreversible loss of proliferative potential, we plan to continue our studies on the two excellent model systems described in this review. Our goal will be to identify specific factors that affect cancer cells and thereby prevent their further division. We also plan to establish the molecular basis that mediates the irreversible loss of proliferative potential especially the role of BNP-36. Our goal in these studies will be to discover new therapeutic approaches that can make cancer cells undergo terminal growth arrest while protecting the proliferative potential of normal stem cells.

Mechanisms to Induce Anticancer and Cancer Suppressor Activity

The Introduction of this article reviewed our definitions of the terms anticancer activity and cancer suppressor activity. To reiterate, anticancer activity is defined as the process by which cells are made resistant to agents that cause neoplastic transformation and cancer suppressor activity is defined as the process by which cancer cells are induced to revert to a non-transformed state. Although it is possible that these two activities may be mediated by similar molecular processes, they are discussed separately in the following sections because this topic is extremely new and because so much information must still be obtained concerning these processes.

A. Anticancer activity.

Three important questions can be asked about anticancer activity. What is the evidence it really exists? What are the mechanisms that mediate this activity? How is the expression of anticancer activity regulated?

Evidence that anticancer activity exists can be obtained from a variety of experimental studies. First and perhaps most significant is the observation that cultured normal human cells are extremely resistant to experimentally induced carcinogenesis whereas rodent cells are much more easily transformed (4,20). This observation, which has been made by numerous investigators, suggests that certain cell types possess mechanisms that make them resistant to malignant transformation. Second, studies by Anders and Anders (1) have demonstrated that resistance to neoplastic transformation in vivo is acquired during neonatal development. This suggests that anticancer activity is an acquired characteristic. Finally, recent studies have established that specific genes may be involved in conveying resistance to malignant transformation. The hallmark of this type of gene is the Rb-1 gene that appears to convey resistance to the development of retinoblastoma in humans (6). This gene has been cloned and it is thought that the development of defects in related genes may also have a significant role in a variety of other human concerns such as osteosarcoma, Wilm's tumor, and others.

The mechanisms that mediate resistance to malignant transformation are however completely unknown. Since anticancer activity can be demonstrated to a variety of physical and chemical carcinogens and also to oncogenic viruses, a unique mechanism probably is involved in effecting anticancer activity. The mechanisms that regulate the expression of anticancer activity are, however, becoming more clear as a result of our recent studies that are now briefly reviewed.

In order to study the mechanisms for regulation of the expression of anticancer activity we chose to study a cell line that is nontransformed in its native state but which can be efficiently transformed by a variety of carcinogens. Since we wanted to study the role of differentiation in the regulation of anticancer activity, we also chose to employ a cell line whose proliferation and differentiation were well characterized and could be easily controlled, i.e., 3T3 T mesenchymal stem cells.

In this regard, 3T3 T cells can be transformed by UV irradiation and by various chemical carcinogens, including 4-nitroquinoline N-oxide (4NQO), 9,10-dimethyl-1,2-benz-anthracene (DMBA), 20-methyl-cholanthrene (MCA), N-methyl-N'-nitro-N-nitroguanidine (MNNG), and propane sultone (PS). We have therefore asked if the induction of nonterminal differentiation could induce anticancer activity in these cells and make them resistant to transformation. Since the in vitro type III focus transformation assay has been established to show an excellent correlation with the expression of in vivo tumorigenicity with this cell system (13,30), our initial studies employed the in vitro assay method.

We specifically compared the transformation characteristics of cell clones derived from rapidly growing 3T3 T stem cells and clones derived from nonterminally differentiated 3T3 T adipocytes. We also studied cell clones derived from pre-differentiation growth arrested 3T3 T cells and cell clones derived from 3T3 T cells that were growth arrested due to growth factor deficiency. Cell populations were prepared at each state and maintained thereat for 4 to 8 days. Thereafter, they were passaged at low density into petri dishes containing cloning microchips (32) and chips containing single cells were

subsequently grown as clonal cell lines. In the case of nonterminally differentiated adipocytes, the differentiated morphology
persisted for approximately 2 to 4 population doublings but then
such cells reverted, i.e., dedifferentiated, to an undifferentiated state. Each clonal line was then grown until approximately
1×10^7 cells were available to evaluate for their transformation
characteristics. Since the most potent carcinogen for native
3T3 T stem cells involves exposure to 90 erg/mm^2 UV irradiation
or 100 ng/ml 4NQO treatment for 24 hours, we required that the
cell clones designated to express anticancer activity had to show
no evidence of transformation with either of these agents nor any
evidence of spontaneous transformation.
    The results of these studies clearly establish that
nonterminal differentiation can induce the expression of
anticancer activity and make cells resistant to neoplastic
transformation. Whereas only 1% of clones derived from
undifferentiated cells were resistant to transformation, >25%
of clones derived from nonterminally differentiated adipocytes
expressed anticancer activity (Figure 4).

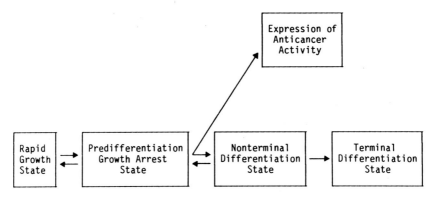

FIG. 4. Model for the induction of anticancer activity by
nonterminal differentiation.

    The reason that only 25% of clones derived from nonterminally
differentiated cells express anticancer activity rather than 100%
is still under investigation. Our working hypothesis is that
100% of nonterminally differentiated cells may actually express
anticancer activity at the molecular level but that this activity
gradually decays during the 20 to 25 population doublings that
are required to grow enough cells to perform a type III focus
assay. In support of this conclusion we have evaluated
sequentially the expression of anticancer activity in specific
cell clones and have found that, although this activity is stable
for >50 population doublings, it subsequently decays so that most
such cell clones that were initially resistant to transformation
become transformable with one or more carcinogens before
100 population doublings.

To determine if those clones that do express differentiation-induced anticancer activity are resistant to additional carcinogens, we evaluated cell clones to test their response to exposure to DMBA, MCA, MNNG, and PS. The results of these assays demonstrated that all anticancer clones are resistant to multiple carcinogens and some clones are resistant to all physical and chemical carcinogens tested. Preliminary studies also suggest that clones expressing anticancer activity can be resistant to "Ej-ras" oncogene-induced transformation and that nonterminal differentiation can also turn off the expression of the large "T" antigen of the oncogenic SV40 virus (Tzen et al. and Minoo et al., manuscripts in preparation). Finally, we have demonstrated that clones that are resistant to carcinogens as determined by in vitro focus transformation assays are also nontransformed when evaluated by in vivo tumorigenicity using nude mice (Scott et al., manuscript submitted).

These results therefore establish for the first time that the expression of anticancer activity can be physiologically regulated by differentiation-dependent mechanisms. These data require that once again we ask the question concerning what mechanisms may be involved in mediating anticancer activity. Using the experimental system described above we have performed a large series of preliminary studies which suggest but do not prove that the following processes are not involved in mediating anticancer activity: DNA repair, cell-cell communication, modulation in growth factor or growth inhibitor effects, or changes in proliferation characteristics.

Current and future studies therefore will be directed at attempts to clone anticancer genes and to characterize their products. Our main interest in this regard is to determine if anticancer genes encode for specific transacting factors that regulate the expression of transforming genes.

B. Cancer suppressor activity.

The same three questions that were asked about anticancer activity can be asked about cancer suppressor activity. What is the evidence it really exists? What are the mechanisms that mediate cancer suppressor activity? How is the expression of cancer suppressor activity regulated?

The evidence that cancer suppressor activity exists can be derived from a large series of cell fusion studies and embryonic implantation studies. For example, Harris (8), Stanbridge (28), Sager (21), Klinger (9), and Koi and Barrett (10) and their coworkers have demonstrated that when normal cells are fused with cancer cells the vast majority of resulting hybrid cells are nontransformed. In fact, it has been reported that at least two complementation groups of cancer suppressor activity exist and that one specific cancer suppressor gene resides on human chromosome 11 (29).

The treatment of some types of transformed cells with interferon has also been reported to induce stable reversion to a

nontransformed state and the latter results have been implicated
to be mediated by modulation in DNA methylation (22).

Finally, embryonic implantation studies clearly document the
existence of cancer suppressor activity. If cancer cells, such
as, embryonal carcinoma cells (3,12) or neuroblastoma cells (17)
or acute myelogenous leukemia cells (7), are implanted into
specific embryonic microenvironments, the transformed phenotype
is suppressed and the resulting revertant cells then participate
in normal development that ultimately results in the propagation
of an adult animal.

Many of these observations are compatible with the possibility
that cellular differentiation can suppress expression of the
transformed phenotype even without inducing irreversible loss of
proliferative potential. That is, the above results indirectly
suggest that nonterminal differentiation may regulate the
expression of cancer suppressor activity in addition to
regulating the expression of anticancer activity.

To test this possibility directly, we employed
tumorigenic/transformed derivatives of 3T3 T mesenchymal stem
cells which retained their ability to differentiate although at
much reduced rates compared to nontransformed cells. Cell clones
were then developed from undifferentiated transformed cell populations and from nonterminally differentiated transformed cell
populations. Thereafter we evaluated which retained the
transformed phenotype. The results show that 100% of the cell
clones derived from undifferentiated cells remained transformed
whereas 35-60% of clones derived from differentiated cells
were nontransformed. These results were derived by use of two
in vitro transformation assays, i.e., the focus assay and the
soft agar growth assay (13,30). The expression of such cancer
suppressor activity in these clones was stably expressed for >30
population doublings. We also evaluated whether these revertant
clones were as resistant to retransformation. The results show
that 15% to 60% of the clones that express cancer suppressor
activity cannot be retransformed by UV irradiation (90 ergs/mm^2)
or 4NQO treatment (100 ng/ml). These results therefore support
the conclusion that cancer suppressor activity and anticancer
activity can be stably induced in tumorigenic/transformed cells
by the process of nonterminal differentiation. Figure 5
summarizes these results.

These results form the basis for future studies designed to
discover unique physiological and/or pharmacological reagents
that specifically and directly induce the expression of anticancer and cancer suppressor genes. If these studies are
successful, it may be possible to modulate the expression of
anticancer/cancer suppressor activity and thereby to both prevent
and treat cancer. If so we should have the opportunity to
achieve our ultimate goal which is the development of new
approaches to keep normal cells in a normal state and to induce
cancer cells to revert to a normal state.

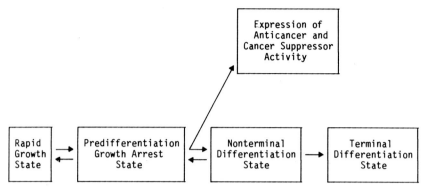

FIG. 5. Model for the induction of anticancer and cancer suppressor activity by nonterminal differentiation.

ACKNOWLEDGEMENTS

The authors thank Mrs. Teresa Hughes and Mrs. Karen Connelly for typing this manuscript and Drs. Bruce Kline and Eric Wieben for helpful scientific discussions. This work was supported in part by the Mayo Foundation and by the following grants to R.E.S.: NIH CA-28240, NIH CA-09441, and CRT-1750.

REFERENCES

1. Anders, A. and Anders, F. (1978): Biochim. Biophys. Acta, 516:61-95.
2. Boman, B. M., Maercklein, P. B., Hoerl, B. J., and Scott, R. E. (1983): Lab. Invest., 48:199-204.
3. Brinster, R. L. (1974): J. Exp. Med., 140:1049-1056.
4. DiPaolo, J. A. (1983): J. Natl. Cancer Inst., 70:3-8.
5. Florine, D. L., Hoerl, B. J., and Scott, R. E. (1982): Cell Differ., 11:195-202.
6. Friend, S. H., Bernards, R., Rogelj, S., Weinberg, R. A., Rapaport, J. M., Albert, D. M., and Dryja, T. P. (1986): Nature, 323:643-646.
7. Gootwine, E., Webb, C. G., and Sachs, L. (1982): Nature, 299:63-65.
8. Harris, H., Miller, O. J., Klein, G., Worst, P., and Tachibana, T. (1969): Nature, 223:363-368.
9. Klinger, H. P. (1982): Cytogenet. Cell Genet., 32:68-84.
10. Koi, M., and Barrett, J. C. (1986): Proc. Natl. Acad. Sci. USA, 83:5992-5996.
11. Krawisz, B. R., and Scott, R. E. (1982): J. Cell Biol., 94:394-399.
12. Mintz, B., and Illmensee, K. (1975): Proc. Natl. Acad. Sci. USA, 72:3585-3589.
13. Mondal, S., and Heidelberger, C. (1976): Nature, 260:710-711.

14. Pardee, A. B., Dubrow, R., Hamlin, J. L., and Kletzien, R. F. (1978): Annu. Rev. Biochem., 47:715-750.
15. Pittelkow, M. R., and Scott, R. E. (1986): Mayo Clin. Proc., 62:771-777.
16. Pittelkow, M. R., Wille, J. J. Jr., and Scott, R. E. (1986): J. Invest. Dermatol., 86:410-417.
17. Podesta, A. H., Mullins, J., Pierce, G. B., and Wells, R. S. (1984): Proc. Natl. Acad. Sci. USA, 81:7608-7611.
18. Sachs, L. (1980): Proc. Natl. Acad. Sci. USA, 77:6152-6156.
19. Sachs, L. (1986): Sc. Am., 254(1):40-47.
20. Sager, R. (1984): Cancer Cells, 2:487-493.
21. Sager, R. (1986): Cancer Res., 46:1573-1580.
22. Samid, D., Flessate, D. M., and Friedman, R. M. (1987): Mol. Cell. Biol., 7:2196-2200.
23. Scott, R. E., Florine, D. L., Wille J. J. Jr., and Yun, K. (1982): Proc. Natl. Acad. Sci. USA, 79:845-849.
24. Scott, R. E., and Maercklein, P. B. (1985): Proc. Natl. Acad. Sci. USA, 82:2995-2999.
25. Scott, R. E., Yun, K., and Florine, D. L. (1983): Exp. Cell Res., 143:405-414.
26. Sparks, R. L., Estervig, D. N., and Scott, R. E. (1987): J. Cell. Biochem. (in press).
27. Sparks, R. L., and Scott, R. E. (1986): Exp. Cell Res., 165:345-352.
28. Stanbridge, E. J. (1984): Cancer Surveys, 3:335-350.
29. Stanbridge, E. J., Flandermeyer, R. R., Daniels, D. W., and Nelson-Rees, W. A. (1981): Somat. Cell Genet., 7:699-712.
30. Terzaghi, M., and Little, J. B. (1976): Cancer Res., 36:1367-1374.
31. Tsao, M. C., Walthall, B. J., and Ham, R. G. (1982): J. Cell. Physiol., 110:219-229.
32. Wier, M. L., and Scott, R. E. (1985): Cancer Res., 45:3339-3346.
33. Wier, M. L., and Scott, R. E. (1986): Am. J. Pathol., 125:546-554.
34. Wier, M. L., and Scott, R. E. (1986): J. Cell Biol., 102:1955-1964.
35. Wier, M. L., and Scott, R. E. (1987): J. Cell. Biochem., 33:137-150.
36. Wille, J. J. Jr., Maercklein, P. B., and Scott, R. E. (1982): Cancer Res., 42:5139-5146.
37. Wille, J. J. Jr., Pittelkow, M. R., Shipley, G. R., and Scott, R. E. (1984): J. Cell. Physiol., 121:31-44.
38. Wille, J. J. Jr., and Scott, R. E. (1982): J. Cell. Physiol., 112:115-122.
39. Wille, J. J. Jr., and Scott, R. E. (1986): Int. J. Cancer, 37:875-881.
40. Yun, K., and Scott, R. E. (1983): Cancer Res., 43:88-96.

Alterations in Control of Terminal Differentiation in Premalignant and Malignant Mouse Keratinocytes

S.H. Yuspa and D.R. Roop

Laboratory of Cellular Carcinogenesis and Tumor Promotion
Division of Cancer Etiology
National Cancer Institute
Bethesda, Maryland 20892

INTRODUCTION

The induction of tumors on mouse skin has been one of the major models from which modern concepts of chemical carcinogenesis have been derived. This model has revealed the multistep nature of the tumor induction process, the irreversibility of early carcinogen-induced changes, the sequential requirements for exposure to initiating and promoting agents, the step wise progression from preneoplastic to neoplastic phenotypes, potential reversibility of preneoplastic lesions, and the ability of sequential carcinogen exposure to enhance malignant progression (10,27). More recently the use of epidermal cell culture systems in association with biochemical and molecular techniques has provided some understanding of the cellular and molecular mechanisms which underlie the biology of tumor development. Exposure of normal mouse skin and normal keratinocytes to chemical carcinogens causes a defect in the program of epidermal differentiation which allows cells to escape some signals for terminal differentiation (27). Tumor promoters appear to selectively expand the clones of these altered cells (28). A subsequent change in these differentiation-altered cells complements the underlying biochemical events in initiation to produce the malignant tumor (10,11). At the gene level it appears that activation of the Harvey ras gene is sufficient to produce the initiated phenotype yielding cells that have both a defect in differentiation and produce a benign tumor (1,14,19). Genetic changes which complement ras activation to affect malignant conversion have not been identified (6).

The association of defective differentiation with epithelial carcinogenesis is not confined to mouse skin. Studies of teratoma cells, bronchial epithelial cells, adipocytes, colonic epithelium and carcinogen-induced hepatic foci have suggested that a defect in differentiation is a general phenomenon early in epithelial carcinogenesis (30). Most importantly, these studies imply that the reversal of this alteration by pharmacological or genetic means might be useful in preventing the progression of preneoplastic lesions to the neoplastic or malignant endpoint. Indeed experimental evidence suggests that reversal of the differentiation defect in neoplastic cells is an uncommon, but reproducible spontaneous change which does lead to tumor regression (5,24). Thus, understanding the fundamental biochemical changes leading to the defect in differentiation could have practical applications in cancer therapy as well as important implications in cancer pathogenesis.

EXPERIMENTAL STUDIES

In order to more specifically evaluate alterations in epidermal differentiation associated with neoplastic change, we have begun to characterize genes and gene products which are uniquely expressed in particular differentiation states of epidermis (16). Among these are keratin proteins, the major cellular products of terminally differentiating keratinocytes. In mouse epidermis, basal cells express primarily a 55 kD type I acidic keratin (K14) and a 60 kD type II basic keratin (K5) as designated in the Moll et al. catalogue (13,17,26). As cells enter their terminal differentiation program, the transcription of these keratins is diminished and a 67 kD type II keratin (K1) and a 59 kD type I keratin (K10) are expressed (3,17). Expression of these latter keratins predominates in the suprabasal cell layers, and these proteins are the major components of the stratum corneum where posttranslational processing also occurs (2). In addition to keratin proteins, suprabasal cells express filaggrin, a complex product of a large gene containing 16 tandem repeat units of 1200 bp. A 20 kb message codes for a large precursor protein of over 700 kD which is processed to multiple monomers of 27 kD (8,20). This protein is a major component of the keratohyalin granule in the granular cell layer of epidermis, and its transcription in normal skin is confined to this layer. Recently a new differentiation-specific protein has been identified as a cystine rich cornified envelope precursor, (CE) (Roop et al., manuscript in preparation). Transcription of this protein is also confined to the granular cell layer in normal skin, and the protein is rapidly cross-linked by epidermal transglutaminase and incorporated into the cornified envelope.

The cloning and sequencing of the epidermal differentiation-specific genes from mouse cDNA and genomic libraries have provided the essential tools to understand the regulation of these genes and to study changes in expression during carcinogenesis (25). This laboratory has provided both structure and sequence data on the mouse epidermal keratins (12,22,23) and similar data are now available for filaggrin and CE (unpublished). Monospecific antibodies to unique peptides of the carboxy terminal portions of individual mouse keratins, filaggrin and CE proteins have been generated (15 and unpublished). These antibodies have been useful probes to study the specific expression of individual keratin proteins within particular cell types (18). Furthermore, gene sequence information has been useful to generate nucleic acid probes specific for the analysis of transcriptional activity by in situ hybridization (19). These tools have been used to study the expression of keratins in both benign and malignant tumors from the epidermis to assess changes in their expression during tumor progression. Furthermore, we propose that these can be useful to assess changes induced by pharmacological agents designed to induce differentiation in tumor cells.

Normal Skin

When monospecific keratin antibodies are used to study frozen sections of normal mouse epidermis by indirect immunofluorescence, K14 staining is found in all basal cells, and the protein persists throughout the suprabasal cell layers but is diminished in the stratum corneum (Fig. 1). In contrast, K1 and K10 are primarily localized to suprabasal cells, although an occasional basal cell is also positive. K10 is detected in the stratum corneum whereas K1 is not since it is processed in this layer to remove carboxy terminal peptides which are the antigenic determinants for the antibodies used in these studies (2,15). Double label immunofluorescence using monospecific antibodies raised in two species (rabbit and guinea pig) indicate that K1 and K10 are coexpressed in suprabasal cells (not shown). In general, K14 positive basal cells do not synthesize K10 and less than 10% express K1. Because of the high stability of keratin proteins, dynamic aspects of expression can better be analyzed by evaluation of keratin gene mRNA content by in situ hybridization. Figure 1 reveals that RNA for K14 is abundant in basal cells, but diminishes in the first suprabasal cell layer. Therefore transcription of this gene is confined to the less differentiated cells although the protein persists into the more differentiated cell layers. Hybridizable transcripts for K1 and K10 are abundant in the first suprabasal cell layer and persist throughout the upper strata diminishing only in the uppermost granular cell layer.

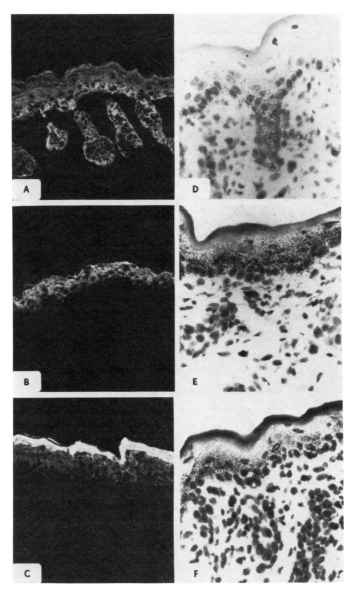

FIG. 1.   Analysis of keratin expression in newborn mouse skin by indirect immunofluorescence and in situ hybridization. Indirect immunofluorescence was performed with the following antisera: A. Guinea pig K14; B. Rabbit K1; C. Rabbit K10. Frozen sections of newborn mouse skin were hybridized with ^{35}S-labeled RNA probes corresponding to K14(D), K1(E) and K10(F). Methods were reported previously for immunofluorescence and in situ hybridization (15,19).

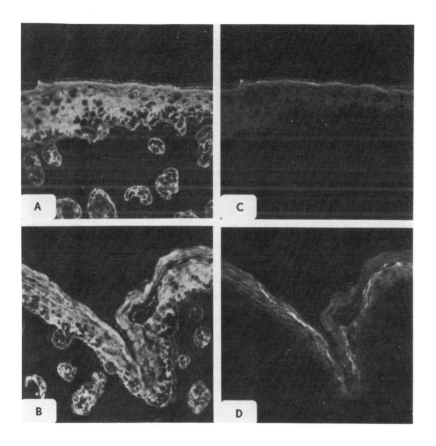

FIG. 2. Analysis of filaggrin expression (C) and CE expression (D) in newborn mouse skin by indirect double label immunofluorescence. K14 staining (A and B) is shown for comparison.

Similar analyses of filaggrin and CE protein and mRNA indicate that these genes are expressed at a later stage of the differentiation program of normal epidermis. The distribution of fluorescence in epidermis probed with antibodies to filaggrin protein. is punctate within cells of the granular cell layer but the pattern is diffuse in the stratum corneum (Fig. 2). Likewise CE protein fluorescence is confined to the granular cell layer and more superficial stratum corneum where the protein assumes a peripheral localization consistent with its function as a major constituent of the cornified envelope (Fig. 2). Analysis of transcript distribution by in situ hybridization reveals that hybridizable mRNA is concentrated in the area around the granular cell layer. This confirms the late activation of gene expression for these products of cells in a more advanced stage of terminal differentiation in normal skin.

Skin Tumors

Similar analyses of protein and mRNA localization were conducted on papillomas and carcinomas. K14 protein staining is prominent in the basal cell layer of papillomas and persists throughout most of the suprabasal layers of the highly stratified lesion (Fig. 3). Both K1 and K10 immunofluorescence are confined to the suprabasal cell layers, and K1 staining is absent from the stratum corneum suggesting that this protein is processed in benign tumors as it is in normal skin. In situ hybridization with a K14 probe indicates a difference in regulation of this keratin from that observed in normal skin. Grain density for hybridizable K14 mRNA (Fig. 4) is greater in papillomas than normal skin and grains persist into the higher suprabasal layers. This is consistent with a diminished responsiveness of papilloma cells to differentiation signals whereby a keratin normally expressed predominately in basal cells continues to be expressed in suprabasal layers. The distribution of hybridizable mRNA for K1 and K10 in papillomas is similar to normal epidermis with transcripts being most abundant in the first and subsequent suprabasal cell layers. Immunostaining with anti K14 antibody in carcinomas reveals a diffuse staining pattern in virtually all tumor cells of epithelial origin. In contrast, K1 and K10 positive cells are rare in carcinomas at any level of stratification (Fig. 5). Double label immunofluorescence confirms that tumor areas negative for K1 and K10 are positive for K14 indicating the epithelial nature of these cells. In situ hybridization analysis reveals intense grain density for K14 transcripts in malignant cells while transcripts for K1 and K10 are essentially undetectable. These data are consistent with the loss of transcriptional activity for the differentiation-specific keratins in the carcinoma phenotype.

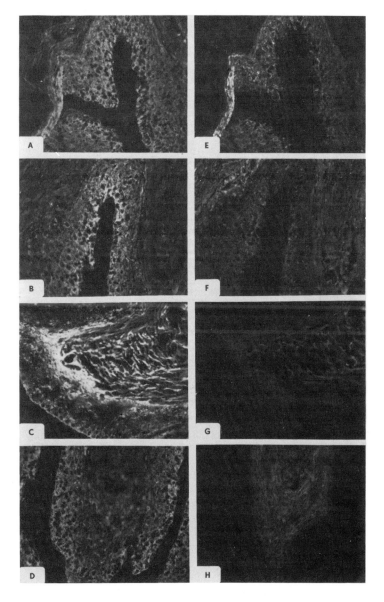

FIG. 3.   Analysis of differentiation-specific gene expression by double staining immunofluorescence in serial sections of chemically induced skin papillomas.   A,B,C and D are stained with guinea pig K14.   The same sections were also stained with rabbit K1(E); rabbit K10(F); rabbit filaggrin(G); rabbit CE(H).

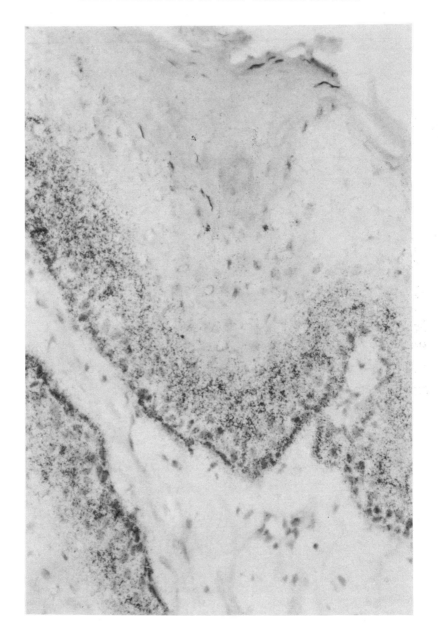

FIG. 4. In situ hybridization of skin papilloma using an ^{35}S-labeled RNA probe to K14.

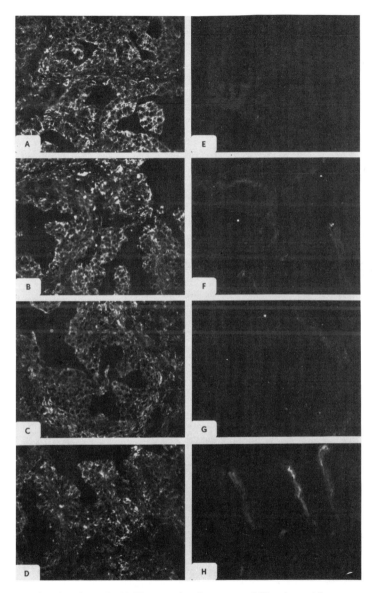

FIG. 5. Analysis of differentiation-specific keratin gene
expression by double label immunofluorescence of serial sections
of chemically induced skin carcinoma. Antibodies are the same as
in Fig. 3. (A,B,C and D are guinea pig K14; E,F,G, and H are
rabbit K1, K10, filaggrin and CE respectively.

Papillomas and carcinomas have also been evaluated by specific probes for filaggrin and CE expression. In general, papillomas are rich in both protein and mRNA for filaggrin and CE (Figs. 3&5) and both are localized to suprabasal cell layers as in normal skin. However in benign tumors the strict confinement of filaggrin and CE expression to granular cells seen in normal skin is not observed, and expression is detected in inferior regions of the suprabasal strata. Several hypotheses for the expansion of cells expressing the late differentiation-specific genes can be considered. Cells receiving signals for late gene expression may accumulate by progressing more slowly into the fully mature state where they are recognized as granular and cornified cells. Alternatively, cells may become responsive for late differentiation gene expression earlier in their maturation program, but the processing of these gene products to their functional form for differentiation may be delayed. CE and filaggrin protein expression is very limited in carcinomas (Figs. 3&5). Only focal expression of either transcript is recognized in malignant cells (not shown). In well differentiated tumors, these gene products are occasionally found in areas of histological differentiation such a keratin pearls.

The loss of K1,K10, filaggrin and CE expression in malignant keratinocytes, relative to their abundance in the benign precursor lesion, is sufficiently reproducible so as to serve as a negative marker for malignant conversion. Exceptions have been noted where K1 is expressed in carcinomas arising from in vivo transplantation of cultured malignant cell lines (4). Nevertheless, in the situation where tumors are induced by initiation-promotion protocols in vivo, these changes appear to be consistent. As such these markers may be useful in studies designed to induce terminal differentiation as a form of chemotherapy. In such cases, the reinduction of K1, K10, CE or filaggrin in treated carcinomas would serve as an indicator of biological response.

The mouse skin model offers other advantages for studies of differentiation therapy. There are well defined stages of neoplastic progression with characteristic pathological lesions of varying biological potential. The superficial locations of the tumors offers an opportunity to test compounds topically or systemically and observe effects directly. The model can be used to distinguish among agents which may affect benign tumors or malignant tumors preferentially. Since squamous cell tumors represent a major form of cancer in internal organs, such as the lung and esophagus, studies performed in the mouse skin model may have direct relevance for therapy of certain forms of human cancer.

Differentiation therapy offers a unique approach to cancer treatment. It could represent a first attempt at cancer therapy which is designed to counteract a fundamental defect in the biology of the cancer cell, a defect which is likely to occur early in the carcinogenesis process and be rate limiting in cancer development. Cell hybridization studies have proven definitively that the induction of terminal differentiation can reverse the cancer phenotype (7,21). However, hybridization studies are unlikely to reveal the molecular changes required for a therapeutic effect. Such information can come only from a fundamental understanding of the signals which regulate normal differentiation and the factors which regulate expression of the differentiation-specific gene products. The mouse skin model is appropriate for such studies as well. The factors which regulate epidermal differentiation have been studied in detail(9,29). A number of differentiation-specific genes have been cloned and reagents produced for their detection, including specific antibodies and unique sequence cDNA probes. Aberrant expression in tumors has now been defined. These elements of the mouse skin model can provide the research base required to define rational pharmacological methods to specifically reverse the cancer phenotype by differentiation therapy.

REFERENCES

1. Bizub, D., Wood, A.W., and Skalka, A.M. (1986): Proc. Natl. Acad. Sci. USA, 83:6048-6052.
2. Bowden, P.E., Quinlan, R.A., Breitkreutz, D., and Fusenig, N.E. (1984): Eur. J. Biochem., 142:29-36.
3. Breitkreutz, D., Bohnert, A., Herzman, E., Bowden, P.E., Boukamp, P., and Fusenig, N.E. (1984): Differentiation, 26:154-169.
4. Breitkreutz, D., Hornung, J., Pahlmann, J., Brown-Bierman, L., Bohnert, A., Bowden, P.E., and Fusenig, N.E. (1986): Eur. J. Cell Biol., 42:255-267.
5. Burns, F.J., Vanderlaan, M., Sivak, A., and Albert, R.E. (1976): Cancer Res., 36:1422-1427.
6. Harper, J.R., Roop, D.R., and Yuspa, S.H. (1986): Mol. Cell. Biol., 6:3144-3149.
7. Harris, H. and Bramwell, M.E. (1987): J. Cell Sci., 87:383-388.
8. Haydock, P.V. and Dale, B.A. (1986): J. Biol. Chem., 261:12520-12525.
9. Hennings, H., Michael, D., Cheng, C., Steinert, P., Holbrook, K., and Yuspa, S.H. (1980): Cell, 19:245-254.
10. Hennings, H., Shores, R., Wenk, M., Spangler, E.F., Tarone, R., and Yuspa, S.H. (1983): Nature, 304:67-69.

11. Hennings, H., Spangler, E.F., Shores, R., Mitchell, P., Devor, D., Shamsuddin, A.K.M., Elgjo, K.M., and Yuspa, S.H. (1986): Env. Health Perspect., 68:69-67.
12. Krieg, T.M., Schafer, M.P., Cheng, C.K., Filpula, D., Flaherty, P., Steinert, P.M., and Roop, D.R. (1985): J. Biol. Chem., 260:5867-5870.
13. Moll, R., Franke, W.W.,Schiller, D.L., Genyer, B., and Krepler, R. (1982): Cell, 31:11-24.
14. Quintanilla, M., Brown, K., Ramsden, M., and Balmain, A. (1986): Nature, 322:78-80.
15. Roop, D.R., Cheng, C.K., Titterington, L., Meyers, C.A., Stanley, J.R., Steinert, P.M., and Yuspa, S.H. (1984): J. Biol. Chem., 259:8037-8040.
16. Roop, D.R., Cheng, C.K. Toftgard, R., Stanley, J.R., Steinert, P.M., and Yuspa, S.H. (1985): Ann. N.Y. Acad. Sci., 455:426-435.
17. Roop, D.R., Hawley-Nelson, P., Cheng, C.K., and Yuspa, S.H. (1983): Proc. Natl. Acad. Sci. USA, 80:716-720.
18. Roop, D.R., Heutfeldt, H., Kilkenny, A., and Yuspa, S.H. (1987): Differentiation, in press.
19. Roop, D.R., Lowy, D.R., Tambourin, P.E., Strickland, J., Harper, J.R., Balaschak, M., Spangler, E.F., and Yuspa, S.H. (1986): Nature, 323:822-824.
20. Rothnagel, J.A., Melviel, T., Idler, W.W., Roop, D.R., and Steinert, P.M. (1987): J. Biol. Chem., in press.
21. Stanbridge, E.J., Der, C.J., Nishimi, R.Y., Peehl, D.M., Weissman, B.E., and Wilkinson, J. (1982): Science, 215:252-259.
22. Steinert, P.M., Parry, D.A.D., Racoosin, E.L., Idler, W.W., Steven, A.C., Trus, B.L., and Roop, D.R. (1984): Proc. Natl. Acad. Sci., USA, 81:5709-5713.
23. Steinert, P.M., Rice, R.H., Roop, D.R., Trus, B.L. and Steven, A. C. (1983): Nature, 302:794-800.
24. Tatematsu, M., Nagamine, Y., and Farber, E. (1983): Cancer Res., 43:5049-5058.
25. Toftgard, R., Yuspa, S.H., and Roop, D.R. (1985): Cancer Res., 45:5845-5850.
26. Winter, H. and Shweizer, J. (1983): Proc. Natl. Acad. Sci. USA, 80:6480-6484.
27. Yuspa, S.H. (1986): J. Amer. Acad. Dermatol., 15:1031-1044.
28. Yuspa,S.H. (1986): In: Accomplishments in Cancer Research 1986, edited by J.G.Fortner and J.E.Rhoads, pp. 169-182, Lippincott Co., Philadelphia.
29. Yuspa, S.H., Ben, T., and Hennings, H. (1983): Carcinogenesis, 4:1413-1418.
30. Yuspa, S.H. and Poirier, M.C. (1987): Adv. Cancer Res., in press.

Differentiation of Normal and Cancerous Colon Cells

Y.S. Kim

Gastrointestinal Research Laboratory (151M2),
Veterans Administration Medical Center, San Francisco, CA 94121,
and the Departments of Medicine & Pathology, University of California,
San Francisco, San Francisco, CA 94143

Although the precise relationship between cellular
differentiation and neoplasia is not clear, neoplasia is thought
to be the result of disordered cellular differentiation arising
from an aberrant programming of normal gene function (49,50,56).
Cancer of the colon and rectum is both common and fatal in the
Western world. However, despite much effort, the overall 5 year
survival rate for colorectal cancer has changed little during
the past three decades and remains at 40-45% (74). Furthermore,
because of the limited effectiveness of cytotoxic agents in colon
cancer chemotherapy, it is attractive to consider an alternate
approach to therapy based not only upon killing of colon cancer
cells, but on controlling growth through the induction of more
differentiated phenotypes.

To achieve this goal, it is important that we understand
the pathways of cell lineage development, cell lineage and
differentiation associated markers as well as the factors
regulating differentiative programs in normal and cancerous
colonic cells.

Although relatively little is known about colonic cell
differentiation compared to the progress that has been made in
other specialized tissues such as the hematopoietic system (36,
52,70,79), some interesting progress has been made recently.
Some of these observations will be reviewed.

Histopathology of normal and cancerous colon.

The normal colonic mucosa is composed of many tubular glands
called crypts of Lieberkuhn which are lined by several types
of epithelial cells. The lower three-fourths of the crypt in
the human colon constitutes the proliferative compartment
consisting of immature dividing cells. Stem cells are thought
to be located in the lower colonic crypt. As cells migrate
upward along the tubular crypt, they differentiate into mature

absorptive columnar cells or goblet cells. The turnover times
for mucosal cells of the colon and rectum are 72-97 hours and
96-192 hours respectively (47). The studies on three dimensional
architecture of the human colonic crypt indicate that several
types of cells line the luminal aspect of the crypt, and there
is a basal lamina and pericryptal fibroblast sheath beneath them
(16,39,53,61). This complex array of structural patterns would
suggest the important role of homotypic and heterotypic cellular
interactions as well as epithelial-mesenchymal interaction in
growth regulation and differentiation of colonic cells in the
colonic crypt.

There are at least three principal colonic cell types.
The main cell types are absorptive columnar epithelial cells,
mucus producing goblet cells and endocrine cells (15,71). In
addition, other minor cell types have been described whose
functions and relationships to the other major cell lineages
is not known. These include paneth cells, tuft (or caveolated
cells), cup cells (48) and deep crypt secretory cells (1).

COLONIC CELL DIFFERENTIATION

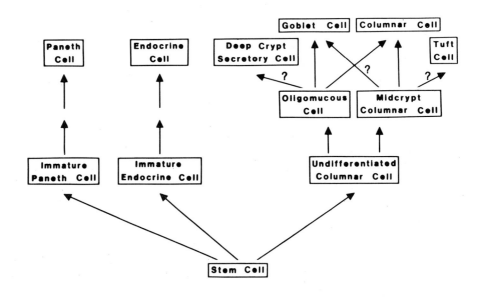

FIG. 1. Hypothetical cell lineage differentiation scheme in
human colon.

Most investigators agree with the unitarian concept that
all intestinal epithelial cell types arise from a progenitor

stem cell as suggested in mouse intestine by Chang and Leblond in 1971 (15). The hypothetical cell lineage differentiation scheme shown in Figure 1 is based on their data and the recent data of other investigators. In this scheme, for example, stem cells differentiate into undifferentiated columnar cells which further differentiate into oligomucus and mid crypt columnar cells which are still proliferating. These cells eventually undergo terminal differentiation to goblet cells and absorptive columnar epithelial cells.

In terms of colon cancer, these tumors can be histologically divided into three main groups (Table 1) (73). The most common group, adenocarcinoma, consisting of columnar epithelial cells, can be subdivided according to the degree of histological differentiation. The second most common group, mucinous carcinoma, can be subdivided according to the pattern of mucin secretion. The larger subgroup, colloid carcinoma, presumably derived from goblet cells is characterized by large extracellular "lakes" of mucin. The "signet ring cell" carcinoma subgroup is characterized by an intracellular accumulation of mucin.

TABLE 1. Histological Classification of Colorectal Carcinoma

Histological Type	Subtype
Adenocarcinoma (80%)a	Well-differentiated (grade 1)b
	Moderately-differentiated (grade 2)b
	Poorly-differentiated (grade 3)
Mucinous Carcinoma (15%)	Colloid Carcinoma (extracellular mucin)
	Signet Ring Cell Carcinoma (intracellular mucin)
Undifferentiated, Anaplastic Carcinoma (<5%)	
Carcinoid, Adenosquamous or Squamous Carcinoma (<1%)	

a. Percent (%) of total colon cancer cases.
b. Intraglandular mucin may be present to variable extents

Although the term "mucinous" is generally used for colloid and signet ring carcinomas, mucin may also be found to variable extents in malignant glands of well- or moderately differentiated adenocarcinomas. Therefore, the cells of origin for adenocarcinoma of the colon are not clear at the present time.

Obviously this classification is a rather simplified one, since most colon cancers consist of more than one cell type. It is likely that during the evolution and progression of colonic carcinogenesis, several lineages of differentiation may be expressed in the clones of one tumor or even in single clones of colon cancer cells. Consistent with this view, Pierce and Cox in 1978 (63), demonstrated in an experimental rat colonic adenocarcinoma of mixed cell types, that when a single clone of cells from this tumor was injected into the rat to form tumors, each tumor displayed mixed cell types. This observation led them to suggest that the undifferentiated colonic cell is a multipotential stem cell capable of differentiating into each of several differentiated colon cell types.

However, most colon cancers display a predominant histological type and therefore the availability of the markers of cell lineage and differentiation will be useful in identifying the subsets of histological types of colorectal tumors that may have prognostic and/or therapeutic importance.

The cell lineage-associated colonic cell differentiation markers in normal and cancerous colonic cells are summarized in Table 2. For the normal columnar absorptive cells, the brush border membrane hydrolases, such as alkaline phosphatase, and basolateral components, such as secretory component and Na-K ATPase appear to be present in differentiated cells (42). In well- to moderately differentiated adenocarcinoma cells, increased levels of onco-fetal forms of antigens and enzymes such as carcinoembryonic antigen (CEA) (77,78), Le^X (38) and Le^y antigens (43), colon associated antigens (60), other antigens (68), placental-like alkaline phosphatase (PLAP) (57,33), and sucrase-isomaltase, γ-glutamyltranspeptidase and aminopeptidase (18,78,83) have been observed. Recent immunohistochemical studies indicate that two distinct groups of cytokeratin recognized by monoclonal antibodies AE1 and AE3 are present in the columnar epithelial cells in the upper crypt but not in the lower crypt (31). However, cytokeratin expression in colon cancer of different degrees of differentiation has not been examined. The content of villin, a major protein in the microvillus core of the brush border in intestinal epithelial cells was found to be much higher in a differentiated colon cancer cell line than in undifferentiated cancer cells (25). The ability to transport fluid and electrolytes is a function of differentiated columnar absorptive cells. However, neither electroneutral or electrogenic Na absorption has been observed in colon cancer cells regardless of the degree of differentiation. For mucous cells, quantitative and qualitative characteristics of mucin may serve as markers in both the normal and malignant states. For example, mucous cells in the upper colonic crypt show reduced binding to ricinus communis agglutinin (RCA) but increased binding to dolichos biflorus agglutinin (DBA) compared to mucous cells in the lower colonic crypt (9).

At least 4 types of enteroendocrine cells have been described and many peptide hormones are synthesized and secreted by these cells (19). These include bombesin, enteroglucagon, serotonin, somatostatin, vasoactive intestinal polypeptide (VIP), peptide YY and substance "P" (58). Because of the close proximity of these cells to stem cells in the normal colon, and because of the frequent presence of endocrine cells in colonic adenocarcinoma, investigation of these cells and their products in normal and cancerous mucosa may lead to new insights concerning growth regulation and differentiation.

TABLE 2. Cell Lineage Associated Colonic Cell
Differentiation Markers

Cell Types	Normal	Cancer

Columnar Cells:

BB Hydrolases (AP) — CEA ↑↓, PLAP ↑↑
Secretory Component — BB Hydrolases (S-I) ↑
Hormone Receptors — Le^X, Le^y ↑↑
— CAA (200 Kd), villin ↑
Villin (95 Kd) — Hormone Receptors
AE1, AE3 — Secretory Component
Le^X, Le^y↓↓↓ — UDP-Nacetylhexosamine ↑↑
— 52Kd soluble proteins

Na absorption
 electroneutral (proximal)
 electrogenic amiloride sensitive and
  aldosterone stimulatable (distal)   not
Cl absorption   determined
 Na dependent Cl-HCO exchange (proximal)
 Na independent Cl-HCO exchange (distal)
 K secretion
  potential dependent
  active electrogenic

Mucous Cells:

Mucins ↑ — Mucins ↑
Qualitative Changes — Qualitative Changes
Altered Sialyation
 & sulfation
RCA↓, DBA ↑

Entero-endocrine cells:

Bombesin, Enteroglucagon
Serotonin, Somatostatin
VIP, peptide YY, substance "P"   present
Chromogranin A (68 Kd)
Synaptophysin (38 Kd)

Paneth Cells:

Lysozyme   present

Deep Crypt Secretory cells:

VIP induced Cl Secretion   present
(Na ,K ,Cl cotransport system)

Tuft (caveolated cells) Cells:

?   ?

Cup Cells:

?   ?

Enteroendocrine cells and paneth cells when present in colon
tumor tissues or colon cancer cell lines express these cell
lineage associated markers. VIP induced Cl secretion is observed
in some colon cancer cell lines after differentiation induction.

In vitro models of normal colonic cell differentiation

The in vitro models of normal colonic cell
differentiation are listed as follows. The viability of normal
colonocytes in organ culture and primary explant culture of
colonic mucosa is very limited (28). Recently Whitehead has
described increased viability and continued proliferation of
epithelial cells from colonic crypts cultured in collagen gels
which are in close contact with a viable feeder layer of bovine
aortic endothelial cells (80,81,82).

It has also been reported that scraped mucosal cells can
grow as suspensions, if enzymatic disruption of cell aggregates
is avoided. However, it appears that the viable cells in such
culture are in intact crypts containing both absorptive and
goblet cells as well as stromal cells and that the cells lose
viability when the crypt structure begins to degenerate after
two weeks (58).

Although epithelial cell lines have been established from
rat small intestine (66), definitive normal human colon cell
lines are not yet available (despite much effort). Further
effort should be made on developing defined growth media with
various growth factors or agents and on improving the growth
conditions of normal colon cells using extracellular matrix or
feeder layer of cells (13,54). Alternatively, attempts should
be made to immortalize the normal colon cells by viral
transformation or insertion of "immortalizing" sequences.

Models for studying colon cancer cell differentiation

The various models that have been used for studying colon
cancer cell differentiation are outlined in Table 3. These
include induction of differentiation, spontaneous differentiation
based on degree of confluency, nutrient manipulation, effect
of peptide growth factors, lymphokines, or extracellular matrix
components, and comparison of cancer cells with different degrees
of differentiation.

TABLE 3. Models for Studying Colon Cancer Cell Differentiation

---

A. Chemical Inducers:
     DMF, NMF, DMSO, Butyrate, HMBA
     Short term treatment (reversible)
     Long Term treatment ("stable" differentiation)
        (HT-29 cells differentiate to mucous & columnar cells)

B. Spontaneous Differentiation:
     Confluent or post-confluent cells:
        (CaCo-2 cells differentiate to columnar cells)
        (T84 cells differentiate to columnar secretory cells)

C. Nutrient Manipulation
    Glucose deprivation
        (HT-29 differentiate to columnar cells)

D. Polypeptide growth inhibitors and lymphokines
    TGFβ, INFα, INFγ

E. Extracellular Matrix

F. Cancer cells with different degree of differentiation

The chemical agents that have been used for induction of differentiation of colon cancer cells include N, N-dimethylformamide (DMF), N-methylformamide (NMF), dimethylsulfoxide (DMSO), hexamethylene bisacetamide (HMBA), and sodium butyrate.

Using these chemical inducers for up to 10 days, several groups have been successful in inducing morphological, functional and biochemical differentiation in some colon cancer cells (34,41,57,78). The short term treatment with these agents caused reduction in the growth rate, marked reduction in saturation density and loss of anchorage independent growth in soft agar, in vitro growth properties that are considered to be more consistent with normal cell growth. Concomitant with these changes in the growth properties, a significant alteration in the level of expression of oncodevelopmental antigens and/or enzymes occurred (34,41,77). For example, when we treated a colon cancer cell line with 2 mM Na butyrate, a thousand fold increase in placental-like alkaline phosphatase activity was observed over an 8 day period with a lag period of 2-3 days before enzymatic activity began to rise (33). We also observed dome formation which is indicative of differentiation of absorptive epithelial cells. Dome formation also required 3 days to develop. "Northern" blot analyses indicated that treatment of these cells with butyrate caused marked induction of 2.7 Kb mRNA that hybridized to a cDNA probe for placental alkaline phosphatase. We concluded from this study that a PLAP-like protein and mRNA are induced by butyrate in a colon cancer cell line with a time course consistent with cellular differentiation (33). Similar results were obtained with CEA (77).

Induction of oncodevelopmental antigens or enzymes in colon cancer cells treated with chemical inducers is interesting since these markers are usually expressed in well-differentiated colon cancer cells but not in poorly-differentiated cancer cells (42). However, the changes produced by short-term treatment of the colon cancer cells is reversible after removal of the chemical inducers (41).

Several investigators treated the colon cancer cell line HT-29 with Na butyrate for longer periods and was able to obtain differentiated cell clones either with distinct mucous morphology with abundant mucin granules or with columnar cell morphology (microvilli, tight junction and desmosomes) (6,37). These differentiated colon cancer cell clones had much lower tumorigenicity in nude mice compared to the parental cell lines (5). When the expression of protooncogenes of the myc and ras family was investigated in these differentiated clones, there was no change in expression of the myc gene family. However, ras gene expression was increased in mucous cells but not in columnar cells. Ha-ras was increased to a greater extent than Ki-ras. From these data they suggested that a high level of ras gene expression is a marker for a particular differentiated state in colon cells, rather than being directly related to transformation or tumorigenicity (5). This observation is of interest since the ras protein detected with a monoclonal antibody using immunohistochemical method was present in highest levels in the most differentiated cells at the top of the crypt in normal colonic mucosa (17).

Colon cancer cells can also be made to differentiate spontaneously depending on cell density (Table 3). For example, post confluent Caco-2 cells show prominent microvilli and high brush border membrane sucrase isomaltase activity (65). This indicates that absorptive columnar cell type of differentiation has occurred.

In confluent well-differentiated T84 colon cancer cells, VIP caused an increase of net Cl secretion which accounted for an increase in short circuit current (22). It was further shown that VIP-induced Cl secretion required a functional Na, K, Cl cotransport system localized in the basolateral membrane for the Cl uptake step (23).

As an example of a model of colon cancer cell differentiation involving nutrient manipulation, when HT-29 colon cancer cells are grown in the absence of glucose, these cells express a typical enterocytic differentiation with prominent brush border microvilli and intestinal brush border membrane hydrolase activities which are normally present in adult small intestine and fetal small intestine and colon (64). Using differentiated and undifferentiated HT-29 cells, fluorograms of SDS-PAGE of sucrase-isomaltase were performed (76). In the differentiated cells, there are 2 bands of the immunoprecipitated labeled enzymes; the lower band being the high mannose form and the upper band, the complex form of the enzyme. Undifferentiated cells show only high mannose forms. The pulse-chase study also suggests that in the undifferentiated cells there is impaired glycosylation of the enzyme, resulting in a rapid degradation of the enzyme. This would partially explain the very low enzyme activity in the undifferentiated colonic cells.

Polypeptide growth inhibitors and lymphokines have also been demonstrated to induce differentiated phenotypes in some colon cancer cells. Recently, interferon$^\alpha$ and γ (INF$^\alpha$ and INF$^\gamma$) were found to have differentiation modulatory activities on a colon cancer cell line. Both INF$^\alpha$ and INF$^\gamma$ caused an increase in cell surface CEA expression in the cells by both an accumulation of more antigen per cell and an increase in the percentage of cells expressing the antigen (32). Since an increased level of CEA expression in colon cancer cells is considered to be suggestive of more differentiated phenotypes, these lymphokines appear to have differentiation inducing properties in colon cancer cells. Similarly, exposure of a colon cancer cell line, Moser, to transforming growth factor (TGF caused both an inhibition of growth, increased secretion of CEA and increased synthesis of laminin and fibronectin (14,35).

Another model involves the use of mesenchyme and extracellular matrix which have been demonstrated to play an important role in embryonic morphogenesis and morphological and functional differentiation. Recently, the rat intestinal crypt cell line, IEC-17 or fetal rat intestinal endodermal cells were layered over fetal gut mesenchyme and grafted under the kidney capsule of adult rats (40). Morphogenesis of crypt cells into villus epithelium with four epithelial cell types (absorptive, goblet, endocrine, and Paneth cell) occurred. This study indicates that fetal rat gut mesenchyme enables morphogenesis and cytodifferentiation of both crypt and embryonic progenitor cells. When we examined the morphogenic potential of human colon cancer cells by combining human colon cancer cells with fetal rat mesenchyme in organ culture, one of the four cell lines examined, LS174T cells formed glandular structures composed of a single columnar or cuboidal epithelial cell which exhibited cellular polarity with microvilli, tight junctions and desmosomes, and basal lamina (29). Recently, extracellular matrix derived from well but not poorly differentiated colon cancer cells caused a colon cancer cell line, Moser, to induce increased secretion of CEA, reduced secretion of urokinase and increased sensitivity to growth inhibiting effects of TGF- (12).

Several comparative studies have been carried out on the biochemical and immunochemical properties of colon cancer cells with different degrees of differentiation (24,45,75). Although some differences have been observed, the results of these studies are difficult to interpret since the definition of well to poorly differentiated colon cancer cells varies considerably among investigators. The criteria for the degree of differentiation of colon cancer cells that are used by various investigators include morphology (light or ultrastructural), growth properties (anchorage-independence), response to exogenous growth factors, karyotype, level of expression of differentiated colon cell gene products such as antigens or enzymes, invasiveness and metastatic properties and nude mouse xenograft tumor morphology (18,24,45,75). Obviously, standardization of the criteria of differentiation is necessary.

Oncogenes and colonic cell differentiation

Considerable amounts of information are being accumulated on the expression of cellular oncogenes and chromosomal abnormalities in normal, premalignant and malignant colonic mucosal tissues and cells. Although abnormalities of several protooncogenes have been described (55), recent studies employing more sensitive techniques indicate that ras gene mutations (mostly occurring as point mutations at codon 12 of the C-Ki-ras gene) occur in over a third of human colon cancers and in benign colonic adenomatous polyps (11,27). These observations, along with previous report that elevated levels of P21 ras expression are found in Duke's stage A and B colon tumors, but not in later stage or metastatic tumors (30), suggest that ras mutation may be involved in the early stage of human colorectal tumorigenesis rather than in the late stage of tumor progression. However, no data are available on whether the ras mutation is related to colon cancer cell differentiation in human colonic tumors. In this regard, the induction of increased ras gene expression in differentiated clones of HT-29 colon cancer cells and increased ras protein expression in well differentiated mucosal cells in human colonic crypts (see above) are of interest.

The protein products encoded by cellular protooncogenes are thought to play an important role in normal cellular growth and differentiation. Although the biochemical function and role of many protooncogene products are unknown, several have been shown to have polypeptide regions containing tyrosine kinase activity or significant homology to this region. Recently, Bolen and his colleagues (10) reported that the tyrosine kinase specific activity of $pp60^{csrc}$ from human colon carcinoma tissues and colon cancer cell lines was increased over that from normal colon tissues or cells. A similar increase in the specific activity of this enzyme has been reported in human tissues of neuroectodermal origin where it is now thought that this increase in $pp60^{csrc}$ reflects events related to differentiation rather than to oncogenesis (69). Therefore, the precise functional significance and role of the observed increased specific activity of the pp60 protein kinase in colon cancer cells are not clear at the present time.

Recently Bodmer and his colleagues have reported chromosome 5 deletion (mapping near bands 5q21-q22) in familial polyposis coli (FPC), an autosomal dominant disorder which gives rise to multiple adenomatous polyps having high probability of developing colon cancer (8). Solomon and her coworkers (72) also examined sporadic colorectal cancer for loss of alleles on chromosome 5. They used a highly polymorphic "minisatellite" probe which maps to chromosome 5q and found that at least 23% of the 45 highly heterogeneous tumors showed partial or complete loss of one allele at the familial polyposis coli (FPC) locus. From these studies, it was suggested that becoming recessive for the FPC gene favors progression of frank malignancy in a high proportion of spontaneously occurring colon cancers. Since polyps from FPC patients did not show the recessive change, they suggested that polyps were not clonal. If the FPC gene codes for a growth supressing gene product, then loss of one allele could decrease suppressor levels sufficiently to allow localized growth abnormalities such as polyps. Once polyps are formed, it provides the opportunity for the second recessive change to take place, followed by other changes leading to the overt colon cancer. These data are consistent with the suggestion of Knudson (44) that the sporadic and inherited form of a particular cancer may both arise from recessive mutations occurring in the same gene and that in order for the cancer to develop, both copies of the gene must be lost. Several other groups have reported abnormalities of chromosomes 1, 7, 8, 12, 14, and 17 in colon cancer (7,46,67,62, & 26). However, only the 17p somatic loss in colon cancers reported by Fearon et al. (26) appears to affect a significant percentage of tumors. The isolation and cloning of the FPC and 17p genes and elucidation of the mechanisms of action of their gene products should have exciting and far reaching effects on our understanding of normal cell replication and differentiation as well as colorectal carcinogenesis. Strategies for prevention and therapy can then be designed with greater precision.

Clinical applications

There are only a few relevant studies in terms of the potential clinical application of differentiation induction therapy in colon cancer.

Several studies demonstrated that exposure to differentiation inducers such as N, N-dimethylformamide (DMF), N-methylformamide (NMF), dimethylsulfoxide (DMSO) and sodium butyrate both in vitro and in vivo can cause increased sensitivity of some human colon cancer cells to such cytotoxic agents as cis-platinum, mitomycin C (20), and misonidazole (3). In addition, these agents not only enhance radiation sensitivity, but also induce an enhanced recovery from potentially lethal damage after exposure to a single large dose of X-rays (21,2). Recently, exposure of colon cancer cells to combination of nucleoside analogs and sodium butyrate greatly enhanced the recovery of these cells from potentially lethal X-ray damage (4).

Another important area in terms of clinical application is the ability of recombinant interferon to enhance specific tumor associated antigens on the surface of colon cancer cells (32). This approach, if successful in in vivo models, may eventually be used in clinical application for the in situ detection and therapy of metastatic colon cancer by monoclonal antibodies either radiolabeled or conjugated with chemotherapeutic agents or toxins.

Summary and future perspectives

Modest but solid progress has been made with respect to our knowledge concerning differentiation of normal and cancerous colonic cells. So far only a few colon cancer cell lines have been used as models for differentiation. In some of these cell lines, chemical inducers of differentiation can cause reversible as well as "stable" differentiation. Cells of different lineage such as columnar cells and mucous cells can be induced or may develop spontaneously. Each cell line responds somewhat differently to the same inducer, indicating the need for studies using combined or sequential exposure to these agents. Several

models of differentiation induction in colon cancer cells are
now available and with further refinement of these models as
well as the development of new models, considerable progress
in this field can be expected. Furthermore, an exciting
beginning has been made with respect to the possible role of
oncogenes and their products, and chromosome aberrations in
regulation of colonic cell growth and differentiation and of
the processes involved in colonic carcinogenesis. Finally,
although available data are limited, they indicate that
differentiation inducers may play an important role in the
detection and therapy of primary and metastatic colon cancer
either directly or by potentiating the effect of cytotoxic agents
or irradiation.

However, much of the work that has been carried out to date
in the colon cancer differentiation field is descriptive and
phenomenological. Clearly, much work needs to be carried out
in the following areas of research. These are: establishment
of normal colon cell lines so that these cell lines can be
modulated to differentiate into cells of various lineages;
further identification of colonic cell types and elucidation
of cell lineages, development of markers (biochemical,
immunological, and molecular) for colonic stem cells and the
cells of various lineage in different stages of differentiation;
use of colon cancer cell lines to develop stable differentiated
colonic cancer cells of various lineages; application of cell
lineage and differentiation-associated markers to classify
colonic tumors in order to predict prognosis and responsiveness
to various types of therapies; isolation and characterization
of growth factors and cell lineage specific differentiation
factors to elucidate the molecular mechanisms involved in
regulation of growth and differentiation of several colonic cell
types; and finally, elucidation of the mechanisms of action of
differentiation inducers used alone or in combination with
cytotoxic agents.

References

1. Altmann, G.G. (1983): Am. J. Anat., 167:95-117.
2. Arundel, C.M., Glickman, A.S., and Leith, J.T. (1985): Cancer Res., 45:5557-5562.
3. Arundel, C.M., Leith, J.T., Lee, E.S., Leite, D.V., and Glicksman, A.S. (1986): Int. J. Radiat. Oncol. Biol. Phys., 12:1429-1432.
4. Arundel, C.M., and Leith, J.T. (1987): Int. J. Radiat. Oncol. Phys., 13:593-601.
5. Augenlicht, L.G., Augeron, C., Yander, G., and Laboisse, C. (1987): Cancer Res., 47:3763-3765.
6. Augeron, C., and Laboisse, C.L. (1984): Cancer Res., 44:3961-3969.
7. Becher, R., Gibas, Z., and Sandberg, A.A. (1983): Cancer Genet Cytogenet, 8:329-332.
8. Bodmer, W.F., Bailey, C.J, Bodmer, J., Bussey, H.J., Ellis, A., Gorman, P., Lucibello, F.C., Murday, V.A., Rider, S.H., Scambler, P., Sheer, D., Solomon, E., and Spurr, N.K. (1987): Nature, 328:614-616.
9. Boland, C.R., Montgomery, C.K., and Kim, Y.S. (1982): Proc. Natl. Acad. Sci. USA, 79:2051-2055.
10. Bolen, J.B., Veillette, A., Schwartz, A.M., DeSear, V., and Rosen, N. (1987): Proc. Natl. Acad. Sci. USA, 84:2251-2255.
11. Bos, J.L., Fearon, E.R., Hamilton, S.R., Verlaan-deVries, M., van Boom, J.H., van der Eb, A.J., and Vogelstein, B. (1987): Nature, 327:293-297.
12. Boyd, D., Florent, G., Chakrabarty, S., Brattain, D., and Brattain, M.G. (1988): Cancer Res., in press.
13. Brattain, M.G., Brattain, D.E., Fine, W.D., Khaled, F.M., Marks, M.E., Arcolano, L.A., and Danbury, B.H. (1981): Oncodev. Biol. & Med., 2:355-367.
14. Chakrabarty, S., Tobon, A., Brattain, M., and Varani, J. (1987): Proc. Am. Assoc. Cancer Res., 28:231.
15. Cheng, H., and Leblond, C.P. (1974): Am. J. Anat., 141:537-561.
16. Cheng, H., Bjerknes, M., Amar, J., and Gardiner, G. (1986): Anat. Rec., 216:44-48.
17. Chesa, P.G., Rettig, W.J., Melamed, M.R., Old, L.J., and Niman, H.L. (1987): Proc. Natl. Adad. Sci. USA, 84:3234-3238.
18. Chung, Y.S., Song, I.S., Erickson, R.H., Sleisenger, M.H., and Kim, Y.S. (1985): Cancer Res., 45:2976-2982.
19. Christina, M.L., Lehy, T., Zeitoun, P., and Dufougeray, F. (1978): Gastroenterology, 75:20-28.
20. Dexter, D.L., Defusco, D.J., McCarthy, K., and Calabresi, P. (1983): Proc. Am. Assoc. Cancer Res., 24:267.
21. Dexter, D.L., Lee, E.S., Bliven, S.F., Glickman, A.S., and Leith, J.T. (1984): Cancer Res., 44:4942-4946.
22. Dharmsathaphorn, K., Mandel, K.G., McRoberts, J.A., Tisdale, L.D., and Masui, H. (1984): Am. J. Physiol., 246:G204-G208.
23. Dharmsathaphorn, K., Mandel, K.G., Masui, H., and McRoberts,

J.A. (1985): J. Clin. Invest., 75:462-471.

24. Drewinko, B., Yang, L.Y., Leibovitz, A., Barlogie, B., Lutz, D., Jansson, B., Strasand, J.J., and Trujillo, J.M. (1984): Cancer Res., 44:4241-4253.

25. Dudouet, B., Robine, S., Huet, C., Sahuquillo-Merino, C., Blair, L., Coudrier, E., and Louward, D. (1987): J. Cell Biol., 105:359-369.

26. Fearon, E., Hamilton, S.R., and Vogelstein, B. (1987): Science, 238:193-197.

27. Forrester, K., Almoguera, C., Han, K., Grizzle, W.E., and Perucho, M. (1987): Nature, 327:298-304.

28. Friedman, E., Thor, A., Horanhand, P. and Schlom, J. (1985): Cancer Res., 45:5648-5665.

29. Fukamachi, H., Mizuno, T., and Kim, Y.S. (1987): J. Cell Sci., 87:615-621.

30. Gallick, G.E., Kurzrock, R., Kloetzer, W.S., Arlinghaus, R.B., and Gutterman, J.U. (1985): Proc. Natl. Acad. Sci. USA, 82:1795-1799.

31. Garin Chesa, P., Rettig, W.J., and Melamed, M.R. (1986): Am. J. Surg. Pathol., 10:829-835.

32. Greimer, J.W., Hard, P.H., Noguchi, P., Fisher, P.B., Pestka, S., and Schlom, J. (1984): Cancer Res., 44:3208-3214.

33. Gum, J., Kam, W., Byrd, J., Hicks, J., Sleisenger, M.H., and Kim, Y.S. (1987): J. Biol. Chem., 262:1092-1097.

34. Hager, J.C., Gold, D.V., Barbosa, J.A., Fligiel, Z., Miller, F., and Dexter, D.L. (1979): J. Natl. Cancer Inst., 64:435-439.

35. Hoosein, N.M., Brattain, D.E., McKnight, M.K., Levine, A.E., and Brattain, M.G. (1987): Cancer Res., 47:2950-2954.

36. Hozumi, M. (1982):In: Cancer Cell Biology Reviews, Vol. 3, edited by J.J. Marchalonis and M.C. Hanna, Jr., pp. 153-211. Marcel Dekker, Inc., New York.

37. Huet, C., Sahuquillo-Merino, C., Coudrier, E., and Louvard, D. (1987): J. Cell Biol., 105:345-357.

38. Itzkowitz, S.H., Yuan, M., Fukushi, Y., Palekar, A., Phelps, P.C., Shamsuddin, A.M., Trump, B.F., Hakomori, S.I., and Kim, Y.S. (1986): Cancer Res., 46:2627-2632.

39. Kaye, G.I., Lane, N., and Pascal, R.R. (1986): Gastroenterology, 54:852-865.

40. Kedinger, M., Simon-Assmann, P.M., Lacroix, B., Marxer, A., Hauri, H.P., and Haffen, K. (1986): Dev. Biol., 113:474-483.

41. Kim, Y.S., Tsao, D., Siddiqui, B., Whitehead, J.S., Arnstein, P., Bennett, J., and Hicks, J. (1980): Cancer, 45:1185-1192.

42. Kim, Y.S., Boland, C.R., and McIntyre, L.J. (1984): In: Markers of colonic cell differentiation, Progress in cancer research and therapy, Vol. 29, edited by S.R. Wolman and A.J. Mastromarino, pp. 221-236. Raven Press, New York.

43. Kim, Y.S., Yuan, M., Itzkowitz, S.H., Sun, Q., Kaizu, T., Palekar, A., Trump, B.F., and Hakomori, S.I. (1986): Cancer

Res., 46:5985-5992.
44. Knudson, A.G. Jr. (1971):Proc. Natl. Acad. Sci. USA, 68:820-823.
45. Leibovitz, A., Stinson, J.C., McCombs, W.B., McCoy, C.E., Mazer, K.C., and Marry, N.D. (1976): Cancer Res., 36:4562-4569.
46. Levin, B., and Reichmann, A. (1986): Cancer Genet Cytogenet, 19:159-162.
47. Lipkin, M. (1986): In: Physiology of the Gastrointestinal Tract, edited by L.R. Johnson, M.J. Jackson, E.D. Jacobson, and H. Walsh, pp. 255-284. Raven Press, New York.
48. Madara, J.L., and Trier, J.S. (1987): In: Physiology of the Gastrointestinal Tract, edited by L.R. Johnson, M.J. Jackson, E.D. Jacobson, and J.H. Walsh, pp. 1209-1249. Raven Press, New York.
49. Markert, C.L. (1968): Cancer Res., 28:1908-1914.
50. Markert, C.L. (1978): In: Cell Differentiation and Neoplasia, edited by G.F. Saunders, pp. 9-22. Raven Press, New York.
51. Marks, M.E., Danbury, B.H., Miller, III, C.A., and Brattain, M.G. (1983): J. Natl. Cancer Inst., 71:664-671.
52. Marks, P.A., Sheffery, M., and Rifkind, R.A. (1987): Cancer Res., 47:659-666.
53. Maskens, A.P., Rahier, J.R., Meersseman, F.P., Dujardin-Loits, R-M, and Hoat, J.G. (1981): Gut, 20:775-779.
54. McBain, J.A., Weese, J.L., Meisner, L.F., Wolberg, W.H., and Willson, J.K.V. (1984): Cancer Res., 44:5813-5821.
55. Meltzer, S.J., Ahnen, D.J., Battifora, H., Yokota, J., and Cline, M.J. (1987): Gastroenterology, 92:1174-1180.
56. Mintz, B., and Illmensee, K. (1975): Proc. Natl. Acad. Sci. USA, 72:3585-3589.
57. Morita, A., Tsao, D., and Kim, Y.S. (1982): Cancer Res., 42:4540-4545.
58. Moxey, P.C. (1978): Gastroenterology, 75:147-149.
59. Moyer, M.P., and Aust, J.B. (1984): Science, 224:1445-1447.
60. Muraro, R., Wunderlich, D., Thor, A., Cunningham, R., Noguchi, P., and Schlom, J. (1987): Int. J. Cancer, 39:34-44.
61. Neal, J.V., and Potten, C.S. (1981): Gut, 22:19-24.
62. Paraskeva, C., Buckle, B.G., Sheer, D., and Wigley, C.B. (1984): Int. J. Cancer, 34:49-56.
63. Pierce, G.B., and Cox, W.F. Jr. (1978): In: Cell Differentiation and Neoplasia, edited by G.F. Saunders, pp. 57-66. Raven Press, New York.
64. Pinto, M., Appay, M.D., Simon-Assmann, P., Chevalier, G., Dracopoli, N., Fogh, J., and Zwerbaum, A. (1982): Biol. Cell, 44:193-196.
65. Pinto, M., Robine-Leon, S., Appay, M.D., Kedinger, M., Triadou, N., Dussaulx, E., Lacroix, B., Simon-Assmann, P., Haffen, K., Fogh, J., and Zweibaum, A. (1983): Biol. Cell, 47:323-330.
66. Quaroni, A., Wands, J., Trelstad, R.L., and Isselbacher,

K.J. (1979): J. Cell Biol., 80:248-265.

67. Reichmann, A., Martin, P., and Levin, B. (1981): Int. J. Cancer, 28:431-440.

68. Richman, P.I., and Bodmer, W.F. (1987): Int. J. Cancer, 39:317-328.

69. Rosen, N., Bolen, J.B., Schwartz, A.M., Cohen, P., DeSeau, V., Israel, M.A. (1986): J. Bio. Chem., 261:13754-13759.

70. Sachs, L. (1987): Cancer Res., 47:1981-1986.

71. Shamsuddin, A.M., Phelps, P.C., and Trump, B.F. (1982): Hum. Pathol., 13:790-803.

72. Solomon, E., Voss, R., Hall, V., Bodmer, W.F., Jass, J.R., Jeffreys, A.J., Lucibello, F.C., Patel, I., and Rider, S.H. (1987): Nature, 328:616-619.

73. Spjut, H.J. (1984): In: Neoplasms of the Colon, Rectum, and Anus, edited by J.S. Spratt, pp. 159-204. W.B. Saunders Co., Philadelphia.

74. Sugerbaker, P., Gunderson, L.L., and Wittes, R.E. (1985): In: Cancer: Principles and Practice of Oncology, Vol. 1, edited by V.T. DeVita, Jr., S. Hellman, and S.A. Rosenberg, pp. 795-884. J.B. Lippincott Co., Philadelphia.

75. Taylor, C.W., Brattain, M.G., and Yeoman, L.C. (1984): Cancer Res., 44:1200-1205.

76. Trugnan, G., Rousset, M., Chantret, I., Barbat, A., and Zweibaum, A. (1987): J. Cell Biol., 104:1199-1205.

77. Tsao, D., Shi, Z., Wong, A., and Kim, Y.S. (1983): Cancer Res., 43:1217-1222.

78. Tsao, D., Morita, A., Bella Jr., A.M., Luu, P., and Kim, Y.S. (1982): Cancer Res., 42:1052-1058.

79. Whelton, A.D., and Dexter, T.M. (1986): Trends Biochem. Sci., 11:207-212.

80. Whitehead, R.H., Jones, J.K., Gabriel, A., and Lukies, R.E. (1987): Cancer Res., 47:2683-2689.

81. Whitehead, R.H., and Gardner, J. (1987): J. Gastroentero. Hepatol., 59-66.

82. Whitehead, R.H., Brown, A., and Bhathal, P.S. (1987): In Vitro, in press.

83. Zweibaum, A., Hauri, H.P., Sterchi, E., Chantret, I., Haffen, K., Bamat, J., and Sordat, B. (1984): Int. J. Cancer, 34:591-598.

STRATEGIES FOR MODIFYING GENE EXPRESSION DURING DIFFERENTIATION

Perspectives on the Feasibility of Differentiation Therapy Through Direct Intervention in Processes that Regulate Expression of Genes Involved in Transformation and Tumorigenicity

J.K. Christman

Department of Molecular Biology, Michigan Cancer Foundation,
110 East Warren Avenue, Detroit, Michigan 48201

INTRODUCTION

Before considering a therapeutic intervention in malignancy that would rely on affecting expression of tumor-related genes and inducing differentiation or response to normal restraints on growth, a number of critical questions must be answered.

What genes should be targeted? Will the primary aim be to activate or inhibit gene expression? How can gene expression be affected equally in all cells in a tumor? Can methods be developed that are relatively specific for tumor cells? How will the genetic heterogeneity of tumor cells affect their response to the proposed therapy?

This chapter will briefly review the current status of evidence indicating the extent of influence of oncogenes and suppressor genes on tumor development and then present a summary of recent contributions toward understanding the regulation of these genes and their role in development and differentiation as communicated by members of subgroup 2.

EVIDENCE OF A GENETIC BASIS FOR CANCER AND REVERSAL OF TUMORIGENIC PHENOTYPES THROUGH DIFFERENTIATION

The role of heredity in oncogenesis has long been recognized and a number of forms of cancer clearly occur in a familial pattern (41, 46). The remainder occur sporadically, with causality generally ascribed to exposure to environmental carcinogens (33). Since the majority of compounds identified as rodent carcinogens are also mutagens in bacterial screens (48), it is further assumed that the bulk of cancers arise as a result of heritable changes in the genome. This concept is supported by the observation of major genetic damage in tumor cells, which can be detected as karyotypic abnormality, amplification of segments of chromosomes [homogeneous staining regions or double minutes], rearrangement of chromosomes or obvious deletions.

If alterations in expression of specific genes lead to cancer, it should follow that reversal of the effects of these changes would lead to reversal of the oncogenic process. The problem, however, is the difficulty in sorting out relevant changes in genetic information from changes that are a result of transformation. At its most extreme, the genetic diversity of human tumor cells would seem to preclude the possibility of identifying causal genetic lesions and reversing them. For example, Shapiro (70) described an enormous variation in chromosome complement of cells from a single freshly isolated human malignant glioma. Chromosome number ranged from 35-200/cell with rearrangements, and loss or overrepresentation of specific chromosomes. At the level of single restriction fragments, Dracopoli, et al. (20) detected loss of heterozygosity in 10 out of 24 autosomal loci and 3 out of 3 loci on the X-chromosome of cells isolated from different metastatic melanomas in a single patient.

Nevertheless, there are numerous examples that indicate the feasibility of reversing the tumorigenic phenotype. The pioneering work of Armin Braun and his colleagues (7), which demonstrated that normal plants could be derived from cells of crown gall tumor, provided the first experimental system where reliable differentiation of tumor tissue could be studied. The acceptability of the idea that cancer therapy might be based on induction of differentiation rather than cell killing required the demonstration that this phenomenon was not limited to plants. This was in great part provided by the studies of Charlotte Friend and her colleagues. They showed that murine erythroleukemia cells which maintained their tumorigenicity in syngeneic hosts could be triggered to express differentiated functions and undergo terminal cell division in vitro (24, 68). Other observations supporting the idea that tumor cells could be induced to behave in a manner indistinguishable from normal cells included demonstrations 1) that highly malignant mouse teratocarcinoma cells introduced into normal blastocysts contributed to the tissues (including germline tissue) of normal, genetically mosaic mice (52), 2) that embryonic fields capable of organizing stem cell differentiation could regulate normalization of tumors of related origin (27, 56), 3) that exposure of tumor tissue to normal adult stroma could result in apparently normal development (22, 63), 4) that contact between malignant and non-malignant cells in vitro could suppress the malignant phenotype (43, 54, 58) and 5) that fusions between normal and tumor cells usually resulted in hybrids that maintained a transformed phenotype in vitro but failed to form tumors on injection into appropriate hosts (40, 76). These results suggest the existence of natural factors, acting humorally or requiring direct contact between the surfaces of the tumor cell and normal cells (or normal extracellular matrices), that are capable of neutralizing or reversing the changes in gene expression that lead to malignant transformation.

IDENTIFICATION OF GENES INVOLVED IN ONCOGENESIS

Dominant Acting Genes

In recent years, studies on the genetic basis of cancer have primarily focused on identification of genes that would act in a dominant manner to transform cells, the oncogenes. Originally identified as the transforming genes of retroviruses, oncogenes have cellular homologues (proto-oncogenes) that have been implicated by association in causing malignant transformation (5, 82). In a variety of tumors, at least one of these genes can often be found to be amplified or translocated to a site which leads to an alteration in the regulation of its expression, or mutated in ways that alter the stability of its transcripts or the function of its protein products. Although to some extent a result of the mechanisms of selection, it is of interest that all of the known proto-oncogenes code for proteins that are involved in signal reception at the cell membrane (hormones, hormone receptors with protein kinase activity), in transmitting signals from the surface (G or N- like signal transduction proteins, protein kinases) or are DNA binding proteins capable of regulating transcription of specific genes or replication of DNA. Thus, malfunction or overabundance of any one of these genes has the potential to affect normal growth regulation and or differentiation. However, it is arguable whether overproduction of any single proto-oncogene is sufficient to transform a normal cell (21). Transgenic mouse studies, in fact, suggest that although expression of transforming proteins such as SV-40 T antigen (8, 31) or even a combination of v-ras and c-myc (44, 72) can increase the probability that an animal will develop tumors to greater than 90%, tumors form in a tissue-specific and stochastic manner. Expression of transforming proteins is not sufficient to cause tumors although it may be sufficient to induce tissue-specific hyperplasia. However, high levels of transforming proteins are found in some organs which do not develop hyperplasia or malignancy and normal cells adjacent to focal tumors in susceptible organs often express similar levels of activated oncogenes to the tumor cells. Several studies of hybrids between normal and tumorigenic cells derived after transformation with activated oncogenes also indicate that elevated levels of oncogene expression persist in non-tumorigenic hybrids and that reversion to tumorigenicity is the result of subsequent loss of specific chromosomes rather than an increase in oncogene expression (15, 55, 74, 76).

Recessive Genes

There is evidence that a variety of familial human tumors are associated with the loss of both functional alleles of a gene whose role is presumably to produce proteins that act as

suppressors of tumor development.   As will be discussed in the
chapter by E. Solomon, major progress has been made in the last
year in cloning and analysis of several of these genes.   This
should soon give clues as to their function.   Introduction of
suppressor genes into different types of tumor cells will allow
a direct test of how their products influence the effects of
oncogene expression and the breadth of their ability to reverse
the tumorigenic phenotype.
     It is already clear that the role of suppressor genes in
regulating oncogenesis and differentiation is not likely to be
any simpler to elucidate than the role of oncogenes.   Karyotypic
and genetic analysis would suggest a minimum of 6 human suppressor loci on different chromosomes, each affecting development
of a different type of cancer (4).   However, it should also be
noted that a single suppressor may have the capacity for affecting more than one tumor type.   More than 65% of retinoblastoma
patients develop secondary osteosarcoma or fibrosarcoma (32,
49) whereas a common locus on chromosome 11 is associated with
Wilm's tumor, hepatoblastoma and rhabdomyosarcoma (42).   Recessive mutations in 24 separate genes have been associated with
the development of malignancy in Drosophila melanogaster, suggesting that many "suppressors" remain to be discovered (25).
The one Drosophila suppressor gene that has been cloned, 1(2)gl,
is expressed in a developmental-stage and tissue specific manner
(50).   Its homozygous inactivation leads to tumors that can be
induced to cease growth by transplantation into normal larvae.
However, the cells do not differentiate (26).
     In summary, there is evidence that both proto-oncogenes and
suppressors are involved in normal development and, at least
for proto-oncogenes with protein-kinase activity, that these
genes are part of multigene families, with each member being
activated and functioning during development of a different
cell lineage (36).   Thus, even without introducing the role of
the immune system, it must be considered that the probability
that expression of a transforming gene or loss of a suppressor
gene will lead to tumor formation may depend on many factors.
These could include 1) the presence of appropriate biochemical
targets that appear only at specific stages of development or
differentiation, 2) the activation of additional oncogenes, or
3) the loss of multiple functions that are capable of blocking
the action of oncogene products at different steps.   In addition, complete expression of the transformed phenotype may well
be influenced by molecules synthesized by adjacent normal cells.

STRATEGIES FOR MODIFYING TUMOR-ASSOCIATED GENE EXPRESSION

     Several strategies for inducing transformed or malignant
cells to differentiate and/or cease unregulated growth were
proposed and critiqued by members of the subgroup during the
First Conference on Differentiation Therapy. Among them were:

1. Inducing differentiation or terminal cell division through use of naturally occurring factors or chemicals that modulate growth and differentiation.

2. Inducing expression of genes that suppress the transformed phenotype and or act as master genes regulating cell differentiation.

3. Suppression of critical oncogene expression through introduction of anti-sense RNAs.

4. Introduction of active tumor suppressor genes.

At present, the most successful therapeutic intervention is likely to result from local or systemic introduction of naturally occurring factors that have been shown to modulate growth and differentiation of tumor cells *in* *vitro* or chemicals that have the potential to activate suppressor genes or genes regulating cell differentiation. The technology does not yet exist for effectively introducing functional suppressor genes or genes that produce antisense RNAs into cells of solid tumors *in* *situ*, no less to get them expressed in every cell. With recent improvements in vectors (47) and use of promoters that should be expressed in all cells regardless of the stage of development (45), it is possible to introduce genes into murine hematopoietic stem cells *in* *vitro* with high efficiency and have them expressed. It remains to be demonstrated that expression of genes introduced with these vectors and promoters will exhibit greater stability in the marrow of recipients than has been found with other constructs (17, 38). However, use of retroviral or other vectors to introduce genes or antisense RNAs into cultured cells is obviously a powerful tool for understanding the contribution of specific gene products to tumor progression, maintenance of the transformed phenotype and loss of normal growth control. A determination of the types of defects in gene regulation that lead to loss of the ability to differentiate or to respond to normal mediators of growth control and of the various mechanisms by which these defects can be corrected or bypassed should eventually form the basis for rational differentiation therapy.

STATUS REPORT

Changes in Oncogene Expression during Transformed Cell Differentiation

The extensive literature on differences in expression of oncogenes during myelopoiesis *in* *vivo* and *in* *vitro* has recently been reviewed (65). The review presents a complex picture of changes in oncogene or proto-oncogene expression at different stages in normal cell development, in leukemic cells, and in

leukemic cells undergoing differentiation in vitro (Also discussed in the chapter by R. Dalla-Favera).

The main emphasis of members of this group has been on determining the relevance of these changes either through altering
the expression of specific oncogenes or through comparison of
cell lines that differentiate with differentiation defective
variants.

Effect of antisense RNAs.

*Holt**, Nienhuis and colleagues found that anti-sense c-fos RNAs
inhibited proliferation and retinoic acid induced differentiation of F9 cells (34) and that anti-sense c-myc RNA inhibited
proliferation of mouse fibroblasts (60). Most interestingly,
an oligonucleotide complementary to c-myc not only inhibited
growth of HL-60 cells but induced differentiation as indicated
by ability to reduce nitroblue tetrazolium dye. Non-specific
oligonucleotides had no effect (35). This indicates that both
c-fos and c-myc proto-oncogenes have important roles in differentiation and cell proliferation.

Effects of enhanced oncogene expression.

Alitalo and his coworkers examined the effects of gene dosage
of c-Ha-ras$^{Val 12}$ on expression of the transformed phenotype
in transfected 3T3 cells. Expression of c-Ha-ras increased
with increased gene dosage and was accompanied by increasing
disruption of cytoskeleton, alterations in growth in culture and
increased levels of ornithine decarboxylase, suggesting that
amplification of mutated oncogenes could play a role in tumor
progression (73).

Roop, Yuspa and co-workers have reported evidence that an
activated c-Ha-ras gene driven by a Mo-MLV LTR was regulated in
primary epidermal cells grafted onto nude mice (64). Benign
tumors developed that had c-Ha-ras transcripts in the basilar
portions of the tumors but not in the more differentiated areas.
Their focus will be on determining whether regulation accounts
for the benign phenotype by placing the c-Ha-ras gene under
control of promoters expressed at different differentiation
states within the epidermis. A strong keratin gene promoter
expressed only under hyperproliferative conditions will also be
used to direct ras anti-sense RNA production and study its
effect on the phenotype of benign and malignant epidermal cell
lines containing an activated c-Ha-ras gene after grafting onto
nude mice.

Fusenig, Stanbridge and their associates have collaborated
on studies of the effects of activated human c-Ha-ras on two
human keratinocyte lines obtained after SV40 transformation,
one with high and the other low degree of differentiation (6).

*Names in italics were participants in the First Conference on
Differentiation Therapy. They reported the information abstrac-
ted here to the Co-chairpersons, J. Christman and E. Stanbridge.
If two participants were collaborators, their names are given
in alphabetical order.

These lines were both converted to malignancy by transfection with activated c-Ha-ras and formed highly differentiated squamous cell carcinomas, leading to the conclusion that malignant cells do not necessarily show major defects in control of proliferation and differentiation. The major emphasis of future work will be on the analysis of regulation of differentiation of normal and transformed human keratinocytes by factors in culture medium, extracellular matrix and mesenchyme under in vitro and in vivo conditions. Single chromosome transfer will be used to identify specific genes controlling malignant conversion.

During studies aimed at determining whether SV-40 T antigen could inhibit differentiation of HL-60 cells, *von Melchner* and his colleagues found that expression of the neomycin phosphotransferase gene introduced for selection purposes delayed differentiation by itself and that expression of T-antigen did not enhance the delay (83). This finding indicates the necessity for careful consideration of the potential effects of an exogenously introduced activity that could phosphorylate cellular proteins. Dr. von Melchner is now focusing on his finding of a GM-CSF mediated reversibility of apparent commitment to terminal differentiation in HL-60 cells (84). He plans to use these cells as a source for subtractive cDNA libraries for isolation of proliferation-specific cDNA sequences.

Oncogene expression in differentiation defective variants.

Verma and his co-workers have concentrated on the role of c-fos. Increased fos gene expression occurs within minutes of exposing cells to a variety of agents that induce cell growth or differentiation and recent studies have shown that c-fos or a c-fos-like protein, participates directly in a nucleoprotein complex that regulates the aP2 gene during adipocyte differentiation (18). However, Mitchell et al. (53) found that c-fos expression could be induced in U937 cells without triggering differentiation. They further found that two HL-60 variants, that were resistant to 12-0-tetradecanoyl phorbol-13-acetate (TPA) as an inducing agent, failed to show an increase in fos expression in response to TPA. However, the variant cells also failed to show increased fos expression on exposure to 1,25-$(OH)_2D_3$ which induced differentiation. These results indicated that fos expression was neither sufficient nor necessary for differentiation of monomyelocytes to macrophages. The group is proceeding with the use of antisense RNA and methylphosphonoate oligonucleotides to determine the effects on differentiation of blocking the synthesis of proto-oncogene products.

We (*Christman* and Calderon) have compared oncogene expression in HL-60 cells and a variant HL-60TR derived in our laboratory (9). HL-60TR cells are resistant to both dimethylsulfoxide (DMSO) and TPA as inducers of differentiation but respond to cis-retinoic acid as an inducer of myeloid differentiation and cis-retinoic acid in combination with TPA as inducers of monocytoid differentiation (51). These cells retain the capability of responding to TPA as evidenced by increased c-fos expression. They also respond to DMSO with decreased c-myc expression. There was no correlation between whether or not they responded to a given inducer by differentiating and shifts in expression of fos and myc. There was even an increase in myc expression in the presence of TPA and cis-retinoic acid. However, c-myb expression in the two lines was markedly different. Although the myb gene was not amplified in HL-60TR cells, myb mRNA was present in at least a 5 fold higher concentration than in HL-60 cells. Myb mRNA levels dropped after treatment with both effective and ineffective inducing agents. However, they only fell below the level found in untreated HL-60 cells with a combination of TPA and cis-retinoic acid. This finding is of some interest in light of the high levels of myb expression in immature hematopoietic cells and human hematopoietic tumors (65) and its apparent importance in commitment of murine erythroleukemia cells to differentiation (59). Further investigations will focus on comparing the structure of the myb transcripts in the two cell lines and the effects of antisense myb RNA on their ability to respond to inducers of differentiation.

Studies of Suppressor Genes and Genes Involved in Normal Development

Suppressor Genes.
Stanbridge and colleagues made an elegant demonstration of the ability of a gene (or genes) on chromosome 11 to suppress the tumorigenic phenotype of a Wilm's tumor cell line (85). A single copy of chromosome 11 [t(X;11)], whose q arm terminus was replaced by the Xq26-Xqter portion of an X chromosome with a functional hypoxanthine phosphribosyltransferase (HPRT) locus, was introduced into cells of an HPRT- variant of the G401 Wilms' tumor line with two cytogenetically normal copies of chromosome 11. This was sufficient to suppress tumorigenicity of the cells in nude mice. Tumorigenicity was regained in cells selected in 6-thioguanine for loss of t(X;11). There was no difference between the tumorigenic and suppressed cells in expression of any of the 8 oncogenes tested.

Homeo box genes.
The homeotic genes that specify organization and diversity of segmental development in Drosophila contain highly homologous regions coding for a strongly conserved domain of 60 amino acids with analogous properties to DNA-binding proteins. These regions, or homeo boxes, have been highly conserved in mammalian genomes. *Kessel* and coworkers have recently cloned cDNAs for two murine homeo box domain proteins, Hox 1.3 (m2) and 1.1 (m6) and prepared antibodies against Hox 1.1 peptides (39, 86). Their results indicate that the genes are expressed during differentiation of F9 embryonal carcinoma cells. Conversely, Hox 1.3 expression was reduced in 3T3 cells after transformation by methylcholanthrene, src or fos oncogenes or SV-40 T antigen. Planned studies will determine the effects of Hox 1.1 and Hox

1.3 proteins on development of transgenic mice by introducing the genes under control of enhancer/promoters that will allow their expression at inappropriate times or locations.

Activation of Genes that Regulate Differentiation

Methylation as a Regulator of Differentiation.
   There is a large body of evidence that methylation of cytosine residues in regulatory regions of genes can inhibit their transcription and that agents that interfere with DNA methylation can activate either whole programs of differentiation or expression of specific genes (12, 19, 37). Further, it is evident that patterns of methylation of specific genes in tumor cells differ from those found in the normal tissues from which they were derived. These differences, which may be either a decrease or an increase in degree of methylation, are found at an early stage of tumor development (3, 28). Loss of methyl groups from genes does not, however, necessarily lead to activation of the genes in tumor cells, presumably because the cells lack appropriate trans-acting regulatory factors or other molecular components necessary for responding to signals that would elicit their production.
Allele specific methylation. Recently, several groups have demonstrated that the methylation pattern of genes in transgenic mice can vary depending on whether the chromosomes carrying the transgene have passed through the male or female germ line (30, 61, 66, 77). In two reports, activity of the transgenes was also determined (30, 77). Methylation of a transgene due to passage through the female germ line was associated with lack of expression, while the relatively unmethylated gene passed through the male germ line was active. The phenomenon of allele specific methylation is not restricted to exogenously introduced genes. *Fusenig, Jones* and coworkers, have demonstrated that autosomal allele-specific methylation of the human c-Ha-ras-1 gene can be detected in fetal tissues and immortal cell lines but not in sperm or normal leukocytes (10).
   These findings suggest that, just as DNA methylation has been linked with X-chromosome inactivation, methylation of individual genes on autosomal chromosomes could lead to differential expression of specific alleles. One intriguing aspect, in terms of development of malignancy, is that damage to a single locus in a gene involved in regulating growth or expression of the transformed phenotype could lead to disruption of normal growth patterns if the other allele had been silenced through methylation. Methylation could occur either during the normal course of development or as a result of disruption of DNA methylation in initiated cells. Assuming that other components of response system are intact, activation of these genes subsequent to treatment with an agent that inhibits methylation would then be predicted to lead to differentiation and/or restoration of growth control.

Methylation and response to inducers of differentiation.   Our
(*Christman*, Schneiderman, Chang) recent studies have focused on
methylation of a set of murine middle-repetitive sequences
[50,000/haploid genome] detected by the probe pMR150 (57).
These sequences are flanked by CCGG sites so that methylation
of regions containing these sequences is readily detected
through use of HpaII and MspI.   The sequences are unmethylated
in both sperm and oocytes, but become fully methylated in the
embryo by 7.5 days of development and remain methylated in
adult somatic tissues (11).   In Friend erythroleukemia (FL)
cells that can be induced to differentiate (Clones 745A and DS-
19), these sites are unmethylated, while in a differentiation
resistant clone (DR-10), they are highly methylated (13).   Since
methylation levels at sites in other genes of these clones did
not reflect this difference, it seemed likely that expression
of some gene in the highly methylated regions detected by the
pMR150 probe might be involved in regulating the ability of the
cells to respond to inducers of differentiation.   In support of
this hypothesis, we have found 1) that the reversal of DR-10 to
inducibility after multiple rounds of treatment with 5-azacyti-
dine is accompanied by loss of methylation in pMR150 sequences
and 2) that a polyadenylated RNA transcript containing pMR150
sequences is expressed in DS-19 but not in DR-10 cells. Treatment with hexamethylene-bis-acetamide (HMBA) increased the level
of this transcript in DS-19 cells but had no detectable effect
on its expression in DR-10 cells (69).   Future work will concen-
trate on cloning this transcript and determining whether its
expression is related to terminal differentiation in other
murine cell lines.

5-azacytidine as an agent for differentiation therapy.
      Although 5-azacytidine (5-azaCR) has been used as a cytotoxic
agent in treating leukemias (62), its ability to trigger differentiation programs or specific gene expression in cultured cells
is striking (12, 37).   5-azaCR has also been used therapeutically to induce fetal globin gene expression in thalassemics,
although there has been some question as to whether the enhanced
expression was the result of gene activation or stem cell selection (78).

      Silverman and colleagues are participating in a trial of
repeated cycles of low-dose 5-azaCR for treatment of patients
with myelodysplastic syndrome (71).   Although results have not
yet been fully analyzed, in a number of cases, response to the
drug as evidenced by increased platelet counts and morphological
normalization of marrow and circulating lymphocyte populations
did not occur until 4-5 cycles of treatment had been completed.
This suggests that multiple rounds of inhibition of methylation
are required before the cells become responsive to signals for
differentiation.   Whether this indicates that multiple genes
must activated, that only part of the tumor cell population is
affected with each round of treatment or that relevant genes
are so heavily methylated as to require multiple rounds of

"demethylation" remains to be determined.

RNA methylation and differentiation. *Tsiftsoglou* and coworker shave found that the naturally occurring nucleoside analog, N^6-methyl adenosine and its derivatives, inhibit initiation of commitment of DMSO-treated murine erythroleukemia cells (79). Since treatment decreases both accumulation of globin-mRNA and methylation of RNA in general without affecting the rate of RNA synthesis, it can be inferred that methylation of critical RNA species is one of the requirements for cell maturation.

Other Related Studies

Evaluation of the association of specific chromosomal abberations with development of human tumors.
Banks-Schlegel has been analyzing the chromosomal abnormalities in human esophageal carcinoma cell lines. Preliminary analysis indicates defects in chromosomes 1,3 and 11, with a consistent location of the defect only on the p arm of chromosome 11 (2). Examination of primary tumors for this defect is underway. It should be noted that reduction to homozygosity in loci of 11p has also been associated with human breast and bladder neoplasia (1, 23).

Since multiple copies of chromosome 1q have been found in 75% of human breast tumors, *Schaefer* is evaluating the role of genes on chromosome 1 in human breast cancer. He has succeeded in cloning 7 fragments from chromosome 1 and is in the process of using these as probes for 1q dosage in human tumors (81).

Development of transgenic mice via blastocyst-derived embryonic stem cell lines.
Kemmler has demonstrated that foreign genes transfected into embryonic stem cells by calcium phosphate DNA precipitation can participate in embryonic development and colonize the germ line of chimeric mice formed by injection of the cells into blastocysts (29). This technique has the advantage of allowing characterization of the transfected genes and their expression during in vitro differentiation prior to blastocyst injection.

Effects of differentiation on tumor development.
Schaefer has shown that dibutyryl cAMP, papavarine and prostaglandins inhibit normal lactogenic differentiation of mouse mammary glands in organ culture (67). Both normal and neoplastic tissue respond with development of squamous metaplasia. With the aid of monospecific antisera to keratins expressed at different differentiation stages (obtained from D. R. Roop), Dr. Schaefer finds induction of new keritin species as the mammary cells become cornified. Future studies will be aimed elucidating how mammary cells become committed to this alternate differentiation pathway.

Effects of differentiating agents on cytotoxicity.
Tsiftsoglou (80) has found that hemin, which induces hemoglobin synthesis in a variety of hemopoitic cell lines, decreases anthracycline-induced cytotoxicity toward cells from a variety

of hemopoietic lines as well as erythroid-burst forming cells from normal human marrow. Hemin failed to protect a number of non-hemopoietic cell lines, leading to the suggestion that hemin might protect the marrow from anthracyclines used during therapy for nonhemopoietic tumors.

IMPLICATIONS FOR THERAPY

The most available compounds for differentiation therapy are those that have been shown to cause cell differentiation in vitro such as retinoids, HMBA, 5-azaCR or naturally occurring biological modifiers such as interferons. However, it is difficult to predict whether effective levels of these agents can be maintained in the patient and, if they are, what their effect will be on normal tissues. Since these agents also have so many effects not related to differentiation, it will be of great importance to determine what is the most biologically effect dose for differentiation, as opposed to the highest dose tolerated by the patient. As yet there are no agents available that can specifically trigger cessation of oncogene expression or activation of suppressor genes.

If, as suggested by the studies discussed here, most tumors result from a combination of enhanced expression of altered proto-oncogenes and inactivation of dominant suppressor genes, then a drug with the potential for activating a wide spectrum of genes such as 5-azaCR or its deoxy-derivative might indeed be an agent of choice. This assumes 1) that at least some genes required for expression of a normal phenotype have been inactivated by methylation, 2) that there are multiple points at which the action of an oncogene can be blocked, i.e., that more than one suppressor has the potential for blocking the malignant phenotype in a given tumor and 3) that treatment can be modulated to enhance the probability of activating genes that can reverse the tumor phenotype rather than genes that will enhance malignancy. In vitro studies support some of these assumptions.

5-azaCR does not activate differentiation programs randomly in cultured cells, even though its mode of action should lead to random inhibition of methylation. 5-azaCR incorporated into DNA causes hypomethylation by tightly binding and inactivating DNA methyltransferase (14). Many sites in newly synthesized DNA become hypomethylated as a result, but subsequent remethylation restores original levels of methylation in all but a few sites (16). Since these sites are often present in genes activated by treatment, it would appear that cellular or extracellular factors that allow the "demethylated" genes to be expressed may also aid in preventing their remethylation (12). Thus, a combined therapy with 5-azaCR, to make genes that regulate growth and differentiation accessible for active transcription, and agents known to mediate normal differentiation in the tissue from which the tumor arose, could be specific and effective.

REFERENCES

1. Ali, I.U., Liderau, R., Theillet, C., and Callahan, R. (1987): *Science*, 238: 185-187.
2. Banks-Schlegal, S.P. *(personal communication)*.
3. Baylin, S.B., Hoppener, J.W.M., deBusto, A., Steinbergh, P.H., Lips, C., and Nelkin, B.D. (1986): *Cancer Res.,* 46: 2917-2922.
4. Benedict, W.F. (1987) In: *Advances in Viral Oncology,* Vol. 7, Raven Press, New York. (in press).
5. Bishop, J. M. (1987): *Science*, 235: 305-311.
6. Boukamp, P., Stanbridge, E.J. Cerrutti, P.A., and Fusenig, N.E. *(ms. submitted)*.
7. Braun, A. (1961) In: *The Harvey Lectures,* Series 56, pp. 191-210. Academic Press, Inc.
8. Brinster, R.L., Chen, H.Y., Messing, A., Van Dyke, T., Levine, A.J. and Palmiter, R.D. (1984): *Cell,* 37: 367-379.
9. Calderon, T. and Christman, J.K. *(ms. in preparation)*.
10. Chandler, L.A., Ghazi, H., Jones, P.A., Boukamp, P., and Fusenig, N.E. (1987): *Cell,* 50: 711-717.
11. Chapman, V., Forrester, L., Sanford, J., Hastie, N., and Rossant, J. (1984): *Nature,* 307: 284-286.
12. Christman, J.K., (1984) In: *Current Topics in Microbiol. and Immunol.,* 108: edited by T.A. Trautner, pp. 49-78. Springer-Verlag, Berlin.
13. Christman, J.K., Karpen, S., and Schneiderman, N. (1986): *Procedings of the Amer. Assoc. of Cancer Res.,* 27: 179A.
14. Christman, J.K., Scheiderman, N., and Acs, G. (1985): *J. Biol. Chem.,* 260: 4059-4068.
15. Craig, R.W. and Sager, R. (1985): *Proc. Natl. Acad. Sci., U.S.A.* 82: 2062-2066.
16. Creusot, F., Acs, G., and Christman, J. (1982): *J. Biol. Chem.,* 257: 2041-2048.
17. Dick, J.E., Magli, M.C., Huszar, R.A., Phillips, A., and Bernstein, A. (1985): *Cell,* 42: 71-79.
18. Distel, R.J., Ro, H-S., Rosen, B.S., Groves, D.L., and Spiegelman, B.M. (1987): *Cell,* 49: 835-844.
19. Doerfler, W. (1983): *Annu. Rev. Biochem.,* 52: 93-124.
20. Dracopoli, N.C., Alhadeff, B., Houghton, A.N., and Old, L.J. (1987): *Cancer Res.,* 47: 3995-4000.
21. Duesberg, P.H. (1985): *Science,* 228: 669-677.
22. Ethier, S.P. and Cundiff, K.C. (1987): *Cancer Res.,* 47: 5316-5322.
23. Fearon, E.R., Feinberg, A.P., Hamilton, S.R., and Vogelstein, B. (1985): *Nature,* 318: 377-380.
24. Friend, C., Patuleia, M.C., and DeHarven, E. (1966): *Natl. Cancer Inst. Monogr.,* 22: 505-522.
25. Gateff, E. (1982): *Adv. Cancer Res.,* 37: 33-74.

26. Gateff, E. and Schneiderman, H.A. (1969) *Natl. Cancer Inst. Monogr.,* 31: 365-397.
27. Gerschenson, M., Graves, K., Carson, S.D., Wells, R., and Pierce, G.B. (1986): *Proc. Natl. Acad. Sci., U.S.A.,* 83: 7307-7310.
28. Goelz, S., Vogelstein, B., Hamilton, S., and Feinberg, A.P. (1985): *Science,* 228: 187-190.
29. Gossler, A., Doetschman, T., Serfling, E., and Kemmler, R. (1986): *Proc. Natl. Acad. Sci., U.S.A.,* 9065-9069.
30. Hadchouel, M., Farza, H., Simon, D., Tiollais, P., and Pourcel, C. (1987): *Nature,* 329: 454-456.
31. Hanahan, D. (1985): Nature, 315: 115-122.
32. Hansen, M.F., Koufos, A., Gallie, B.L., Phillips, R.A., Fodstad, O., Brogger, A., Gedde-Dahl, T., and Cavenee, W.K. (1985): *Proc. Natl. Acad. Sci., U.S.A.,* 82: 6216-6220.
33. Higginson, J. and Muir, C.S. (1973) In: *Cancer Medicine* edited by J.F. Holland and E. Frei pp. 241-263. Lea and Febiger, Philadelphia.
34. Holt, J.T., Moulton, A.D., and Nienhuis, A.W. *(ms in preparation).*
35. Holt, J.T., Redner, R.L., Moulton, A.D., and Nienhuis, A.W. *(ms. in preparation).*
36. Hunter, T., (1987): *Cell,* 50: 823-829.
37. Jones, P.A., Taylor, S.M., and Constantinides, P. (1984): In: *Current Topics in Microbiol. and Immunol.,* 108: edited by T.A. Trautner, pp. 115-127. Springer-Verlag, Berlin.
38. Keller, G., Paige C., Gilboa, E., and Wagner, E.F. (1985): *Nature,* 318: 149-154.
39. Kessel, M., Schulze, F., Fibi, M., and Gruss, P. (1987): *Proc. Natl. Acad. Sci., U.S.A. (in press).*
40. Klinger, H.P. (1980): *Cytogenet. Cell. Genet.,* 27: 254-256.
41. Knudson, A.G., Jr. (1975): *Cancer,* 35: 1022-1026.
42. Koufos, A., Hansen, M.F., Copeland, N.G., Jenkins, N.A., Lampkin, B., and Cavanee, W.K. (1985): *Nature,* 316: 330-334.
43. Kyner, D., Christman, J., Acs, G., Silagi, S., Newcomb, E.W., and Silverstein, S.C. (1978): *J. Cell. Physiol.,* 95: 159-168.
44. Leder, A., Pattengale, P.K., Kuo, A., Stewart, T.A., and Leder, P. (1986): *Cell,* 45: 485-495.
45. Lim, B., Williams, D.A., Orkin, S.H. *(1987): Mol. Cell Biol.,* 7: 3459-3465.
46. Lynch, H.T. (1976): *Cancer Genetics,* Thomas, Springfield.
47. Magli, M.C., Dick, J., Huszar, D., Bernstein, A., and Phillips, R.A. (1987): *Proc. Natl. Acad. Sci., U.S.A.,* 84: 789-793.
48. McCann, J., Choi, E., Yamasaki, B., and Ames, N. (1975): *Proc. Natl. Acad. Sci., U.S.A.,* 72: 5135-5139.

49. Meadows, A.T., Braun, E., Fossati-Belani, F., Green, D., Jenkin, R.D.T., Mursden, B., Nesbit, M., Newton, W., Oberlin, O., Sallan, S.G., Siegel, S., Strong, L.C. and Voute,P.A. (1985): *J. Clin. Oncol.*, 3: 352-538.
50. Mechler, B., McGinnis, W., and Gehring, W.J. (1985): *EMBO Journal*, 4: 1551-1557.
51. Mendelsohn, N., Calderon, T., Acs, G., and Christman, J.K. (1983): *Exp. Cell Res.*, 148: 514-519.
52. Mintz, B. and Illmensee, K. (1975): *Proc. Natl. Acad. Sci., U.S.A.*, 72: 3585-3589.
53. Mitchell, R.L., Henning-Chubb, C., Huberman, E., and Verma, I.M. (1986): *Cell*, 45: 497-504.
54. Newcomb, E.W., Silverstein, S., and Silagi, S.(1978): *J.Cell Physiol.*, 95: 169-177.
55. Oshimura, M., Gilmer, T.M., and Barret, J.C. (1985): *Nature*, 315: 636-639.
56. Pierce, G.B., Pantazis, C.G., Caldwell, J.E., and Wells, R.S. (1982): *Cancer Res.*, 42: 1082-1087.
57. Pietras, D.F., Bennet, K.L., Siracusa, L.D., Woodworth-Gutai, M., Chapman, V.M., Gross, K.W., Kane-Haas, M., and Hastie, N.D. (1983): *Nucleic Acids Res.*, 20: 6965-6983.
58. Poste, G., Doll, J., and Fidler, I.J. (1981): *Proc. Natl. Acad. Sci., U.S.A.*, 78: 6226-6230.
59. Ramsay, R.G., Ikeda, K., Rifkind, R.A., and Marks, P.A. (1986): *Proc. Natl. Acad. Sci., U.S.A.*, 83: 6849-6853.
60. Redner, R.L., Holt, H.J., and Nienhuis, A.W. *(in press)*.
61. Reik, W., Collick, A., Norris, M.L., Barton, S.C., and Surani, M. (1987): *Nature*, 328: 248-251.
62. Rivard, G.E., Momparler, R.L., Demers, J., Benoit, P., Raymond, R., Lin, K.T., and Momparler, L.F. (1983): *Leukemia Res.*, 5: 453-462.
63. Rivera, E.M. and Vijayaraghavan, S. (1982): *J. Natl. Cancer Inst.*, 69: 517-525.
64. Roop, D.R., Lowy, D.R., Tambourin, P.E., Strickland, J., Harper, JR., Balaschak, M., Spangler, E.F., and Yuspa, S.H. (1986): *Nature*, 323: 822-824.
65. Rowley, P.T. and Skuse, G.R. (1987): *Int. J. Cell Clon.*, 5:255-266.
66. Sapienza, C., Peterson, A.C., Rossant, J., and Balling, R. (1987): *Nature*, 328: 251-254.
67. Schaefer, F.V. (1986): *Differentiation*, 32: 238-242.
68. Scher, W., Preisler, H.D., and Friend, C. (1973): *J. Cell Physiol.*, 81 63-76.
69. Schneiderman, N., Chang, Z-F., and Christman, J. *(ms. in preparation)*.
70. Shapiro, J.R. (1986): *Seminars in Oncology*, 13: 4-15.
71. Silverman, L.R. *(personal communication)*.
72. Sinn, E., Muller, W., Pattengale, P., Tepler, I., Wallace, R., and Leder, P. (1987): *Cell*, 49: 465-475.

73. Sistonen, L., Keski-Oja, K., Ulmanen, I., Holtta, E., Wilkgren, B.J., and Alitalo, K. (1987): *Exp. Cell Res.,* 168: 518-530.
74. Srivatsan, E.S., Benedict, W.F. and Stanbridge, E.J. (1986): *Cancer Res.,* 46: 6174-6179.
75. Stanbridge, E.J., Der, C.J., Doersen, C-J., Mishimi, R.Y., Puhl, D.M., Weissman, B.E., and Wilkenson, J.E. (1982): *Science,* 215: 252-259.
76. Stanbridge, E.J., Flander Meyer, R.R., Daniels, D.W., and Nelson-Rees, W.A. (1981): *Somat. Cell. Genet.,* 7: 699-712.
77. Swain, J.L., Stewart, T.A., and Leder, P. (1987): *Cell,* 50: 719-727.
78. Torrealba-DeRon, A., Papayannopoulou, T., Knapp, M.S., Fu, M.F., Knitter, G., and Stamatoyannopoulos, G. (1984): *Blood,* 63: 201-210.
79. Tsiftsoglu, A.S. *(personal communication).*
80. Tsiftsoglu, A.S., Wong, W., Wheeler, C., Steinberg, H.N., and Robinson, S.H. (1986): *Cancer Res.,* 46: 3436-3440.
81. van Peer, C.M.J. and Schaefer, F.V. *(ms. submitted).*
82. Varmus, H.E. (1984): *Ann. Rev. Genet.,* 18: 553-612.
83. von Melchner, H. and Hoffken, K. (1985): *Blood,* 66: 1469-1472.
84. von Melchner, H. and Housman, D.E. (1987): *(ms. submitted).*
85. Weissman, B.E., Saxon, P.J., Pasquale, S.R., Jones, G.R., Geiser, A.G., and Stanbridge, E.J. (1987): *Science,* 236: 175-180.
86. Zink, B., Kessel, M., Colberg-Poley, A.M., and Gruss, P. (1987): *(ms. submitted).*

Induction of Altered Oncogene Expression and Differentiation of Squamous Cell Carcinoma *In-Vitro*

E.H. Chang[1] , J. Ridge[2], Z. Yu[1], W.J. Richtsmeier[3],
J.B. Harford[4] and R. Black[1]

*[1]Department of Pathology, Uniformed Services University of the Health Sciences,
Bethesda, Maryland, 20814;
[2]Bureau of Biologics, FDA, Bethesda, Maryland, 20892;
[3]Department of Otolaryngology-Head and Neck Surgery, The Johns Hopkins
Medical Institutions, Baltimore, Maryland, 21205;
[4]National Institute of Child Health, National Institute of Health,
Bethesda, Maryland, 20892*

ABSTRACT

Treatment of A431 cells in a monolayer or three dimensional
culture system with interferon-gamma (IFN-γ) resulted in rapid
morphological changes, cell death, elevated expression of <u>ras</u>
and epidermal growth factor receptor (EGFR), and enhanced
expression of a differentiation-specific keratin (67KD). It
appeared that the killing by (IFN-γ) of A431 cells resulted
from an induction of terminal differentiation. The tumoricidal
activity of a synergism between tumor necrosis factor-α
(TNF-α) and IFN-γ has been demonstrated in many cell culture
systems. A number of squamous cell carcinoma (SCCA) cell lines
have also been examined in our laboratory in this regard. The
majority of the cell lines were sensitive to the cytostatic and
cytolytic effects of IFN-γ . TNF-α alone had little or no
effect on most of the cell lines. However, a synergistic effect
was clearly observed. To more closely resemble <u>in-vivo</u> tumor
conditions, the 3-dimensional culture systems was used to
maintain primary explants of surgically removed human SCCA
tumors from the head and neck regions. The tumor pieces,
treated with IFN-γ and/or TNF-α at various durations, were
examined for viability, necrosis, degeneration and degree of
cellular differentiation. Over 80% of the tumors responded to
the treatment in a manner supporting our previous findings that
IFN-γ and TNF-α caused SCCA cell death through induction of
terminal differentiation.

*To whom correspondence should be addressed

Interferons function as antiviral agents, cell growth inhibitors and antitumor factors (13). The antitumor, antiproliferative activity of interferon-gamma (IFN-γ) have been demonstrated in a variety of human tumor cells lines (3,48,50,55). These observations suggest that this naturally occuring immunomodulatory protein may be a potential therapeutic agent for cancer and have led to the recent phase I and II clinical studies involving recombinant IFN-γ (5,12,26,29,40,57). Another cytokine, tumor necrosis factor-α (TNF-α), a product of activated lymphocytes and monocytes, has cytolytic and cytostatic effects on murine and human tumor cell lines (20,32,52), and causes hemorrhagic necrosis in-vivo (38). The synergistic antitumor effect of TNF-α and IFN-γ has also been demonstrated in model systems in-vitro and in-vivo (1,2,39,49). The tumor cell lines not responsive to the antiproliferative effect of TNF-α often respond to the combination of these two cytokines. Studies by Philip and Epstein, demonstrated that IFN-γ induces TNF and the latter is responsible for mediating the monocyte cytotoxicity (39). The molecular mechanisms by which IFN-γ and TNF-α exert their antitumor effects remain obscure. Modulation of the expression of the oncogene by IFN's and/or TNF-α has been observed concurrently with cell growth inhibition or phenotypic reversion (10,23,24,31,51). We have examined the effects of IFN-γ and/or TNF-α on various human squamous cell carcinoma cell lines including A431. These cells maintain large numbers of epidermal growth factor receptors (EGFR) on their surface and contain amplified copies of the EGFR gene (11,17,33,34). In addition to this amplification, evidence has been presented suggesting that gene rearrangement has also occured in a portion of the EGFR gene copies contained in A431 cells (58). There are four EGFR transcripts detected in A431 cells that are 10 kb, 5.6 kb, 4.6 kb and 2.9 kb in size. Although the EGFR gene shares homology with the v-erb B, it is not known whether the amplified or the rearranged EGFR genes are involved in the transformed state of A431 cells. Upon treatment of A431 cells with IFN-γ , expression of the 10 kb EGFR mRNA species and the c-Ha-ras message were increased. In addition, we have found a relationship between treatment of A431 cells with IFN-γ and induction of differentiation leading to extensive cell death, concomitant with the increased EGFR and c-Ha-ras expression (6,7). A system has been developed in which human tumor tissue can be maintained "alive" for periods exceeding 6 weeks and with which tumoricidal effects of potential therapeutic agents can be tested. Treatment of fresh primary explants of squamous cell carcinomas of the head and neck with IFN-γ and/or TNF-α results in tumor cell differentiation as well as tumor degeneration and necrosis.

Cytoplasmic RNA was isolated from cells that were pelleted (1000 x g) after being washed in cold 1 x PBS. The cell pellet was resuspended in lysis buffer (0.5% Triton X 100; 150 mM NaCl, 3 mM MgCl$_2$, 0.25 M sucrose and 10 mM Hepes/NaOH pH 8.0) by gentle pipetting. Nuclei and cells were removed from the lysate by low speed centriguation (1000 x g). The supernatant was extracted once with an equal volume of phenol saturated with extraction buffer (0.5% SDS, 1 mM EDTA, 100 mM Tris pH 9.0) once with an equal volume of phenol: chloroform: isoamyl alcohol (25:24:1) and then with chloroform: isoamyl alcohol (24:1) until the interface was clear. RNA was precipitated overnight at -20°C with 2 volumes of absolute ethanol plus 0.2 M sodium acetate pH=5.5. The RNA was centrifuged at 15,000 x g for 30 min, dissolved in diethyl pyrocarbonate-treated H$_2$0 and frozen at -70°C.

Hybridization were performed at 40°C in a solution of 50% formamide, 0/1% Denhardts solution, 5 x SSC, 0.01 M Tris pH=7.5, 0.25 mg/ml salmon sperm DNA and 10% dextran sulfate for 16–18 hrs. Blots were washed with 2 x SSC-0.1% SDS three times at room temperature followed by 1 or 2 washes at 50°C in 0.1 x SSC-0.1% SDS then autoradiographed at -70°C (30,53).

Cell lysis, immunoprecipitation of 2 x 10^7 cpm TCA-precipitable protein, SDS–PAGE and autoradiography were as described previously (19).

Methodologies for cell culture and processing for microscopy have been described (18).

Recombinant human IFN-γ and TNF-α were the generous gifts of Drs. H. Michael Shepard and Christine Czarniecki (Genentech Inc.)

RESULTS AND DISCUSSION

IFN-γ treatment of A431 cells yielded striking results. Cells exhibited an altered morphology prior to extensive cell death within 72 hrs of treatment with 200 u/ml of IFN-γ . This effect was seen with both immune IFN-γ and recombinant IFN-γ . Untreated A431 cells grew as compact colonies. With IFN-treatment, flattened cells appeared within 24 hrs. By 48 hrs floating and pyknotic cells and bare areas of the culture dish were observed. At 72 hrs approximately 60-70% of the cells appeared rounded and detached from the culture substrate. The remaining, adherent cells were elongated and many had extended processes. These effects were even more pronounced at 96 hrs. The cytolytic effect of IFN-γ and/or TNF-α on A431 cells can clearly be shown to be dose dependent (Fig. 1). The synergistic effect of the combined treatment is readily seen at concentrations of IFN-γ of 100 units per ml and with TNF-α at 10 ng per ml. Combinations of lower concentrations of each individual cytokine may also result in a total cytolytic effect on A431 cells.

TNF (ng/ml)

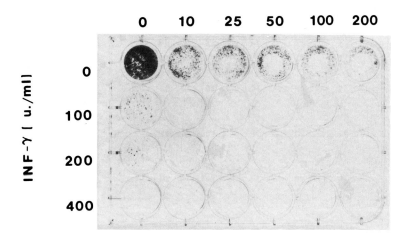

FIG. 1 Effect of IFN-γ and/or TNF-α treatment on A431 cell growth. A431 cells were cultured for 6 days in DMEM plus 10% FBS with the indicated concentration of IFN- γ and/or TNF- α . Every 48 hrs fresh media containing IFN- γ and/or TNF- α were replenished. The 24 well plate was fixed and stained with Gram stain in 25% ETOH and 2.5% formaldehyde.

We have examined the expression of several cellular genes during the course of the IFN-γ treatment described above. Using an EGFR cDNA probe, 4 transcripts (10 kb, 5.6 kb, 4.8 kb and 2.9 kb) were detected in total cytoplasmic RNA extracted from treated and untreated A431 cells. These multiple EGFR transcripts have been previously reported in A431 cells (56,58,60). After 24 hrs of IFN-γ treatment, we observed an elevation specifically in the expression of the 10 kb transcript (Fig. 2). The effect of IFN-γ on the level of 10 kb EGFR mRNA was time dependent. The kinetics of maximal effect (24 to 48 hrs) and the magnitude of the effect (up to 10-fold) varied depending upon the IFN-γ preparation but the effect was observed with several preparation of human immune IFN-γ as well as recombinant IFN-γ . The level of c-Ha-ras specific mRNA was also elevated by IFN-γ treatment albeit to a lesser extent than that seen with the EGFR mRNA (data not shown). The

24 hr

C IFN

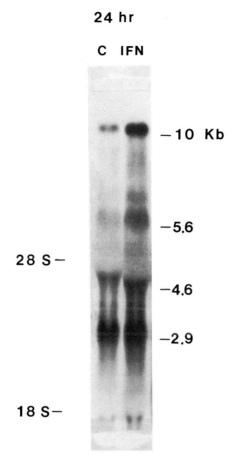

FIG. 2 Effect of IFN-γ on expression of EGFR in A431 cells. A431 cells were treated for the indicated times with 200u/ml IFN-γ . Cytoplasmic RNA was extracted and 30 µg subjected to Northern analysis using a nick translated ^{32}P-EGFR cDNA probe.

increase and subsequent decrease in H-ras p21 expression occurs more rapidly than that of the EGFR after IFN- γ treatment. There is a 2-3 fold increase in ras mRNA at 2 hrs post IFN-γ treatment which decreases to very low levels at times of treatment exceeding 24 hrs. These results are consistent with the hypothesis that these genes may be influenced by related control mechanisms due to similarities between the promotor regions of the EGFR and Ha-ras p21 genes (21).

To establish that the significant increases in the transcript levels of both EGFR and Ha-ras were manifested at the protein level, biosynthetic labeling of A431 cells with ^{35}S-methionine was undertaken. Specific immunoprecipitation of the EGFR revealed that the alterations in the level of the 10 kb transcript were reflected in elevated 170 kd EGFR synthesis (Fig. 3A). The biosynthetic rate for the 21 kb Ha-ras product was also elevated reflecting the higher p21 mRNA levels (Fig. 3B). In contrast, biosynthesis of the tranferrin receptor was shown to be unaffected by IFN- γ treatment in this time frame. It has been reported that elevation in EGF binding sites per cell accompanies increasing density of A431 cells (15). It would appear unlikely that the increase seen with IFN- γ treatment in our study is a result of increasing cell density as the density is decreased by IFN- γ induced cell death.

To examine further the biological effects of IFN- γ on A431, cells were grown in a long term, 3-dimensional culture system which we have previously shown permits tumor cell suspensions inoculated onto agar discs (1 x 10^6 cells per disc) to form aggregated tumor masses or "tumoroids" with in-vivo-like histotypic architecture and expression of cellular functions not found in monolayer (44-46). Cultures were grown up to 29 days with (1200 u/ml) and without IFN- γ ; media were changed 3 times weekly with respective IFN levels maintained throughout the incubation periods. Tumoroids were removed at specific times, fixed in Bouin's solution, paraffin embedded and serial sections prepared for histological staining (44). Hematoxylin and eosin stained sections showed elements reminiscent of in vivo squamous cell carinoma, i.e., keratin pearls and intercellular bridges (Fig. 4B arrow). Compared to controls, IFN-treated cultures exhibited increased cellular stratification similar to that observed in stratifying squamous epithelia and were consistently reduced in both thickness and diameter (Fig. 4C-F). Moreover, increased areas of pyknosis were seen in treated cultures (Fig. 4D and F).

Since cytokeratins have been shown to be useful markers for epithelial cell differentiation (35), immunohistochemical staining (46) with anti-keratin antibodies (Abs) was done to determine if the effects observed were connected with the state of differentiation of the A431 cells. Two monospecific, anti-keratin Abs were used: one to a 50 kd keratin, associated with proliferating epithelia; the other, to a 67 kd keratin, considered differentiation-specific (8,47). Both treated and

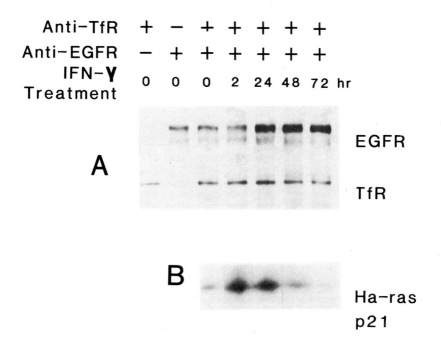

FIG. 3 Effect of IFN-. γ on the biosynthesis of EGFR and
Ha-ras p21 in A431 cells. A431 cells were treated for the
indicated times with 200u/ml human IFN- γ before being
incubated with 50uCi/ml of ^{35}S-methionine in methionine-free
growth medium. Immunoprecipitations were performed on
detergent lysates of the radiolabled cells. In panel A,
anti-EGFR (a gift from Dr. M. Waterfield) and/or
anti-transferrin receptor (TfR) (B3/25, Boehringer-Mannheim)
were employed as indicated and samples analyzed on a 10%
acrylamid gel. In a panel B, anti-p21 (14) (Y13-259, a gift
of Dr. M. Furth) was used and a 12% acrylamid gel employed.
The relevant regions of the resultant autoradiographs are
shown.

untreated tumoroids were found to express the two keratins. However, the control cultures (Fig. 4C) expressed significantly more 50 kd keratin than those treated with IFN- γ (Fig. 4D), whereas the controls (Fig. 4E) expressed less 67 kd keratin than the IFN-treated cultures (Fig. 4F). These initial results suggest that in this system IFN-γ enhances and accelerates squamous cell differentiation in A431 cells, leading to terminal differentiation and subsequent cell death (6,7). Further characterization of this biological effect is currently underway.

The question of a relationship between the IFN-γ alteration in expression of EGFR and the induction of the terminal differentiation of the A431 cells remains open. It has been reported by Jetten that treatment of mouse 3T6 cells with retinoic acids resulted in an increase in the number of EGFR (22) and a similar increase in EGFR was found to accompany retinoic acid-induced differentiation of mouse teratocarcinoma stem cells (41). These studies tend to support the connection between increased EGFR numbers and the process of differentiation. Two classes of EGFR's exist on A431 cells, with "low-affinity" receptors comprisin 90% of the total (25,42). Boonstra, et al., (4) have suggested that the ability of epidermal cells to commit to differentiation is inversely proportional to their number of low affinity EGFR. King and Sartorelli (25) have isolated variants of A431 that differ in their numbers of EGFR and their sensitivity to growth inhibition by the ligand EGF. Variants having lower numbers of EGFR appeared more likely to differentiate in response to serum starvation than were lines with higher numbers of EGFR. The complexity of the process of differentiation may account for what appears to be a variance between our studies and those of King and Sartorelli (25), i.e., they argue that lower numbers of EGFR correlate with the tendency to differentiate whereas we observe increased EGFR expression accompanying differentiation.

We have examined a number of other squamous cell lines and have found a positive correlation between EGFR expression and susceptibility to killing by IFN-γ (data not shown). In the case of A431 cells, treatment with IFN-γ has been shown to result in higher levels of EGFR-mRNA, enhanced EGFR synthesis, and keratin immunohistochemistry consistent with an induction of differentiation. These results are in agreement with those of Nickoloff, et. et., who demonstrated that differentiation in normal keratinocytes in culture was accelerated by IFN-γ (37). Terminal differentiation and cell death are the normal course of events in normal skin cells. The derangement of these events may result in skin diseases including squamous cell carcinomas. From our findings, it would appear that IFN-γ is capable of redirecting a carcinoma cell line along the course of terminal differentiation.

In order to evaluate the therapeutic potential of IFN-γ and/or TNF-α treatment in a system more closely approximating

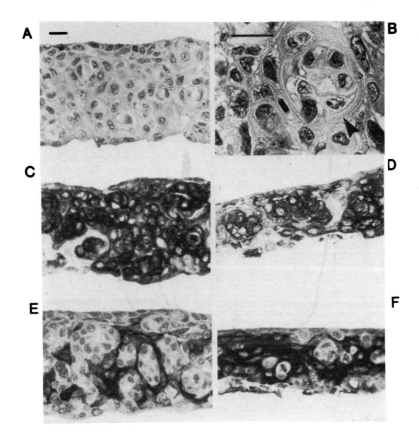

FIG. 4 Features of squamous differentiation in A431 cells grown
in 3-dimensional culture. A431 cells were grown as
3-dimensional agar cultures for 5 days with no IFN (panels A, B,
C, E) or with 1200u/ml IFN-γ   (panels D and F).
Immunohistochemistry was performed with preimmune rabbit serum
(panel A), rabbit anti 50kd keratin (panels C and D), or anti
67kd keratin (panels E and F). Panel B was stained with
hematoxylin and eosin to reveal keratin pearls and intercellular
bridges (arrow). Bars in panels A and B represent 20um and
panels C-F are of the same magnification as panel A.

the in vivo situation, the 3-dimensional agar disc culture system has been employed to maintain primary explants of fresh human tumors during treatment. The tumor tissue can be maintained for periods exceeding 6 weeks. A tumor-associated antigen that is expressed in carcinoma biopsy material but not in carcinoma cell lines grown in monolayers was expressed at significant levels when these cell lines were grown under the conditions of this agar-disc assay (18).

Fresh biopsies from a poorly differentiated squamous cell carcinoma of the larynx were maintained on the agar discs. Tumor pieces of similar size were treated with IFN-γ (1200 u/ml) and/or TNF-α (10 ng/ml). At various times, samples were fixed, embeded, sectioned and stained with hematoxylin and eosin. This specific neoplasm was of a fairly undifferentiated, infiltrating type (Fig. 5A). Three weeks after IFN-γ treatment alone, the tumor piece exhibited a more fibrous and differentiated appearance, developing keratin pearls (Fig 5B). This was not observed in the TNF-α treated samples (Fig 5C). The combination treatment with both cytokines has led to tissue necrosis and degeneration and a great deal of fibroblastic activity can be seen (Fig. 5D).

In this manner, we have studied several fresh tumor biopsies of squamous cell carcinomas. In general, IFN-γ has a greater effect on tumor necrosis, differentiation and degeneration than TNF-α. However, the combination of the two cytokines has shown a synergistic effect on these tumor samples, even with concentrations of TNF-α that alone have no apparent effect.

The tumor samples have also been examined with regard to their expression of EGFR, HLA-DR and keratin. Approximately 40% of the tumors we have studied exhibited elevated levels of EGFR compared to normal epithelium. IFN-γ and/or TNF-α were found to induce an even greater expression of EGFR in these tumors. Using this system for maintaining and treating fresh tumor biopsies in 3-dimensional culture, we hope to correlate the results in vitro with the patients' responses in clinical trials.

We thank Drs. D. Roop, M. Waterfield and M. Furth for monoclonal antibodies against keratins, EGFR, and ras p21 respectively; Dr. J. Schlessinger for EGFR cDNA clone; Ms. R. Garner for excellent technical support, Ms. S. Taylor for manuscript preparation. This work was supported in part by grants from NIH (CA45158) and USUHS (CO7488) to EHC.

The opinions or assertions contained herein are the private views of the authors and should not be construed as official or necessarily reflecting the views of the Uniformed Services University of the Health Sciences or Department of Defense.

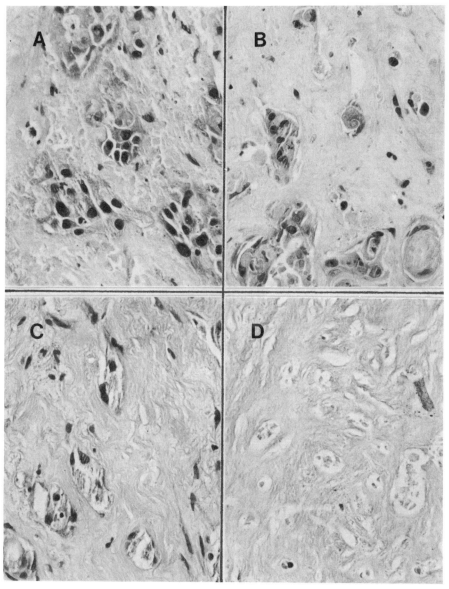

FIG. 5 Effect of IFN-γ   and/or TNF-α   on fresh human SCCA
tumor biopsies. The tumor piece was maintained in culture for 3
weeks (A). Tumor pieces of similiar size were treated with
either IFN-γ (1200u/ml) (B), TNF-α   (10ng/ml) (C), or the
combination of IFN-γ   (1200u/ml) and TNF-α   (10ng/ml) (D) for
3 weeks. Fresh medium and the appropriate cytokines were
replenished twice per week. The samples were fixed, embeded,
sectioned and stained with hematoxylin and eosin as described
(44).

REFERENCES

1. Aggarwal, B.B., Eessalu, T.E., and Hass, P.E. (1985): Nature, 318:665-667.

2. Balkwill, F.R., Fiers, W., and Ward, B.G. In: Ciba Symposium on Tumor Necrosis Factor and Related Cytokines, 1987 In Press.

3. Baron, S., Tyring, S., Albrecht, C., Fleischmann, Jr., W.R., Klimpel, G., Bennett, A., Sarzotti, M., Sanchez, R., Voss, W. (1985). Edited by Dianzani, F., and Rossi, G.B. The Interferon System. Serono Symposia Publication, New York: Raven Press, Vol. 24: pp 333-343.

4. Boonstra, J., DeLatt, S.W., and Ponec, M. (1985): Exptl Cell Res, 161:421-433.

5. Brown, T.D., Koeller, J., Beougher, K., et al (1987): J Clin Oncol, 5:790-798.

6. Chang, E.H., Black, R., Zou, Z-Q., Masnyk, T., Ridge, J., Noguchi, P., and Hanford, J.B. (1986). In: Interferons as Cell Growth Inhibitors and Antitumor Factors. Edited by R.M. Friedman, T. Merigan and T. Sreevalsan. pp 335-349. Alan R. Liss., Inc., New York.

7. Chang, E.HJ., Ridge, R., Black, R., Zou, Z.Q., Masnyk, T., Nogachi, P., and Harford, J.B. Proc Soc Expl Biol Med. In Press.

8. Cooper, D., Schermer, A., and Sun, T.T. (1985): Lab Invest 52:243-256.

9. Downward, J., Yarden, Y., Mayes, E., Scrace, G., Totty, N., Stockwell, P., Ullrich, A., Schlessinger, J., and Waterfield, M.D. (1984): Nature 307:521-527.

10. Einat, M., Resnitzky, D., and Kimchi, A. (1985): Nature, 313:597-600.

11. Fabricant, R.N., DeLarco, J.E., and Todaro, G.J. (1977): Proc Natl Acad Sci USA 74:565-569.

12. Foon, K.A., Sherwin, S.A., Abrams, P.G., et al. (1985): Cancer Immunol Immunother, 20:193-197.

13. Friedman, R.M., Merigan, T., and Sreevalsan, T., eds. Interferons as Cell Growth Inhibitors and Antitumor Factors. New York: Alan R. Liss, Inc., 1986.

14. Furth, M.E., Davis, L., Fleurdelys, B., and Scolnick, E.M. (1982): J Virol 43:294-304.

15. Gill, G.N., and Lazar, G.S. (1981): Nature 293:305-307.

16. Gonda, T.J., and Metcalf, D. (1984): Nature, 310:249-251.

17. Haigler, H., Ash, J.F., Singer, S.J., and Cohen, S. (1978): Proc Natl Acad Sci USA 75:3317-3321.

18. Hand, P.H., Colcher, D., Salomon, D., Ridge, J., Noguchi, P., and Schlom, J. (1985): Cancer Res 45:833-840.

19. Harford, J.B. (1984): Nature, 311:673-675.

20. Helson, L., Green, S., Carswell, E., and Old., L.J. (1975): Nature, 258:730-732.

21. Ishii, S., Merlino, G.T., and Pastan, I. (1985): Science 230:1378-1381.

22. Jetten, A.M. (1980): Nature, 284:626-629.

23. Jonak, G.J., and Knight, E. (1984): Proc Natl Acad Sci USA, 81:1747-1750.

24. Kimchi, A., Yarden, A., and Resnitzky, D. (1986): Interferons as Cell Growth Inhibitors and Antitumor Factors. Edited by R.M. Friedman, T. Merigan and T. Sreevalsan. pp 391-402. Alan R. Liss, Inc., New York.

25. King, I.C.L., and Sartorelli, A.C. (1986): Biochem Biophy Res Comm, 140:837-843.

26. Kurzrock, R., et al. (1986): Blood, 68:225a.

27. Kurzrock, R., Quesada, J.R., Rosenblum, M.G., et al: (1986) Cancer Treat Rep, 70:1357-1364.

28. Kurzrock, R., Rosenblum, M.G., Quesada, J.R., et al. (1986): J Clin Oncol, 4:1677-1683.

29. Kurzrock, R., Rosenblum, M.G., Sherwin, S.A., et al. (1985): Cancer Res, 45: 2866-2871.

30. Lehrach, H., Diamond, D., Wozney, J.M., and Boedeker, H. (1977): Biochemistry, 16:4743-4751.

31. Lin, S.L., Garber, E.A., Wang, E., Caliguiri, L.A., Schellekens, H., Goldberg, A.R., and Tamm, I. (1983): Mol Cell Biol, 3:1656-1664.

32. Matthews, N., and Walters, J.F. (1978): J. Cancer, 38:302-309.

33. Merlino, G.T., Ishii, S., Whang-Peng, J., Knutsen, T., Xu, Y., Clark, A.J.L., Stratton, R.H., Wilson, R.K., Ma, D.P., Roe, B.A., Hunts, J.H., Shimizu, N., and Pastan, I. (1985): Mol Cell Biol 5:1722-1734.

34. Merlino, G.T., Xu, Y.H., Ishii, S., Clark, A.J.L., Semba, K., Toyoshima, K., Yamamoto, T., and Pastan, I. (1984): Science, 224:417-419.

35. Moll, R., Franke, W.W., Schiller, D.L., Geiger, B., and Krupler, R. (1982): Cell 31:11-24.

36. Muller, R., Curran, T., Muller, D., and Guilbert, L. (1985): Nature, 314:546-548.

37. Nickoloff, B.J., Mahrle, G., and Morhenn, V. (1986): Ultrastructural Pathology, 10:17-21.

38. Old, L.J. (1985): Science, 230:630-632.

39. Philip, R., and Epstein, L.B. (1986): Nature 323:86-89.

40. Quesada, J.R., Kurzrock, R., Sherwin, S.A., et al. (1986): Proc Am Soc Clin Oncol, 5:226.

41. Rees, A.R., Adamson, E.D., and Graham, C.F. (1979): Nature, 281:309-311.

42. Rees, A.R., Gregoriou, M., Johnson, P., and Garland, P.B. (1984): EMBO J, 3:1843-1847.

43. Resnitzky, D., Yarden, A., Zipori, D., and Kimchi, A. (1986): Cell, 46:31-40.

44. Ridge, J., Cunningham, R.E., and Noguchi, P.D. (1986): J Tissue Culture Methods, 9(4):211-216.

45. Ridge, J., and Noguchi, P.D. (1983). TCA Report 17:5.

46. Ridge, J., Noguchi, P., Muller, J., and Chang, E. (1986). J Cell Biol 103:206a.

47. Roop, D.R., Hawley-Nelson, P., Cheng, C.K., and Yuspa, S.H. (1983): J Invest Dermatol 81:144s-149s.

48. Rubin, B., Gupta, S.L. (1980): Proc Natl Acad Sci USA, 77:5928-5932.

49. Ruggiero, V., Tavernier, J., Fiers, W., and Baglioni, C. (1986): J. Immunol, 136:2445-2450.

50. Salmon, S.E., Drurie, B.G.M., Young, L., et al (1983): J Clin Oncol, 1:217-221.

51. Samid, D., Chang, E.H., and Friedman, R.M. (1984): Bioch Bioph Res Comm, 119:21-28.

52. Sugarman, B.J., Aggarwal, B.B., Hass, P.E., Figari, I.S., Palladino, Jr., and Shepard, H.M. (1985): Science, 230:943-945.

53. Thomas, P.S. (1980): Proc Natl Acad Sci USA, 77:5201-5206.

54. Ucer, U., Bartsch, H., Scheurich, P., and Pfizenmaier, K. (1985): Int J Cancer, 36:103-108.

55. Ucer, U., Vehmeyer, K., and Nagel, G.A. (1985): Cancer Res, 45:3503-3509.

56. Ullrich, A., Coussens, L., Hayflick, J.S., Dull, T.J., Gray, A., Tam, A.W., Lee, J., Yarden, Y., Libermann, T.A., Schlessinger, J., Downward, J., Mayes, E.L.V., Whittle, N., Waterfield, M.D., and Seeburg, P.H. (1984): Nature 309:418-425.

57. Vadhan-Raj, S., Al-Katib, A., Bhalla, R., et al. (1986): J Clin Oncol, 4: 137-146.

58. Weber, W., Gill, G.N., and Spiess, J. (1984): Science 224:294-297.

59. Westin, E.H., Wong-Staal, F., Gelmann, E.P., Dalla Favera, R., Papas, T.S., Lautenberger, J.A., Eva, A., Premkum, A.R., Reddy, E., Tronick, S.R., Aaronson, S.A., and Gallo, R.C. (1982): Proc Natl Acad Sci USA, 79:2490-2494.

60. Xu, Y., Ishii, S., Clark, A.J.L., Sullivan, M., Wilson, R., Ma, D.P., Roe, B.A., Merlino, G.T., and Pastan, I. (1984): Nature 309:806-810.

Human Myeloid Leukemia Cells: Studies of Proto-oncogene Expression and Cell Differentiation In Vitro

H.D. Preisler, A. Raza, Z. Wang, X.Z. Gao and P. Yang

Department of Hematologic Oncology
Roswell Park Memorial Institute
666 Elm Street, Buffalo New York 14263

There is a growing appreciation of the importance of the biological characteristics of leukemic cells in determining both the course of the disease and response to therapy. In addition, there is increasing evidence that at least a part of the efficacy of cytotoxic therapy may be ascribable to the ability of cytotoxic agents to induce the differentiation of the leukemic cells which survive chemotherapy (2,15). Since it will soon be possible to alter the behavior of leukemic cells by administering recombinant hemopoietins (5) or biologically active noncytotoxic agents (11,17) we must rapidly develop an understanding of the biologic characteristics and potentials of acute leukemic cells and of the potential responsiveness of these cells to these bioactive agents and to cytotoxic agents as well. For these reasons we have been studying the clinical characteristics of AML and the behavior of AML cells in vitro and attempting to relate these to the pattern of gene expression in the leukemic cells. In this paper we will provide a brief overview of our studies.

Studies of Leukemic Cell Differentiation in Vitro

The existence of acute leukemia and the clinical character-istics of this disease attest to the fact that the spontaneous differentiation of AML cells in vivo is an uncommon event. On the other hand, observations of in vivo differentiation associa-ted with cytotoxic therapy strongly suggest that the proportion of leukemic cells which differentiate can be increased. Since it is axiomatic that mature cells of the myeloid series do not proliferate, any substantial increase in the proportion of leukemic cells which mature is likely to reduce the malignancy of the leukemia.

We are conducting in vitro studies of leukemic cell proliferation and differentiation to better define the conditions in which leukemic cell differentiation is facilitated.   Bone marrow and peripheral blood cells obtained from patients with either AML or chronic myelogenous leukemia (CML) are processed by density cut centrifugation over Ficol-Hypaque (sp.g 1.077) and the light density cells recovered. These cells are rosetted with sheep erythrocytes to remove T cells and following which phagocytic cells are removed (8). AML cells are studied at this point while CML cells are subjected to another Ficol Hypaque density cut centrifugation (sp.g. 1.063) to increase the proportion of immature cells to >50%.

Table 1 provides data regarding the behavior of 15 AML specimens placed into liquid culture (RPMI 1640, 20% FCS). During the first week of culture cell numbers fell by > 25% for 8 specimens, there was no change in cell numbers in 4 cultures, and a > 25% increase in cell numbers was observed in 3 cultures. Between weeks 1 and 2 of culture, cell numbers either fell or were unchanged in 12 specimens and increased in 3 cultures. Cell viability was poor with <50% of the cells in the majority of cultures excluding trypan blue after 7 or 14 days of culture. Prior to culture, and after 7 and 14 days of culture, the proportion of immature cells (blast cells plus promyelocytes), maturing myeloid cells (myelocytes, metamyelocytes, and granulocytes) and monocyte/macrophages were assessed with the latter two groups of cells being classified as differentiating cells. All cultures at t=0 contained <10% differentiated cells. As seen in Table 1 evidence for differentiation was seen only in 3 of 15 cultures at week 1 while at week 2 differentiation was noted in almost two-thirds of the cultures.

TABLE 1a. Studies of AML Cells In Liquid Suspension Culture

a)	Cell Counts in Culture					
	7 days+			14 days++		
	↓>25%	NΔ	↑>25%	>75%	NΔ	↑>25%
Control	9	4	3	6	6	3
1L1 α	5	3	4	4	5	3
GM-CSF	5	4	3	4	4	4

+ Relative to number of cells placed into culture.
++ Relative to 7 day culture.

TABLE 1b. Studies of AML Cells In Liquid Suspension Culture

b)	**Percentage of Differentiated Cells in Culture***					
	7 days			**14 days**		
	NΔ	≥10% ≤50%	>50%	NΔ	≥10% ≤50%	>50%
Control	12	3	3	5	5	3
1L1 α	6	6	2	2	7	3
GM-CSF	7	6	2	1	7	5

* % differentiated cells at t=0 = <10%.

Table 2 provides similar data for studies of immature cells obtained from 5 patients in the chronic phase of CML and 8 patients in the blastic phase of CML. In contrast to the AML cultures, in the majority of cases cell counts increased over the two week period of culture with maintenance of excellent cell viability. Further, substantial differentiation was observed in the majority of cultures at both 7 and 14 days.

TABLE 2a. Studies of CML Cells In Liquid Suspension Culture

a)	**Cell Counts in Culture**					
	7 days			**14 days**		
	↓≥25%	NΔ	↑≥25%	↓≥25%	NΔ	↑≥25%
Control C-CML[+]	1	0	4	1	0	4
1L1 α	1	0	3	1	0	2
GM-CSF	1	0	3	0	0	4
Control Bl-CML[++]	2	2	4	2	1	5
1L1 α	2	2	4	1	1	5
GM-CSF	3	1	4	2	0	5

+ Relative to number of cells placed into culture.
++ Relative to 7 day culture.

TABLE 2b. Studies of CML Cells In Liquid Suspension Culture

b)	Percentage of Differentiated Cells in Culture					
	7 days			14 days		
	NΔ	>10% ≤50%	≥50%	NΔ	≥10% ≤50%	≥50%
Control C-CML	1	1	2	0	2	2
1L1 α	1	0	2	0	1	2
GM-CSF	1	1	2	1	0	3
Control B1-CML	2	3	3	1	3	3
1L1 α	2	3	2	1	3	3
GM-CSF	2	3	3	1	2	4

C-CML = chronic phase of CML.
B1-CML = accelerated or blastic phase of CML.

Tables 1 and 2 also provide information on the effects of 1L1α and GM-CSF on the proliferation and differentiation of AML and CML cells in vitro. Neither recombinant hemopoietin had a clear cut effect on cell proliferation. On the other hand, with respect to AML cells, these factors increased both the proportion of cultures showing differentiation and also accelerated the appearance of differentiating cells. In contrast, these growth factors had no demonstrable effects on CML cells in culture.

In summary, cells obtained from the majority of patients with AML will mature to a significant degree in vitro with this process being accelerated and increased by the presence of either 1L1α or GM-CSF. AML cells, however, do not proliferate well in vitro and viability is poorly maintained. CML cells differ from AML cells in that CML cells proliferate well in vitro, maintain excellent viability, and manifest a greater ability to differentiate. With respect to CML cells, proliferation and differentiation does not appear to be dependent upon the addition of exogenous growth factors to the cultures.

Studies of Proto-oncogene Expression in AML Cells

The differences in acute leukemic cell behavior in vitro and in vivo are undoubtedly a reflection of differences in the pattern of gene expression in leukemic cells growing in the two different environments. An important part of our studies are our attempts to define the pattern of gene expression in leukemic cells in vivo and to relate these to the clinical characteristics of the disease.

Leukemic cells obtained from patients at the time of presentation of their leukemia and Northern blot analysis of whole cell RNA performed as previously described (9). Table 3 provides a list of the proto-oncogenes and genes being studied. To date these studies have demonstrated that the level and pattern of proto-oncogene RNA transcripts differ substantially among leukemic patients (9,12,13). The level of expression of the 3 proto-oncogenes associated with cell differentiation (fos, fms, and fes) appear to be correlated with each other and are not correlated with the level of expression of the genes associated with proliferation(myc, myb, histone H_3). With respect to the latter 3 genes, there may be a weak correlation between the level of myc and myb RNA but histone H_3 RNA levels are not correlated with the RNA levels of either myc or myb.

TABLE 3. <u>Genes Being Studies</u>

c-myc	—	associated with proliferation
c-myb	—	associated with proliferation and perhaps differentiation
c-fos	—	associated with proliferation and differentiation
c-fes	—	associated with differentiation
c-fms	—	cell membrane receptor for CSF-1
histone H_3	—	associated with S-phase

Our initial studies demonstrated that the RNA transcript levels for different genes differ depending on the level of maturation of the cells being studied. For example, c-myc RNA levels are highest in immature myeloid cells and low or absent in mature cells (10). c-fos and histone H_3 RNA levels are highest in mature myeloid cells and lowest in immature cells. Therefore comparisons of RNA levels present in different cell populations must take into account differences in the cellular compositions of the populations. A comparison of c-myc RNA levels in acute leukemic bone marrow cells with that present in normal or remission marrow illustrates this point. While myc RNA levels are substantially higher in leukemic marrows, if one corrects for the greater proportion of immature cells present in the leukemic marrows most of the quantitative differences in myc RNA levels between normal and leukemic marrows disappears. With respect to bone marrow and peripheral blood AML cells, proto-oncogene transcript levels in these two cell populations are generally related in terms of either absolute transcript levels or with respect to correlations of the transcript levels present (13).

We have not as yet recognized any relationship between level or pattern of gene expression and FAB type of leukemia (9,12). A weak positive correlation between the level of c-fos RNA and both the percentage of monocytic cells present in a leukemic cell population and the height of the white blood cell count has been detected (13). Preliminary analyses of in vivo cell cycle data (16) and simultaneous gene transcript levels suggest a direct correlation between histone H_3 RNA levels and the percentage of S phase cells present in a population and between c-fms RNA levels and the duration of S phase.(Table 4) The correlations are weak, perhaps as a result of the methodological difficulties with Northern blot analyses described below. With respect to treatment outcome, the data suggest a possible relationship between c-myc RNA levels and treatment outcome (12). Patients whose leukemic cells contain high levels of c-myc RNA appear to have a reduced likelihood of entering complete remission. Preliminary studies have demonstrated that protooncogene transcript levels are affected by cytotoxic therapy and that a fall in c-myc RNA levels after the first 24 hours of treatment may be associated with an increased likelihood of both response to remission induction therapy as well as a long duration of remission (12).

Northern blot analysis can provide useful information regarding the size of RNA transcripts, the number of RNA species present, and the relative level of expression of each species. On the other hand it is difficult to interpret the significance of differences in transcript levels if the differences are small (<2-3 fold). Hence many of the clinical relationships described above must be considered to be tentative. A further limitation with respect to data derived from Northern blot analyses is due to the fact that mean population values are obtained. Consequently the presence of subpopulations of cells whose properties differ substantially than the mean population value will be undetected. Finally, a one to one relationship between RNA transcript level and gene expression in terms of cellular behavior may not be present since gene expression may be regulated at both the translational and post translational level.

For these reasons we have initiated studies of gene expression using antibodies directed against the protein products of the oncogenes. Our initial studies have focused on c-myc expression (14) using a polyclonal antibody kindly provided by Dr. R. Watt (18). Our initial studies have demonstrated differences in both the distribution of cells containing c-myc protein and in the amount of c-myc protein within the leukemic cells of patients whose AML cells have similar appearances and similar RNA transcript levels . Further, by performing double label studies using [3]HTdR autoradiography simultanously with the anti-myc antibodies we have found that not all S-phase cells contain detectable c-myc protein (Fig 1). One can speculate that these cells are perhaps in their last S-phase before leaving the cell cycle. Fig 2 illustrates the effects of chemotherapy on c-myc protein levels in leukemic cells of a patient with AML. Chemotherapy reduced c-myc protein levels but recovery is seen 12 hours after chemotherapy.

TABLE 4. <u>Relationship Between Cell Cycle Characteristics and Gene Expression In AML Cells</u>

			Blot 1[@]	Blot 2[@]
Histone H_3 RNA Level vs % S phase Cells	Pearson	r[+]	.34	.54
		p[++]	.06	.01
	Kendal	r	.23	.46
		p	.08	.005
	Spearman	r	.32	.56
		p	.074	.002
c-fms RNA level vs duration of S phase	Pearson	r	.42	.51
		p	.05	.01
	Kendal	r	.31	.28
		p	.05	.04
	Spearman	r	.41	.36
		p	.06	.06

[@] Duplicate Northern blots of the same RNA specimens.

[+]r = Correlation coefficient.

[++]p = Statistical significance.

FIG. 1. Double Label Study of Bone Marrow Cells Obtained From a
Patient with Newly Diagnosed AML

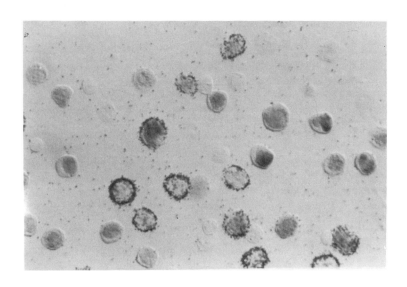

Dark nuclei indicate presence of c-myc protein. Grains around
the cell indicate that the cell has incorporated ^{3}HTdR and
therefore is in S phase. Note that cell containing c-myc
protien may or may not be in S phase. The same is true for
cells not containing detectable c-myc protein.

The introduction of these antibody methodologies will complement the Northern blot analyses in that gene expression at
the single cell level can be quantitated using a method which
has fewer potential sources of quantitative errors. Northern
blot analyses will continue, however, to provide important
qualitative information regarding the size and number of RNA
transcripts.

FIG 2a. Effects of High Dose Cytosine Arabinoside on c-myc Expression in Peripheral Blood AML Cells in Vivo

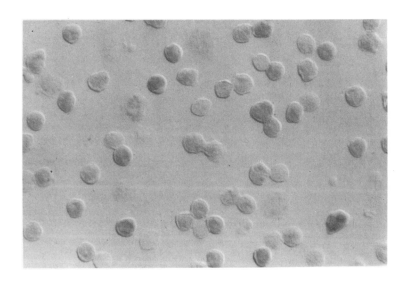

a) Pretherapy - 85% of the cells contain c-myc protein. Note dividing cell in center of field with distribution of c-myc protein to both daughter cells.

FIG 2b.

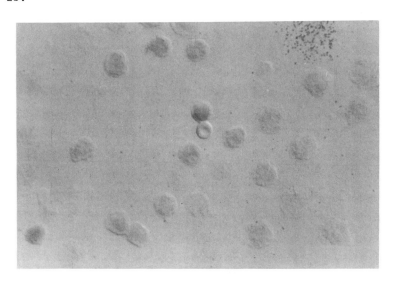

b) Peripheral blood cells obtained 3 hours after the end of administration of dose #1 of cytosine arabinoside. Note intact strongly positive cell immediately above on erythrocyte. Also note cells with poor integrity and a shower of grains from a burst [3]HTdR labeled cell and that c-myc protein levels within cells appears to be reduced.

FIG 2c.

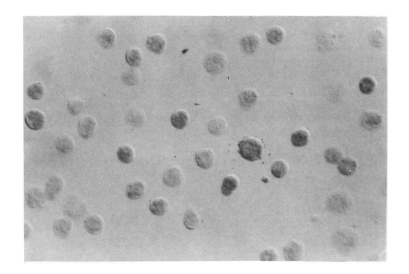

c) Peripheral blood cells obtained 12 hours after the administration of dose #2 of cytosine arabinoside. Note that cell integrity has returned, that c-myc RNA levels are similar to that noted prior to therapy. An S phase cell can be seen.

Leukemic Cell Behavior in vitro - Studies of Proto-oncogene Expression

The observation that leukemic cells differentiate to a much greater extent in vitro than they appear to in vivo is not a unique observation (1,3,4,6). Hence this phenomenon is a general characteristic of AML cells. These observations raise the critical question as to why leukemic cells behave differently in vitro than in vivo. We have initiated studies designed to identify the changes in gene expression which are associated with and possibly responsible for the changes in cell behavior.

Northern blot analyses have been performed on RNA specimens obtained prior to the leukemic cells being placed into culture

and after 24 hours of culture. In 2/3 of the studies to date c-myc RNA levels have fallen after 24 hours of culture. In fact reduced levels can be seen after as little as 3 hours in vitro (7). Fos RNA levels generally fall as well. The reduction in RNA transcript levels are not reflective of a general running down of cellular metabolism since the RNA levels of different proto-oncogenes do not always change in parallel.
Figure 3 illustrates the effects of in vitro culture on gene expression in two leukemic specimens. Changes in myc, myb, and p53 RNA levels parallel each other but vary independently of changes in fos and fms RNA levels. It is of special interest that while RNA transcript levels of some genes fall, for other genes transcript levels which are not detectable in freshly obtained leukemic cells may become detectable after 24 hours of culture (Fig 3b).

Table 5 provides a summary of the changes in gene expression observed when 11 AML specimens were placed into liquid culture for 24 hours. The relationship of these changes to cell proliferation and differentiation at 7 and 14 days are also provided. Note that substantial and uncoordinated changes in gene expression occurred. As noted above, this lack of coordination indicates that the observed changes are not a reflection of cell death but rather they probably reflect the different sensitivities of the expression of different genes to environmental conditions/regulators. There does not appear to be any simple relationship between the changes in gene expression in the population as a whole and cell proliferation and/or differentiation. Despite this lack of correlation in the changes in gene expression, as with leukemic cell differentiation in vitro, these alterations in gene expression are an indication of the profound changes that occur when cells are placed into culture in vitro.

TABLE 5. Changes in RNA Transcript Levels in AML Cells Cultured in Vitro for 24 Hours

Pt No.	myc	H_3	TPI	fos	fms	fes	cell counts	differentiation
1	NC[+]	↑	↑	↓	↑	↑	↑	myeloid - 2 wks[*]
2	NC	↑	NC	↓	ND[++]	↓	NC	myeloid - 1 wk
3	↓	↓	↑	↓	NC	↑	↑	mono/macro - 1 wk
4	NC	NC	↑	↓	↑	↑	↓	none
5	NC	NC	↓	↓	↓	↓	↓	
6	↓	↑	NC	↓	ND	NC	↑	myeloid - 2 wks
7	NC	NC	NC	↓	NC	NC	↓	mono/macro - 1 wk
8 PB	↓	NC	↑	↓	ND	NC	NC	none
BM	↓	↓	NC	↓	ND	NC	↓	
9	↓	NC	NC	↓	↓	↓	↓	mono/macro - 1 wk
10	↑	NC	NC	↓	ND	NC	↓	myeloid - 2 wks

NC[+] = No change. Change = 〉50% ↑ or ↓ in transcript level at t=24 hrs compared to t=0 time.

ND[++] = Not detected at t=o

[*] - Type of differentiation and time when detected

Discussion

A comparison of the behavior of AML and CML cells in vitro demonstrates several significant differences. AML cells proliferate poorly in vitro and quickly lose viability. In contrast, CML cells proliferate well and maintain good viability. The capacity to differentiate is manifested by both forms of leukemia cells but is much more extensive in CML cultures. Several conclusions can be drawn from these observations. The first is that the growth requirements of AML cells are more stringent than those of CML cells at comparable levels of maturation. The observations that AML cells appear to differentiate to a greater extent in vitro than in vivo suggests that in vivo environmental conditions may foster AML cell proliferation while inhibiting the differentiation of these cells. This does not necessarily mean that abnormal conditions exist in vivo in AML patients since the behavior of AML cells in a normal environment is not likely to be "normal". On the other hand, the existence of abnormal environmental conditions which foster abnormal behavior by already abnormal cells cannot be ruled out. The failure of many AML cell populations to maintain c-myc transcript levels in vitro may be due to the absence of growth promoting factors in the in vitro cultures. Attempts to maintain c-myc RNA levels by the addition of either a calcium ionophore, TPA, or the two together failed in most cases to maintain c-myc RNA levels (Fig 3). The fact that on occasion these in vitro manipulations are successful suggests that the rate limiting phenomena responsible for the reduction in gene expression may not be the same in all cases.

With respect to the behavior of CML cells in vitro, the high level of proliferation and differentiation evidenced by these cells suggests that the cells are already preprogrammed in vivo and simply continue their in vivo behavior in vitro without a need for growth and differentiation promoting substances, that they produce their own growth factors, or that very small levels of these regulators are present in the in vitro system (? in fetal calf serum) and that these levels are sufficient to stimulate CML cells but not AML cells. Whatever the reason, CML cells are clearly less stringent in their growth requirements than the majority of AML cells. The cells obtained from patients in advanced blastic crisis continue to proliferate well in vitro but do not differentiate suggesting that high proliferative ability is inherent in CML cells and is independent of the ability of the cells to differentiate. Given that the Ph' chromosome and presumably the bcr-abl fusion protein is present in both chronic phase and blastic phase CML cells, this gene product may be responsible for the enhanced proliferative characteristics of CML cells in vitro.

Recombinant hemopoietins increase both the rate of AML cell differentiation and the degree of differentiation in vitro suggesting that similar effects might be produced in vivo. There is a potential risk, however, of administering these factors to patients with AML since under in vivo conditions proliferation might be stimulated with resultant adverse clinical effects. On the other hand such effects could be beneficial if they served to increase the sensitivity of AML cells to cytotoxic chemotherapeutic agents. Whatever their eventual role, the ability of these hemopoietins to produce biological effects is likely to lead to their being useful in some settings in the treatment of AML.

FIG 3. Proto-oncogene Transcript Levels in AML Cells Before and After 24 Hours of Culture

FIGURE 3

a) Patient # 1

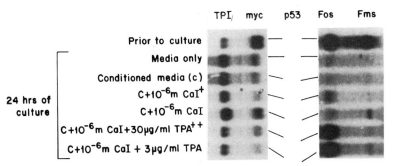

+calimycin
++12-0-tetradecanoyl phorbol-13-acetate

a) c-myc, p53, c-fos and c-fms levels fall while TPI (triose phosphate isomerase) RNA levels are maintained. The presence of TPA in the culture media either maintains or stimulates c-fos expression with no effect on c-fms, c-myc or p53 expression. In contrast calimycin, alone, appears to stimulate c-myc and p53 expression without affecting c-fos expression.

FIG 3b.

FIGURE 3

(b) Patient #2

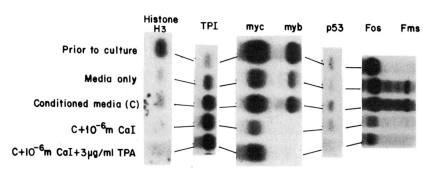

b) c-myc, c-myb, p53, and c-fos expression are maintained in vitro while c-fms expression is detectable only after culture. In this study the presence of calimycin alone or together with TPA appears to reduce both c-fos and c-fms expression.

ACKNOWLEDGEMENT
This work is supported by NCI grant #41285. The authors would like to thank Dr. S. Gilles and the Immunex Company for providing the ILIℓ and GM-CSF used in these studies.

REFERENCES

1. Elias L and Greenberg P. (1977): Blood, 50:263-274
2. Fearon ER, Burke PJ, Schiffer CA, et al. (1986): N. Engl. J. Med., 315:15-24
3. Golde DW, Byers LA, and Cline MJ. (1974): Cancer Res., 34:419-423
4. Golde DW, and Cline MJ. (1973): Blood, 41:45-57
5. Groopman JE, Mitsuyasu RT, DeLeo MJ, et al. (1987): N.Engl. J. Med., 317:593-598
6. Palu A, Powles R, Selby P, et al. (1979): Br. J. Cancer, 40:719-730
7. Preisler HD, Sato H, Yamanchi K, and Kinniburgh A. (1986): Blood 68: abst. #925
8. Preisler HD, and Epstein J. (1987): J. Lab. Clin. Med., 94:414-420
9. Preisler HD, Kinniburgh AJ, Guan W, and Khan S. (1987): Cancer Res., 47:874-880
10. Preisler HD, Kinniburgh AJ, Guan W, and Khan S. (1988) Leuk. Res. (in press)
11. Preisler HD, Li Y, Lam FM, and Raza A. (1987): Proc. Amer. Soc. Hemat., Blood 68: abstr #792
12. Preisler HD, and Raza A. (1987): Semin. Oncol., 14:207-216
13. Preisler HD, Sato H, Li Y, and Stein G. (1987): Cancer Res. 47: 3747-3751
14. Preisler HD, Kaufman C, Watt R, Gao XZ, Wang Z, Wilson M, and Sato H. (1987): Am. Soc. Hemat. Meeting Washington DC. Abstract # H-MO-0009
15. Raza A, and Preisler HD. (1986): J. Cancer, 1:15-18
16. Raza A, Maheshwari Y, and Preisler HD (1987): Blood, 69(6) 1647-1653
17. Talpaz M, McCredie KB, Mavligit G, and Gutterman JU. (1983): Blood, 62:689
18. Watt R, Shatzman A, Rosenberg M. (1985): Molec. Cell. Biol., 5:448-456

CELL BIOLOGY OF DIFFERENTIATION THERAPY: CELL-CELL INTERACTION

Cell-Cell and Cell-Stromal Interactions in Differentiation Therapy

D. Medina and E. Huberman*

*Baylor College of Medicine, Department of Cell Biology,
One Baylor Plaza, Houston, Texas 77030 and
*Division of Biology and Medicine, Argonne National Laboratory, Argonne,
Illinois 60439*

I.   INTRODUCTION

The significance and role of cell-cell and cell-stromal interactions is well established in normal fetal developmental processes. For example, ductal morphogenesis of the mammary gland
during late fetal stages is determined by the interaction of mesenchymal cells, androgens and the recipient epithelial cells
(39,40). Similar interactions occur in the development of the
prostate glandular epithelium (12). Such interactions continue
to play a determinant role in the functional differentiation of
the mature organ. For instance, the functional differentiation
of the mammary gland depends on multiple components of the
cellular and acellular stroma. The interactions between epithelium and stroma occur in both directions, a concept emphasized by
the term "dynamic reciprocity" which has been used to describe
such interactions (4). Functional differentiation depends on
cytodifferentiation which is influenced to a large extent by the
interactions of cell surface molecules with constituents of the
extracellular matrix (2,30). There are numerous examples of such
interactions involving glandular cells, corneal cells, neurons,
and hepatocytes.

Cell-cell and cell-stromal interactions may play a critical
role in neoplastic development since tumor cells are often viewed
as cells with altered developmental fates. It is interesting
that an early pioneer of tumor biology, Leslie Foulds, viewed
neoplastic development in terms of the concepts underlying normal
developmental biology (21). Similarly, Barry Pierce has written
extensively on the theme that "neoplastic development is a cari-
cature of the normal process of tissue renewal" (63). It is
timely to examine the role of such interactions in the possible
differentiation of preneoplastic and neoplastic tissues and
determine if such interactions could play an important role in
differentiation therapy. In this paper, we review some of the
evidence that alterations of epithelial-mesenchymal interactions
or cell-cell interactions can alter the expression of neoplasia.

II.   INTERACTIONS IN NORMAL AND NEOPLASTIC CELLS

A.   Mammary Gland

The importance of epithelial-mesenchymal cell interactions in the development of the primary mammary duct has been elegantly detailed by Kratochwil (39,40). In a series of publications, he documented the existence and nature of reciprocal interactions between the mammary epithelial bud and underlying mesenchyme. The mesenchyme induces the down-sprouting of skin epithelium to form the presumptive mammary bud. Subsequently, the epithelial cells induce the appearance of morphologically unique mesenchyme (mammary mesenchyme) and the formation of androgen receptors (in the male) in this special mesenchyme. In the male, androgens interact with the mesenchyme to cause condensation and migration of the mesenchyme around the epithelial bud, followed by rupture of the epithelial stalk and necrosis of the epithelium. The use of epithelial-mesenchymal recombinants for wild-type and androgen insensitive Tfm mice established the mesenchyme as the androgen-responsive tissue. The "androgen-responsive window" for these events occurs between days 13-14 of fetal life. The significance of mammary mesenchyme in female mice is not clear, although such mesenchyme resides around the nipple and contains estrogen receptors. Additionally, Sakakura (70) has proposed that the mammary mesenchyme determines the ability of the epithelium to interact with the fatty stroma.

In the growing mammary gland, the importance of the stromal component for morphogenesis and functional differentiation is highlighted by several observations. First, mammary epithelial cells exhibit normal morphogenesis only in white adipose stroma, thereby emphasizing the importance of the stroma in providing critical factors for morphogenesis. In branching morphogenesis of the gland, specific interactions occur between the prolif-erating portion of the duct (end buds) and stromal cells, which can be detected by increased ^{3}H-thymidine labeling of stromal cells and differential glycosaminoglycan synthesis around the end buds (92). In the mature mammary gland, disruption of the basal lamina by hyaluronidase leads to epithelial growth reminiscent of ductal dysplasias (75). In addition, Sakakura et al. (70,71) have shown that the morphogenic patterns of the epithelium are directed by the specific type of mesenchyme. Thus, salivary mesenchyme will induce a salivary pattern of duct morphogenesis in mammary epithelial cells. Even dysplastic epithelium is responsive to the inductive influences of salivary mesenchyme (70). Interestingly, functional differentiation specific for the mammary gland is maintained under these conditions. In contrast, in the prostate gland, functional differentiation is not disso-ciated from morphological differentiation.

Secondly, numerous experiments have demonstrated that the expression of many mammary epithelial functions can be regulated by the extracellular matrix (ECM). Morphological differentiation and cell shape of mammary cells in culture depends on the nature of the substratum (16-18,43,45,55,86). Similarly, the regulation of different milk components in mouse mammary epithelial cells is modulated to different extents by the particular constituents of the substratum (43,45,55). For instance, the floating collagen gel membrane supports synthesis and secretion of all caseins but not those of whey acidic proteins and alpha-lactalbumin. The modulation of mammary-specific function by the substratum has also been demonstrated for rat (91) and rabbit mammary gland (81).

Third, specific mammary differentiation may also depend on specific cell types in the mammary gland, as evidenced by the presence of metabolic cooperativity between epithelial and stromal cells in vivo (1). Also, estrogenic effects on proliferation of mammary epithelial cells in vitro require the presence and contact of stromal fibroblasts (29). In vitro, an interaction between mammary epithelial cells and specific 3T3 sublines also promotes maintenance of hormone-dependent differentiation in the absence of exogenous ECM (44).

The above examples illustrate the complex set of interactions involving epithelial cells, stromal cells, ECM and hormones that are involved in mammary gland morphogenesis and differentiation. Are any of these interactions operative in neoplastic development? It is well-documented that a full-term pregnancy and lactation early in life can decrease mammary tumor risk in humans (50). Similarly, full term pregnancy and lactation after treatment of rats (28,69) and mice (51) with known chemical carcinogens can significantly reduce mammary tumor risk. Several investigators have proposed that hormones stimulate differentiation of high risk cells (69) or existing preneoplastic cells (28) into a low risk cell compartment. This hypothesis has never been directly tested and the role of the stromal compartment in this process has not been examined.

In one experiment that examined the link between induced differentiation and tumor potential, no correlation was found between the capacity of preneoplastic cells to exhibit mammary-specific functional differentiation (i.e. milk-protein synthesis) and their subsequent tumor potential (Medina, unpublished results).

Despite the absence of direct proof for an interrelationship between induced mammary differentiation and tumor potential, there is evidence that cell-cell and cell-ECM interactions, similar to that in normal development, also occur in the early stages of neoplastic development. First, preneoplastic but not neoplastic cells are dependent upon the white adipose stroma for growth and spatial organization (20,53). Second, recombinant cell populations comprising normal and preneoplastic cells

exhibit a decreased tumor potential compared to that of preneoplastic cells alone (54). A similar phenomena has been
reported for tracheal cells in vivo (84) and mesenchymal cell
lines in vitro (3. In the reconstituted tracheal grafts, the
growth of preneoplastic and neoplastic cells is inhibited by
normal cells. The growth-inhibitory activity of differentiated
normal tracheal cells was detected in active form in conditioned
medium. In the 10T1/2 cell line, growth of neoplastic transformed 10T1/2 cells was inhibited by nontransformed cells of the
same strain. Inhibition required cell contact suggesting that
diffusable factors were not involved.

Finally, DeCosse et al. (14) reported that embryonic mammary
mesenchyme co-incubated with a transplanted tumor caused the appearance of differentiated ductules, an increase in acid mu-
copolysaccharide deposition in the ECM, and a decrease in DNA
synthesis in the tumors. These events did not require cell
contact. Unfortunately, the tumors did not exhibit any changes
in growth rate when retransplanted back into syngeneic mice.

B. Prostate Gland

Adult urothelium is sensitive to fetal urogenital sinus mesenchyme (UGS) with the result being induction of differentiation
to prostatic glandular epithelium. The induced prostatic cells
express morphological, ultrastructural, histochemical, antigenic
markers and androgen receptors specific for prostate (13,59).
Heterotypic combinations utilizing epithelium other than
urothelium do not result in altered developmental fate of the
epithelium. The inductive influence of UGS upon adult urothelium
is not species-specific but is observed in heterospecific
combinations involving human, rabbit, rat and mouse tissues (11).
Epithelial cells from BALB/cTfm mice, which are devoid of nuclear
androgen-binding sites, in combination with the wild-type stromal
cells (androgen-receptor positive) result in prostatic
development, suggesting that stromal cells have a direct role on
androgen-mediated differentiation in the prostate (82). This
result is seen in both embryonic and adult urothelial cells.
Several reports have suggested that stromal cells synthesize
regulatory molecules that influence prostatic epithelial
proliferation (73,82). Several trophic factors, both of stromal
and epithelial origin have been proposed to regulate prostate
epithelial development in a "stimulation feedback" loop (83).
Cell-stromal interactions can be detected also under in vitro
culture conditions where adult rat ventral prostate will form
three-dimensional differentiated structures in a collagen gel
culture (37).

Are neoplastic bladder epithelial cells responsive to similar
inductive influences by embryonic urogenital sinus mesenchyme?
Hodges et al. (31) showed that carcinogen-induced stromal alterations influenced cell surface architecture of normal urothelium,

however neoplastic epithelial cell surface architecture was not influenced by the normal stroma. Fujii et al. (23) demonstrated the induction of partial acinar differentiation in transitional cell carcinomas of rat urinary bladder in recombinants with UGS mesenchyme. The latter suggests that tumors retain some sensitivity to UGS mesenchyme control. Recently, Rowley and Tindall (68) demonstrated that the NBT-II bladder carcinoma cell line was responsive to conditioned medium from normal rat fetal urogenital sinus. The NBT-II cells exhibited a decreased proliferative index, an increase in protein secretion, a decrease in total cellular protein synthesis, and an altered morphology. The latter may be an excellent model system to examine some of the factors involved in control of differentiation of normal and neoplastic cells.

C. Hematopoetic Differentiation

Hematopoesis in vivo depends on bone marrow, spleen and other related types of stromal cells (72,87,94). The nature of the dependency presumably resides in both cell-cell interactions between stromal and progenitor cells and in diffusable factors and constituents of the extracellular matrix produced by stromal cells (15,62,64,66,94,95). Although some of the diffusable factors (i.e., CSF, IL-3) have been identified, there is evidence that additional diffusable macromolecules and undefined components of the extracellular matrix are important for differentiation and proliferation of hematopoetic cells (7,78-79; Wicha, this volume). Part of the basis for stromal regulation of hematopoesis is the requirement for cell adhesion of progenitor cells to stromal cells and/or their microenvironment. One such adhesion molecule is hemonectin (7; Wicha, this volume). The requirement for adhesion is illustrated in several recent reports (66,77-79,96). In the cell lines developed by Spooncer and coworkers (78,79), adhesion to stromal cells is positively correlated with survival and proliferation on stromal cells in the absence of IL-3.

The importance of marrow stromal cell and blood progenitor cell interactions has been observed with normal, extended life, and leukemic blood cells (87,94,95). With HL-60 myeloid leukemic cells, the differentiative and proliferative responses to 1-alpha, 25-dihydroxy vitamin D_3 are modulated by adhesion to marrow stromal cells (60). The cellular interactions between HL-60 and bone marrow stromal cells required attachment and were specific, since stromal cells from thymus and lymph node were not effective in modulating the response of HL-60 cells to 1-alpha, 25-dihydroxy vitamin D_3. Interestingly, the marrow stromal cells produced a diffusable factor that stimulated vitamin D_3-induced responses of nonattached HL-60 cells; the factor that modulated inhibition of attached cells was not diffusable. One of the differences between normal and leukemic stem cells may reside in their respective abilities to adhere and/or physically interact with marrow stromal cells (27,33). Gordon et al. (27) recently reported that CML progenitor stem cells exhibited altered adhesive properties with marrow stromal cells. The macromolecules of interest are not known yet.

III. MECHANISMS

Several mechanisms have been postulated to play a necessary, albeit insufficient, role in the regulation of tumor growth or differentiation by cell-cell interactions. Five frequently discussed factors include cell-cell communication, diffusable factors, extracellular matrix, cell surface molecules and cyto-differentiation. The latter three factors are probably all interrelated and may represent the phenotypic signature of a cell committed to a differentiated response.

A. Cell-Cell Communication

The importance of cell-cell communication in tumor promotion has been extensively discussed over the past 10 years. Proponents of this mechanism argue that it is central to the control of cell growth and differentiation and that disruption of the communication between cells provides a selective advantage for initiated cells (46,65,88). The understated emphasis in the theory of cell communication is that regulatory molecules from normal cells can influence the behavior of initiated cells. The theory presumes cell-cell contact. It has been postulated to be operative in fibroblast (3,19) and epithelial cell lines (57,88). Basically, nontransformed or premalignant cells exhibit inter-cellular communication in homologous or heterologous combinations whereas transformed or malignant cells do not. In 3T3 cells, cells within carcinogen-induced foci communicate with each other, but not with nontransformed monolayer cells. In an extensive study of this phenomeon, Mehta et al. (56) showed that the level of intercellular communication in heterologous combinations between untransformed and transformed cell lines was proportional to the degree of growth inhibition. Similarly, cell contact was necessary for growth inhibition in this system. Cell-communi-cation occurs via gap junctions (49); tumor promoters which block cell communication also inhibit the presence of gap junctions (34,35).

The relevance of gap junctional communication in drug-induced differentiation of tumor cells is not well defined. Inferential data from retinoid effects on junctional communication and cell differentiation suggest a lack of association between the two parameters (8,56). This relationship holds for embryonal carcinomas (7,61) and 10T1/2 mesenchymal cells (56). However, cell-communication via gap junctions is optimally present in hepatocytes where cyto- and biochemical differentiation is maintained by the appropriate epithelial-mesenchymal cell interactions. Thus, proteoglycans and glycosaminoglycans are critical for the maintenance of intercellular communication (24). Disruption of this association alters normal intercellular communication, which would alter both cellular differentiative and growth properties (93).

B. Diffusable Factors - TGF_B

Some of the most compelling evidence for cell-cell communication operating via paracrine mechanisms comes from the recent study of TGF_B. Contrary to its name, TGF_B inhibits growth in epithelial cells (58,74,80) and is a member of a family of molecules that are involved in growth regulation, including morphogenetic processes (80). With respect to possible cell-cell interactions in the inhibition of growth and induction of differentiation, there are four important recent observations. In the trachea system, Terazagki-Howe (84) has demonstrated that TGF_B is an operative molecule in the inhibition of growth of transformed cells by normal cells. Whether these cells differentiate or not is unclear; however, Masui et al. (52) have shown that TGF_B is an important differentiation-inducing agent for respiratory epithelium. Rowley and Tindall (68) have recently demonstrated that a TGF_B-like molecule appears to play a role in the inhibition of growth and induction of differentiation of a urinary bladder cell line by urogenital sinus mesenchyme, a classical inducer system. Silberstein and Daniel (76) and Knabbe et al. (38) have demonstrated that TGF_B inhibits the growth of mammary duct end bud cells and human breast cancer cells, respectively. One pathway of TGF_B action may be through stimulation of the synthesis of ECM molecules like collagen and fibronectin (32,76). Other growth inhibitors derived from normal mammary gland appear to be unrelated to classical TGF_B (5).

C. Cell-Surface Receptors and Extra-Cellular Matrix

A recurring theme in the regulation of cell differentiation is the importance of the extracellular matrix. The molecular pathways by which information can be transmitted into cells from factors operating via extracellular matrix macromolecules have been hypothesized by several investigators (2,4,30,67,76). A linkage between extracellular macromolecules and intracellular events is mediated by specific cell surface receptors for ECM molecules (6,9,41,67; Wicha, this volume), which in turn are associated with the cytoplasmic cytoskeleton. This relationship has been shown for laminin, fibronectin, hyaluronate, and

proteoglycan molecules. As mentioned above, TGF_B acts to
increase synthesis of extracellular matrix molecules and this in
turn may inhibit growth and/or stimulate differentiation. The
above studies, although few in number, suggest that the induction
and/or maintenance of the ECM-cell surface receptor-cytoskeletal
pathway is an attractive target for differentiation therapy
agents.

A related theme is the induction of altered cell surface properties in response to certain chemopreventive agents. For instance, Lotan and coworkers (47,48) have demonstrated that
retinoids inhibit growth as well as enhance morphological and
biochemical differentiation of murine melanomas and human
squamous-cell carcinomas. These phenomena were associated with
increased glycosylation of cell surface sialoglycoproteins and
altered mobility of cell membrane macromolecules. Other
modifiers of transformation result in altered adhesiveness to
substratum, which presumably reflects modification in linkages of
the cytoskeleton to membrane macromolecules (42,85). For
instance, retinoids increase attachment to laminin and collagen
IV substrates, presumably via alterations of cell surface
receptors (36).

IV. SUMMARY

There are several theoretical mechanisms by which a resident
stromal cell type can modulate the function of tumor cells.
Differentiation and proliferation of tumor cells can be modulated
by direct cell contact and by diffusable macromolecules produced
by stromal cells. The expression of specific functions of stromal as well as epithelial cells can be influenced by specific
inducers (i.e., Vitamin D_3, TGF_B) that can modulate synthesis and
secretion of growth factors, extracellular matrix molecules and
cell surface molecules (which affect adhesion). The end result
of such alterations of stromal cell function is a decrease in
proliferation and/or increase in differentiative properties of
the tumor cell. The important factors in normal prostate gland
differentiation are not well defined, whereas a variety of
molecules have been defined in mammary gland and hematopoetic
growth and differentiation.

It is important to recognize that the induction of differentiation in epithelial systems does not automatically signify an alteration in tumorigenesis, much less prove the importance of
cell-cell interactions in differentiation of epithelial tumors.
Although there are reports of regression of tumors in strong embryonic fields or in regenerating fields (25,26,89,90) and
isolated reports of non-neural epithelial tumors converting to
benign growth when placed in heterotypic cellular interactions
(10,22), what is desperately needed is convincing evidence in

well-documented model systems that specific induction of differentiated function in epithelial tumors occurs and that the phenomenon operates under the same fundamental laws that regulate cell differentiation in normal development. Until such results can be demonstrated and accepted widely, the concept of differentiation therapy will only be applicable to specialized cases like hematopoetic tumors and teratocarcinomas. To simply demonstrate that an inducer generates a differentiated response in a tumor cell population is not sufficient to argue that growth and tumorigenicity will be compromised. Likewise, the knowledge that cell-cell interactions are important in normal development does not guarantee that the same fundamental laws are operative in the tumorigenic process. Indeed, one can speculate that one of the primary alterations in tumors or preneoplasias in a decreased requirement or sensitivity to microenvironment-related signals. Whether tumors can regain sensitivity to these signals is an important and unanswered question.

V. REFERENCES

1. Bartley, J.C., Emerman, J.T., and Bissell, M.J. (1981): *Am. J. Physiol.*, 241:C204-C208.
2. Bernfield, M., Banerjee, S.D., Koda, J.E. and Rapraeger, A.C. (1984): In: "Role of Extracellular Matrix in Development," edited by R.L. Trelstad, pp. 545-572. Alan R. Liss, Inc., New York.
3. Bertram, J.S. and Faletto, M.B. (1985): *Cancer Res.*, 45:1946-1952.
4. Bissell, M.J., Hall, H.G., and Parry, G. (1982): *J. Theor. Biol.*, 99:31-68.
5. Bohner, F.D. Lehmann, W., Schmidt, H.E., Langen, P., and Grosse, R. (1984): *Expt. Cell Res.*, 150:466-476.
6. Brown, S.S., Malinoff, H.L., and Wicha, M.S. (1983): *Proc. Natl. Acad. Sci.*, USA., 80:5927-5930.
7. Campbell, A.D., Long, M.W., Wicha, M.S. (1987): *Nature*, in press.
8. Campione-Piccardo, J., Sun, J-J., Craig, J., and McBurney, M.N. (1985): *Dev. Biol.*, 109:25-31.
9. Chen, W-T., Hasegawa, E., Hasegawa, T., Weinstock, C., and Yamada, K.M. (1985): *J. Cell Biol.*, 100:1103-1114.
10. Cooper, M. and Pinkus, H. (1977): *Cancer Res.*, 37:2544-2552.
11. Cunha, G.R., Sekkingstad, M., and Meloy, B.A. (1983): *Differentiation*, 24:174-180.
12. Cunha, G.R., Chung, L.W.K., Shannon, J.M., Taguchi, O., and Fujii, H. (1983): *Rec. Progr. Hormone Res.*, 39:559-598.
13. Cunha, G.R., Fujii, H., Neubauer, B.L., Shannon, J.M., Sawyer, L., and Reese, B.A. (1983): *J. Cell Biol.*, 96:1662-1670.

14. DeCosse, J.J., Gossens, C., Kuzma, J.F., and Unsworth, B.R. (1975): J. Natl. Cancer Inst., 54:913-922.
15. Dexter, T.M., Whetton, A.D., Spooncer, E., Heyworth, C.M., and Simmons, P. (1985): J. Cell Sci., 3:1-13.
16. Durban, E.M., Medina, D., and Butel, J.S. (1985): Dev. Biol., 109:288-298.
17. Emerman, J.T. and Pitelka, D.R. (1977): In Vitro, 13:316-328.
18. Emerman, J.T., Bartley, J.C., and Bissell, M.J. (1981): Expt. Cell Res., 134:241-250.
19. Enomoto, T. and Yamasaki, H. (1984): Cancer Res., 44:5200-5203.
20. Faulkin, L.J., Jr., and DeOme, K.B. (1960): J. Natl. Cancer Inst., 24:953-969.
21. Foulds, L. (1969): Neoplastic Development. Academic Press, Inc., London.
22. Freshney, R.I. (1985): Anticancer Res., 5:111-130.
23. Fujii, H., Cunha, G.R., and Norman, J.T. (1982): J. Urology, 128:858-861.
24. Fujita, M. (1986): Prog. Clin. Biol. Res., 226:333-360.
25. Gerschenson, M., Graves, K., Carson, S.D., Wells, R.S., and Pierce, G.B. (1986): Proc. Natl. Acad. Sci., USA., 83:7367-7370.
26. Gootwine, E., Webb, C.G., and Sachs, L. (1982): Nature, 299:63-65.
27. Gordon, M.Y., Dowding, C.R., Riley, G.P., Goldman, J.M., and Greaves, M.F. (1987): Nature, 328:342-344.
28. Grubbs, C.J., Hill, D.L., McDonough, K.C., and Peckham, J.C. (1983). J. Natl. Cancer Inst., 71:625-628.
29. Haslam, S.Z. (1986): Cancer Res., 46:310-316.
30. Hay, E.D. (1984): In: "Role of Extracellular Matrix in Development," edited by R.L. Trelstad, pp. 1-31. Alan R. Liss, Inc., New York.
31. Hodges, G.M., Hicks, R.M., and Spacey, G.D. (1977): Cancer Res., 37:3720-3730.
32. Ignotz, R. and Massague', J. (1986): J. Biol. Chem., 261:4337-4345.
33. Islam, A. (1985): Med. Hypoth., 17:69-77.
34. Kalimi, G.H. and Sirsat, S.M. (1984): Carcinogenesis, 5:1671-1677.
35. Kalimi, G.H. and Sirsat, S.M. (1984): Cancer Lett., 22:343-350.
36. Kato, S. and DeLuca, L.M. (1987): FASEB Abstracts.
37. Kawamura, H. and Ichihara, I. (1987): Prostate, 10:153-162.
38. Knabbe, C., Lippman, M.E., Wakefield, L.M., Flanders, K.C., Kasid, A., Derynck, R., and Dickson, R.B. (1987): Cell, 48:417-428.
39. Kratochwil, K. (1977): Devel. Biol., 61:358-365.

40. Kratochwil, K. (1987): In: "Cell and Molecular Biology of Mammary Cancer," edited by D. Medina, W.R. Kidwell, G.H. Heppner, and E. Anderson, (in press). Plenum Publ. Corp., New York.

41. Lacy, B.E. and Underhill, C.B. (1987): J. Cell Biol., 105:1395-1404.

42. Leader, W.M., Stopak, D., and Harris, A.K. (1983): J. Cell Sci., 64:1-11.

43. Lee, E.Y-H., Parry, G., and Bissell, M.J. (1984): J. Cell Biol., 98:146-155.

44. Levine, J.F. and Stockdale, F.R. (1985): J. Cell Biol., 100:1415-1422.

45. Li, M.L., Aggeler, J., Farson, D.A., Hatier, J., and Bissell, M.J. (1987): Proc. Natl. Acad. Sci., USA, 84:136-140.

46. Loewenstein, W.R. (1979): Biochim. Biophys. Acta Cancer Res., 560:1-65.

47. Lotan, R., Neumann, G., and Deutsch, V. (1983): Cancer Res., 43:303-312.

48. Lotan, R., Sacks, P.G., Lotan, D., and Hong, W.K. (1987): Int. J. Cancer, 40:224-229.

49. MacDonald, C. (1985): Essays Biochem., 21:86-118.

50. MacMahan, B., Cole, P., Liu, M., Lowe, C.R., Mirra, A.P., Ravinehar, B., Salber, E.J., Valaoras, V.G., and Yuasa, S. (1970): Bull. W.H.O., 34:209-221.

51. Marchant, J. (1958): Brit. J. Cancer, 12:55-61.

52. Masui, T., Wakefield, L.M., Lechner, J.F., LaVeck, M.A., Sporn, M.B., and Harris, C.C. (1986): Proc. Natl. Acad. Sci., USA, 83:2438-2442.

53. Medina, D. (1973): Methods Cancer Res., 7:3-53.

54. Medina, D., Shepherd, F., and Gropp, T. (1978): J. Natl. Cancer Inst., 60:1121-1126.

55. Medina, D., Li, M.L., Oborn, C.J., and Bissell, M.J. (1987): Expt. Cell Res., 172:192-203.

56. Mehta, P.P., Bertram, J.S., and Loewenstein, W.R. (1986): Cell, 44:187-196.

57. Mesnil, M., Montesano, R., and Yamasaki, H. (1986): Exptl. Cell Res., 165:391-402.

58. Moses, H.L., Tucker, R.F., Leof, E.B., Coffey, R.J., Halper, J., and Shipley, G.D. (1985): Cancer Cells, 3:65-71.

59. Neubauer, B.L., Chung, L.W.K., McCormick, K.A., Taguchi, O., Thompson, T.C., and Cunha, G.R. (1983): J. Cell Biol., 96:1671-1676.

60. Ohkawa, H. and Harigaya, K. (1987): Cancer Res., 47:2879-2882.

61. Papaioannou, V.E., Waters, B.K., and Rossant, J. (1984): Cell Different, 15:175-179.

62. Patt, H.M., Maloney, M.A., and Flannery, M.L. (1982): Exptl. Hemat., 10:738-741.

63. Pierce, B. (1983): Am. J. Pathol., 113:117-124.

64. Piersma, A.H., Brockbank, K.G.M., Ploemacher, R.E. (1984): Exptl. Hemat., 12:617-623.
65. Potter, V.R. (1980): Yale J. Biol. Med., 53:367-384.
66. Quesenberry, P.F., Song, Z., Alberico, T., Gualtieri, R., Stewart, M., Innes, D., McGrath, E., Cranston, S., and Kleeman, E. (1985). In: "Hematopoetic Stem Cell Physiology," edited by E.P. Cronkite, N. Dainiak, R.P. McCaffrey, J. Palek, and P.F. Quesenberry, pp. 247-256, Alan R. Liss, Inc., New York.
67. Rapraeger, A., Jalkanen, M., and Bernfield, M. (1986): J. Cell Biol., 103:2683-2696.
68. Rowley, D.R. and Tindall, D.J. (1987): Cancer Res., 47:2955-2960.
69. Russo, I. and Russo, J. (1986): Cancer Surveys, 5:649-670.
70. Sakakura, T. (1983): In: "Understanding Breast Cancer: Clinical and Laboratory Concepts," edited by M.A. Rich, J.C. Hager and P. Furmanski, pp. 261-284, Dekker, New York.
71. Sakakura, T., Sakagami, Y., and Nishizuka, Y. (1982): Devel. Biol., 91:202-207.
72. Schofield, R. (1978): Blood Cells, 4:7-25.
73. Shannon, J.M. and Cunha, G.R. (1984): Biol. Reprod., 31:175-183.
74. Shipley, G.D., Pittelkow, M.R., Wille, J.J., Scott, R.E., and Moses, H.L. (1986): Cancer Res., 46:2068-2071.
75. Silberstein, G.B. and Daniel, C.W. (1982): Dev. Biol., 90:215-222.
76. Silberstein, G.B. and Daniel, C.W. (1987): Science, 237:291-293.
77. Spooncer, E., Lord, B.I., and Dexter, T.M. (1985): Nature, 316:62-66.
78. Spooncer, E., Gallagher, J.T., Krizsa, F., and Dexter, T.M. (1983): J. Cell Biol., 96:510-514.
79. Spooncer, E., Heyworth, C.M., Dunn, A., and Dexter, T.M. (1986): Differentiation, 31:111-118.
80. Sporn, M.B., Roberts, A.B., Wakefield, L.M., and deCrombrugghe, B. (1987): J. Cell Biol., 105:1039-1045.
81. Suard, Y.M.L., Haeuptle, M-T., Farinon, E., and Kraehenbuhl, J-P. (1983): J. Cell Biol., 96:1435-1442.
82. Sugimura, Y., Cunha, G.R., and Bigsby, R.M. (1986): Prostate, 3:217-225.
83. Tenniswood, M. (1986): Prostate, 9:375-385.
84. Terzaghi-Howe, M. and McKeown, C. (1986): Cancer Res., 46:917-921.
85. Thorne, H.J., Jose, D.G., Zhang, H-Y., Dempsey, P.J., and Whitehead, R.H. (1987): Int. J. Cancer, 40:207-212.
86. Tonelli, Q.J. and Sorof, S. (1982): Differentiation, 22:195-200.
87. Trentin, J.J. (1971): Am. J. Path., 65:621-628.
88. Trosko, J.E., Chang, C-C., Medcalf, A. (1983): Cancer Invest., 1:511-526.

89. Tsonis, P.A. (1984): Can. J. Zool., 62:2681-2685.
90. Wells, R.S. and Miotto, K.A. (1986): Cancer Res., 46:1659-1667.
91. Wicha, M.S., Lowrie, G., Kohn, E., Bagavandon, P., and Mahn, T. (1982): Proc. Natl. Acad. Sci., USA, 79:3213-3217.
92. Williams, C.W. and Daniel, C.W. (1983): Dev. Biol., 97:274-290.
93. Yamasaki, H., Enomoto, T., and Martel, N. (1984): IARC Sci. Publ., 56:217-238.
94. Zipori, D. and Sarson, T. (1980): Expt. Hematol., 8:816-817.
95. Zipori, D., Toledo, J., and Vander Mark, K. (1985): Blood, 66:447-455.
96. Zuckerman, K.S. and Rhodes, R.K. (1985): In: "Hematopoietic Stem Cell Physiology," edited by E.P. Cronkite, N. Dainiak, R.P. McCaffrey, J. Palek, and P.F. Quesenberry, pp. 257-266, Alan R. Liss, Inc., New York.

Extracellular Matrix, Endothelial Cell Shape Modulation, and Control of Angiogenesis: Potential Targets for Anti-Tumor Differentiation Therapy

D.E. Ingber and J. Folkman

From the Department of Surgery, The Children's Hospital,
Department of Pathology, Brigham and Women's Hospital, and
Departments of Pathology, Surgery, and Anatomy & Cell Biology,
Harvard Medical School, Surgical Research-Enders 1021,
The Childrens Hospital, 300 Longwood Ave., Boston, MA 02115

INTRODUCTION

Chemotherapeutic agents used for treatment of cancer are commonly selected based on their ability to inhibit tumor cell proliferation. However, their clinical effectiveness is limited because they also inhibit the growth of normal cells. The most common cause of side effects in tumor therapy is therefore injury to normal tissues which exhibit the most rapid rates of cell turnover. Cytotoxicity within the intestine, immune system, and hair follicles results in nausea, compromised immune response, and hair loss, respectively. Side effects that do not subside often lead to cessation of therapy and treatment failure. Our current methods for design and selection of anti-cancer agents will most likely produce new and more potent anti-mitotic drugs. Yet, their clinical efficacy undoubtedly will be limited in a similar fashion.

One reason for the current emphasis on development of cytotoxic chemotherapy is the commonly held belief that cancer is a disease that results from uncontrolled cell proliferation. While cancer formation requires sustained cell growth, this defect on its own would not result in the formation of a malignant tumor. Rather, cancer may be thought to result from progressive loss of the normal regulatory controls which coordinate cell growth, orientation, differentiation, and tissue boundary expansion. For example, loss of cell-cell relations and

local breakdown of tissue boundaries are usually required for
designation of an epithelial neoplasm as malignant. In addition,
the sustained growth of solid tumors requires that the tumor must
also gain the ability to stimulate ingrowth of new capillaries to
provide a continuous supply of oxygen and nutrients. In this
manner, malignant tumors may be thought to result from
deregulation of the normal developmental processes by which cells
become organized into tissues and tissues into organs (for a
review of cancer as a disease of tissue genesis see ref. 13).

Based on the observation that the sustained growth of tumors
requires continued neovascularization, we previously suggested
that tumors may be "angiogenesis-dependent" and that tumor growth
could be controlled through the use of specific inhibitors of
capillary growth (3,4). Thus, our approach differs from other
investigators in the area of "Differentiation Therapy" in that we
hope to develop an anti-tumor therapy that interferes with
malignant histodifferentiation rather than promoting
cytodifferentiation of individual tumor cells. Nonetheless, we
share a common aim: to develop a non-cytotoxic therapeutic
regimen that can result in effective eradication of malignant
tumors.

INHIBITION OF ANGIOGENESIS

We recently described a new class of steroids, known as
"angiostatic steroids", which inhibit angiogenesis when
administered in combination with heparin (2,6,8). These
compounds are defined as members of a new class of steroids since
their anti-angiogenic activity is independent of all previously
recognized steroid functions including glucocorticoid,
mineralocorticoid, and sex steroid activities. Many of the major
"inactive" steroid metabolites (e.g., the tetrahydrocortisols)
also have been found to be potent inhibitors of capillary growth
when combined with heparin. All of the known angiostatic
steroids induce regression of growing capillaries although they
have no effect on non-growing vessels or nearby epithelium.
Thus, the importance of this specificity for growing (i.e.,
pathologic) capillaries is that clinical use of angiostatic
steroids should be relatively free of any complicating side
effects.

Angiostatic steroids and heparin can inhibit tumor-induced
angiogenesis when administered locally (8). Systemic
administration of heparin-steroid combinations can also induce
complete regression of a variety of solid tumors in rodents (6).
Yet, clinical use of these compounds has been limited by two
major problems: 1) lack of sufficient quantities of active
heparin and 2) insufficient knowledge of the anti-angiogenic

mechanism. A more thorough understanding of the underlying mechanism of action should hopefully allow us to design more potent anti-angiogenic compounds and perhaps circumvent the need for heparin.

MECHANISM OF ANTI-ANGIOGENESIS

Little was known about the mechanism of action of angiostatic steroids since they acted independently of all previously recognized steroid functions. However, we gained a clue to the mechanism of capillary regression from examination of what is known about other epithelial tissues that undergo involution. For example, it is known that physiological regression of mammary gland (27) and Mullerian duct (11) correlates temporally and spatially with breakdown of the epithelial basement membrane (BM).

This was an important coincidence since our own past studies on the mechanism of neoplastic disorganization of normal tissue morphology showed that BM stability is required for maintenance of normal tissue form (12,15,16). We were able to demonstrate that BM serves as a spatial organizer which controls cell shape and orientation and physically coordinates individual cells within a polarized epithelium (16). Based on these studies, we proposed that normal and pathological changes of tissue form may be controlled through directed alterations of BM structure that alter cell shape (12-14). Thus, we thought that the relation between tissue involution and BM dissolution could be more than just a correlation.

Based upon our hypothesis that BM alterations may be central to the anti-angiogenic mechanism, we used immunofluorescence microscopy to determine whether combinations of angiostatic steroids and heparin altered BM as part of their action. To study the relation between BM and anti-angiogenesis, we utilized the chick chorioallantoic membrane (CAM) as a model system. The CAM is the major site for gas exchange in the embryonic chick and is comprised of planar ectoderm and endoderm separated by a highly vascular mesoderm. Chick embryos can be cultivated in vitro if removed from their shells at day 3 of development and placed within petri dishes at 37°C under 3% CO_2. Under these conditions, the chick will develop normally for at least an additional week. During this period, the CAM appears on the surface of the embryo by day 6 and extends to cover its entire surface by day 8. The vascular network of the CAM therefore undergoes rapid lateral extension during this period.

We commonly screen compounds for anti-angiogenic activity by placing the substance within methylcellulose sustained-release

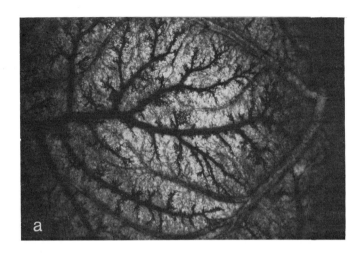

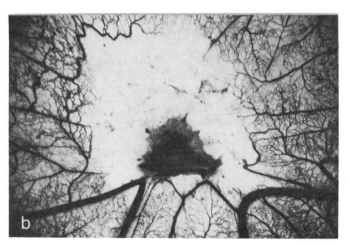

FIG. 1. Inhibition of Angiogenesis in the Chick Chorioallantoic Membrane (CAM). a) Normal 8 day CAM. India ink has been injected into the vascular system to show that the entire surface of the CAM is underlined by a continuous, branching capillary network. b) CAM Treated with Angiogenesis Inhibitors. This CAM was exposed for 48 hr to a combination of heparin (50 µg; Hepar, Franklin, OH) and the angiostatic steroid, 6α-fluoro-17,21-dihydroxy-16β-methyl-pregna-4,9-(11)-diene-3,20-dione (70 µg; UpJohn, Kalamazoo, MI). Inhibition of angiogenesis and induction of capillary involution can be seen within the avascular zone that appears free of india ink-filled capillaries. An abnormally sparse, hexagonal India ink pattern can be seen at the periphery in regions of partial regression.

disks. The disks are applied to the surface of 6 day CAM and the CAM is inspected 48 hr later for the presence of capillary regression or what appears as an avascular zone (FIG. 1). The potency of a compound is measured in terms of the percentage of CAMs that exhibit avascular zones.

Using this method, we have shown that combinations of angiostatic steroids and heparin induce avascular zones in approximately 40% of CAMs tested (2). When BM components, such as fibronectin and laminin, were localized by immunofluorescence microscopy within regions of capillary regression, it became clear that BM dissolution was a major effect of the steroid-heparin combination (17). In addition, we could demonstrate that capillary BM dissolution was directly associated with capillary retraction and endothelial cell rounding (FIG. 2). Interestingly, BM within nearby large vessels and overlying ectoderm were not effected.

Recently, we have used time-lapse video to analyze early capillary development in the CAM. Capillary systems first appear in the CAM as sparse hexagonal cellular networks which are separated by large intercapillary distances. Continued angiogenesis is made possible by formation of side branches that stretch out, cross the tissue interspace, and anastomose with a distance arm of the same hexagon. Continuation of this process therefore results in smaller and smaller hexagons and thus greatly decreased intercapillary distances. It is important to point out that endothelial cell migration is made possible by continued deposition of BM components (23). Immunofluorescence studies confirm that BM molecules surround growing capillaries although although an intact basal lamina does not appear by electron microscopy. The absence of morphologic basal lamina is not uncommon in regions that undergo rapid BM turnover (1) and in vitro studies suggest that capillary cell migration is also associated with elaboration of collagenolytic activity (22). Thus, capillary extension represents a dynamic process in which cells move by repeatedly forming, breaking, and reforming their connections with surrounding matrix.

In this manner, normal CAM becomes maximally vascularized by approximately day 8 to 10 of development. Avascular zones can be produced by steroid-heparin combinations if administered prior to completion of CAM formation. Capillary involution results from progressive capillary retraction beginning with the smallest and probably most recently formed branches (FIG. 2). Continued retraction results in production of larger and larger hexagons until only the largest vessels remain. It is also important to emphasize that only "high turnover" capillaries are effected. Steroid-heparin combinations have no effects on larger vessels or nearby epithelium that exhibit intact BM and thus may be viewed as low turnover or more formalized structures.

Thus, these studies demonstrate that capillary regression induced by angiostatic steroids is a true example of tissue involution. Capillaries regress through reversal of the process by which they developed.

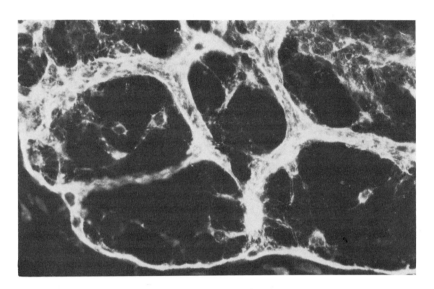

FIG. 2. Fluorescence View of Fibronectin Localized within a Region of Partial Capillary Regression at the Edge of an Avascular Zone. Early retraction of the finest capillaries results in production of rounded endothelial cells which remain associated with wisps of fibronectin staining. The smallest hexagonal capillary arrays are lost first resulting in production of progressively larger hexagonal forms. x 1,100.

EXTRACELLULAR MATRIX AS A SOLID STATE REGULATOR IN ANGIOGENESIS

While initial studies demonstrated a direct correlation between BM dissolution and capillary involution, it remained unclear whether BM breakdown was the cause of capillary regression or a result secondary to endothelial cell injury. To explore the possibility that structural alterations of extracellular matrix (ECM) could be causally involved in the anti-angiogenic mechanism, we asked whether specific modulators of ECM metabolism could alter capillary development.

Perhaps the best characterized modulators of matrix metabolism are the proline analogues, cis-hydroxyproline (CHP)

and L-azetidine-2-carboxylic acid (LACA). CHP and LACA compete
with proline and are incorporated in its place during collagen
biosynthesis. Substitution with proline analogues interferes
with collagen triple helix formation and inhibits deposition of
both interstitial and basement membrane collagens into organized
ECMs.

When CHP and LACA were tested using the CAM system, we found
that these inhibitors of collagen deposition were potent
inhibitors of angiogenesis (20). For example, application of
600 µg CHP resulted in production of avascular zones in 100% of
CAMs. Furthermore, when administered in suboptimal doses,
proline analogues could greatly potentiate the anti-angiogenic
effects of angiostatic steroids and heparin. In fact,
combination of a suboptimal dose of proline analogue with
angiostatic steroid alone could produce avascular zones in 100%
of CAMs, thus circumventing the requirement for heparin. All the
effects of proline analogues could be negated by coadministering
equimolar amounts of L-proline. Again, these anti-angiogenic
compounds had no effect on older non-growing capillaries.

Proline analogues may have some generalized toxicity
secondary to effects on general protein synthesis when
administered in high amounts. However, these results suggest
that modulators of collagen metabolism may be used at suboptimal
concentrations to potentiate angiostatic steroid action. It
appears that the steroid can focus the anti-collagen effect of
the proline analogues so that only growing capillary endothelium
is effected.

These studies also demonstrate that inhibition of collagen
accumulation is sufficient to induce capillary involution in the
growing CAM. Thus, the steroid-induced changes in ECM observed
in our original studies most likely play a causal role in anti-
angiogenesis. The question remains: How do structural changes
of ECM alter capillary growth and development?

Cell Shape as a Physiological Control Element

During capillary involution, BM dissolution was associated
with capillary retraction and endothelial cell rounding. Could
these matrix-dependent changes in cell form be involved in the
mechanism of capillary regression?

We set out to answer this question by developing an in vitro
system for analysis of capillary endothelial cell growth
regulation. Capillary endothelial cells derived from bovine
adrenal cortex were cultured on dishes coated with ECM components
and tested for their ability to respond to the purified
angiogenic factor, basic fibroblast growth factor (FGF), which is
a potent endothelial mitogen. These studies were carried out in

the absence of serum which contains a variety of other growth and attachment factors. ECM molecules were pre-adsorbed onto bacteriological dishes which could not normally support cell attachment. In this manner, we asked whether specific ECM molecules could act locally to modulate the growth responsiveness of capillary endothelial cells.

We found that the growth response of capillary cells differed depending upon the type of ECM molecule used for cell attachment as measured by effects on incorporation of tritiated thymidine into DNA (18). Capillary cells increased their DNA synthetic rates approximately 8 fold when grown on type IV collagen while cells on laminin only doubled their DNA synthetic rates. When computerized morphometry was used to analyze the effects of culture conditions on cell spreading, we found that cell shape varied enormously depending upon the substratum used for cell attachment. Comparison of morphometric data with effects on DNA synthesis demonstrated that DNA synthetic rates were tightly coupled to cell size regardless of the presence of FGF or the substratum used for cell attachment.

In most simple terms, these studies suggested that it was the shape or degree of cell extension that dictated a cell's rate of DNA synthesis. Furthermore, FGF appeared to act by inducing cell spreading. For instance, in the absence of FGF, cells on type IV collagen covered approximately 750 square microns and incorporated about 2 dpm of tritiated-thymidine per cell whereas addition of growth factor induced cell spreading resulting in coverage of 1500 square microns. This corresponded to about a 6 to 8 fold increase in DNA synthesis on a per cell basis. Our results also suggested that ECM could act locally to control GF action by supporting or preventing changes in endothelial cell form. For example, FGF-stimulated cells on laminin only spread enough to cover an area similar in size to that covered by unstimulated cells grown on type III collagen. These similarly sized cells synthesized the same amount of DNA regardless of the presence or absence of FGF. Finally, we found that under all conditions cell extension was associated with changes in nuclear spreading indicating that cell and nuclear form altered in a coordinated fashion.

These studies clearly demonstrated a correlation between capillary endothelial cell growth and ECM-dependent changes in cell and nuclear shape.   However, the question remained: are these cell shape changes the cause or result of alterations in cell growth rates?

To get at this question, we have recently extended these studies by focusing on cell growth modulation by a single matrix component, fibronectin. Our previous results were difficult to interpret because we could only measure the equilibrium shape that a cell displayed on different substrata in the absence or presence of growth factors and thus under different growth conditions. By using fibronectin, we have been able to develop three different methods for modulating capillary endothelial cell shape from the outside independent of the presence of soluble growth factors (19). These studies were carried in a defined, serum-free medium comprised of DMEM supplemented with transferrin (5 μg/ml), high density lipoprotein (10 μg/ml), and saturating amounts of basic FGF (2 ng/ml).

Using one method, capillary endothelial cells were held in different shape configurations by altering the number of fibronectin attachment points. This was done simply by preadsorbing bacteriological plastic dishes with increasing amounts of fibronectin. In the second method, cells were grown on dishes coated with saturating amounts of fibronectin in the presence of increasing concentrations of soluble fibronectin peptides. It has been previously demonstrated that small peptides which contain the Arginine-Glycine-Aspartate (RGD) sequence found within the cell-binding region of fibronectin can cause cell detachment from fibronectin-coated dishes (10). We attempted to use these soluble peptides in low concentrations so as to inhibit cell spreading without causing complete cell detachment. Finally, we could control cell spreading on dishes preadsorbed with fibronectin by overlaying the dishes with increasingly thick coats of the non-adhesive polymer, poly-hydroxyethylmethacrylate (poly-HEMA). We have previously demonstrated that poly-HEMA can be used in this manner to progressively restrict formation of cell contacts and cell spreading on standard tissue culture dishes (5).

We were able to hold endothelial cells in a variety to different shape configurations using these methods. For example, cell spreading could be promoted in a controlled fashion using bacteriological dishes coated with fibronectin at 10, 50, 100, or 1000 ng/cm^2 (FIG. 3). Autoradiography in conjunction with incorporation of tritiated-thymidine demonstrated that over 50% of cells grown on the highest fibronectin concentration were able to enter S phase. Decreases in cell extension associated with lower fibronectin coating densities were paralled by a decrease in the nuclear labelling index. Less than 5% of the endothelial cells that remained in a rounded form on the lowest fibronectin concentration were able to synthesize DNA even though they were exposed to the same FGF-containing medium. In general, DNA synthetic rates and cell proliferation rates increased in an exponential fashion in direct relation to linear increases in cell extension (i.e., projected cell area as measured using computerized morphometry). Similar results were obtained by extracellular restriction of cell spreading using either the RGD-containing peptides or poly-HEMA coatings.

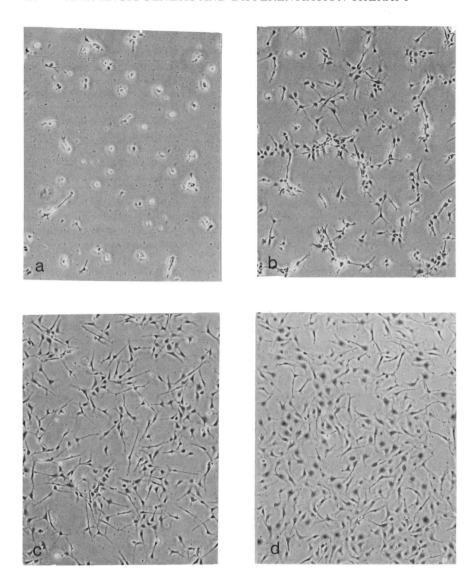

FIG. 3. Effect of Fibronectin Coating Density on Capillary Endothelial Cell Shape. Bacteriological dishes were coated with fibronectin at 10 (a), 25 (b), 100 (c), and 1000 (d) ng/cm^2. Capillary endothelial cells take on dramatically different forms depending upon the number of fibronectin attachment points that are provided. Growth rates directly parallel fibronectin-dependent changes in cell size. All magnifications, x250.

Thus, these studies demonstrated that capillary endothelial cell growth could be finely regulated by supporting or preventing cell extension from outside. In this manner, we have come to think of ECM as a solid state regulator in angiogenesis. Neovascularization may be stimulated by soluble stimuli (7), but pattern formation appears to be regulated through controlled alterations of ECM that modulate cell shape and growth factor responsiveness locally (18).

Theoretical Considerations

How could matrix-dependent alterations of cell shape get transduced into changes of cell metabolism, such as increases in DNA synthesis? One major direction that we are moving in involves analysis of the effect of cell shape modulation on classical systems of signal transduction. For example, we hope to identify the point at which cell rounding uncouples growth factor receptor occupancy from its normal signalling response. Do changes in cell shape alter growth factor receptor number, affinity, or clustering? By rounding the cell, do we inhibit or promote phosphorylation of specific regulatory proteins? Do we alter phophatidylinositide hydrolysis or cell alkalinization? We also hope to investigate signal transduction at the level of the fibronectin receptor.

The other major thrust in our laboratory is to explore the possibility that cell shape changes act to modulate metabolism in a mechanical fashion by altering a structural system of signal transduction within cells. This idea comes out of past studies with inorganic cell models built according to the rules of an architectural system known as Tensegrity (14). Using these models, we have been able to predict many of the alterations of cell form that are observed upon attachment to extracellular substrata including the coordination between cell and nuclear spreading described earlier.

The significance of the tensegrity cell models is that they suggest that cells may contain signal transduction pathways that are structural in nature. For instance, regulatory information may be conveyed directly from the cell's surface to the nucleus in the form of physical forces of tension and compression (12,14). Recent evidence from many laboratories suggests that regulation of DNA replication and gene expression may depend upon physical interactions with the nuclear protein matrix. For example, nuclear matrix contains fixed sites for DNA replication and transcription and is directly involved in DNA packaging (24,25). Thus, any alteration of force distributions that changes nuclear matrix organization could alter the arrangement and function of associated DNA regulatory enzymes.

From studies with tensegrity cell models, we would expect that changes in physical forces that are associated with cell spreading would be transduced intracellularly via alterations of cytoskeletal polymerization and organization (12-14). A tensegrity structure is defined as being comprised of a series of isolated compression-resistant elements that are interconnected and literally pulled up and open by a continuous series of tension elements. Recent studies suggest that microtubules act as compression-resistant struts within cells and that they are interconnected by a continuous series of tension-generating microfilaments (21). These experiments also demonstrated that cell form depends upon maintenance of tensional integrity, thus strongly supporting the concept that cells may actually utilize a tensegrity mechanism to regulate cytoskeletal polymerization as well as cell function.

Thus, our long term goal is to dissect the molecular mechanism by which mechanical signals, exerted on the surface of a cell, can be transduced into intracellular changes of biochemical metabolism.

SIGNIFICANCE FOR DIFFERENTIATION THERAPY

While we are interested in dissecting molecular mechanisms of cell growth regulation, development of an effective means of anti-cancer therapy remains our major focus. We hope that our studies on the mechanism of anti-angiogenesis stimulate other investigators to develop new methods for pharmacological perturbation of ECM turnover as well as cell shape. In fact, we have recently been selecting for anti-angiogenic compounds simply by searching for agents that induce capillary endothelial cell rounding in vitro. At present, our results have been extremely exciting.

Discovery of new methods for modulation of ECM structure may have additional significance for control of cancer development. We have previously suggested that local alterations of ECM turnover may be involved in the disorganization of normal tissue form during early stages of tumor formation that precede onset of malignant invasion (12-16). Recently, we discovered that the potent angiogenic factor, basic FGF, may be stored and sequestered in an inactive form within normal BM (9). This could explain why neovascularization occurs at sites of tumor formation; increased BM turnover could release angiogenic factors. A similar phenomenon could be responsible for coordination between morphogenetic changes in tissue form and vascular ingrowth observed during normal development.

Thus, development of new methods for pharmacological control of ECM metabolism could provide means of attacking cancer at various stages of its development. Suppression of increases in BM turnover could prevent cancer progression and initiation of capillary ingrowth if initiated during early stages of tumor formation. In fact, previous studies have shown that well-differentiated tumor cells remain dependent upon continued deposition of ECM components for their growth whereas more anaplastic tumors grow totally independent of anchorage (26,27).

We believe that more advanced, solid tumors may be effectively treated by taking advantage of their requirement for continued neovascularization. The studies described herein suggest that treatment of solid tumors may require induction of BM dissolution, specifically breakdown of capillary ECM. In this manner, poorly differentiated tumor cells may be thought to exhibit secondary anchorage-dependence, that is, they require the continued presence of anchorage-dependent capillary endothelial cells. Specific induction of capillary ECM dissolution may therefore be an effective means of inducing endothelial cell rounding, inhibiting cell responsiveness to soluble angiogenic factors, and inducing capillary involution. Hopefully, inhibition of angiogenesis within a rapidly growing tumor will be able to produce tumor regression free of systemic toxicity.

REFERENCES

1. Bernfield, M.R. and Banerjee, S.D. (1978): In: Biology and Chemistry of Basement Membranes, edited by N. Kefalides, pp. 137-148. Academic Press, New York.
2. Crum, R., Szabo, S., and Folkman, J. (1985): Science, 230:1375-1378.
3. Folkman, J., Merler, E., Abernathy, C., Williams, G. (1971): J. Exp. Med, 133:275-288.
4. Folkman, J. (1972): Ann. Surg., 175:409-416.
5. Folkman, J. and Moscona, A. (1978): Nature, 273:345-349.
6. Folkman, J., Langer, R., Linhardt, R.J., Haudenschild, C., Taylor, S. (1983): Science, 221:719-725.
7. Folkman, J. and Klagsbrun, M. (1987): Science, 235:442-447.
8. Folkman, J. and Ingber, D.E. (1987): Ann. Surg., 206:374-383.
9. Folkman, J., Klagsbrun, M., Sasse, J., Wadzinski, M., Ingber, D.E. and Vlodavsky, I. Am. J. Pathol., (in press).
10. Hayman, E.G., Pierschbacher, M.D., and Rouslahti, E. (1985): J. Cell Biol., 100:1948-1954.
11. Ikawa, H., Trelstad, R.L., Hutson, J.M., Manganaro, T.F., and Donahoe, P.K. (1984): Dev. Biol., 102:260-264.
12. Ingber, D.E., Madri, J.A., and Jamieson. J.D. (1981): Proc. Natl. Acad. Sci. U.S.A., 78:3901-3905.

13. Ingber, D.E. and Jamieson, J.D. (1982): In: Tumor Invasion and Metastasis, edited by, L.A. Liotta and I.R. Hart, pp. 335-357. Martinus Nijhoff, The Hague, The Netherlands.
14. Ingber, D.E. and Jamieson, J.D. (1985): In: Gene Expression During Normal and Malignant Differentiation, edited by L.C. Andersson, C.G. Gahmberg, and P. Ekblom, pp. 13-32. Academic press, Orlando.
15. Ingber, D.E., Madri, J.A., and Jamieson, J.D. (1985): Am. J. Pathol., 121:248-280.
16. Ingber, D.E., Madri, J.A., and Jamieson, J.D. (1986): Am. J. Pathol., 122:129-139.
17. Ingber, D.E., Madri, J.A., and Folkman, J. (1986): Endocrinol., 119:1768-1775.
18. Ingber, D.E., Madri, J.A., and Folkman, J. (1987): In Vitro Cell Dev. Biol., 23:387-394.
19. Ingber, D.E. and Folkman, J. (1987): J. Cell Biol., 105:219a.
20. Ingber, D.E. and Folkman, J. Lab. Invest. (submitted)
21. Joshi, H.C., Chu, D., Buxbaum, R.E., and Heidemann, S.R. (1985): J. Cell Biol., 101:697-705.
22. Kalebic, T., Garbisa, S., Glaser, B., and Liotta, L. (1983): Science, 221:281.
23. Madri, J.A. and Stenn, K.S. (1982): Am. J. Pathol., 106:180-188.
24. Pardoll, D.M., Vogelstein, B. and Coffey, D.S. (1980): Cell, 19:527-536.
25. Pienta, K.J. and Coffey, D.S. (1984): J. Cell Sci. Suppl., 1:123-35.
26. Vembu, D., Liotta, L.A., Paranjpe, M., and Boone, C.W. (1979): Exp. Cell Res., 124:247-252.
27. Wicha, M.S., Liotta, L.A., Vonderhaar, B.K., and Kidwell, W.R. (1980): Dev. Biol., 80:253-263.

Acknowledgments

This work was supported by USPHS Grants CA-45548 (D.E.I.) and CA-37395 (J.F.), and by a grant to Harvard University from Takeda Chemical Industries, Limited.

MEMBRANE EVENTS REGULATING DIFFERENTIATION AND RELATION TO TERMINAL CELL DIVISION

Membrane Events Associated with Tumour Cell Differentiation

R. Lotan and J.P. Abita*

*Department of Tumor Biology, The University of Texas-M.D. Anderson Hospital and Tumor Institute at Houston, Houston, Texas 77030, USA and *Institute de Recherches sur les Maladies du Sang, Unité Inserm 204, Hôpital Saint Louis, 75010 Paris, France*

INTRODUCTION

The surface membrane is one of the most important organelles of the cell. It is responsible for mediating and controlling various fundamental functions that are essential for cell growth, division, communication with other cells and with the extracellular matrix, movement, differentiation, and death. The diverse membrane functions are carried out by specific proteins, glycoproteins or lipids. Some proteins possess enzymatic activities (e.g., adenylate cyclase, and protein kinase), whereas others are involved in active transport of ions (e.g., Na^+/K^+-ATPase) or nutrients. The binding of various hormones and growth factors to the cell surface depends on the presence of specific receptors [e.g., receptors for epidermal growth factor (EGF), insulin, platelet-derived growth factor (PDGF), and transferrin], which may interact with other membrane components to transduce the signals into the cell interior. Other membrane components (glycoproteins and gangliosides) can serve as binding sites for viruses, bacteria and toxins. Intercellular recognition and adhesion are mediated by cell surface adhesive molecules [e.g., fibronectin, laminin, vitronectin, cell adhesion molecules (CAMs)] and complementary receptors for such molecules on adjacent cells. The immunological identity of cells is also determined by the repertoire of cell surface antigens (e.g., HLA histo-compatibility antigens, and ABO, H, Le, Ia and T blood group substances).

The cell membrane changes its composition and some of its specific functions during normal development as cells differentiate to perform special functions. Such changes may involve the loss of some membrane components and the synthesis of new ones. For example, membrane glycoproteins and glycolipids undergo programmed changes during early embryogenesis as does the expression of histocompatibility antigens and EGF receptors (49, 73, 101, 103).

Malignant transformation is also accompanied by a variety of changes in the structure and function of the surface membrane. Changes were reported in a variety of characteristics including: 1. membrane fluidity, which may alter the lateral mobility of membrane components including hormone receptor clustering and internalization; 2. the amount and activity of surface membrane receptors for growth factors, which may change cell growth regulation and endow the tumor cell with growth advantage over the normal cells; 3. the structure of the oligosaccharide chains of glycolipids and glycoproteins, which may alter cell-cell and cell-extracellular matrix communication, recognition and adhesion; 4. cell surface adhesion mediating molecules, which may have implications on cell motility and invasiveness; 5. cell surface antigens, which may affect the ability of the immune system to recognize and destroy the tumor cells; 6. secretion and shedding of proteolytic enzymes (e.g., collagenase or plasminogen activator), which may influence the invasive capacity of the cells. Many of these changes result from alterations in the expression of mature cell products due to an arrest at an early stage of differentiation or because of other deviations from the normal differentiation pathway (49, 69, 76, 85, 101).

The realization that malignancy can be reversed or suppressed under certain conditions in vivo and in vitro has led to intensive studies using cultured cancer cells to find physiologic and pharmacologic agents that can induce or enhance the differentiation of tumor cells. It is thought that such agents might provide a rational and noncytotoxic approach to cancer therapy (19, 69, 85). A few neoplastic cell types have been found that can be induced to differentiate in culture under defined conditions. These include murine and human embryonal carcinomas, leukemias, neuroblastomas, melanomas, and carcinomas (69, 85). The agents that have been identified as possessing differentiation inducing activity for tumor cells include physiologic regulators of normal cell differentiation [e.g., colony stimulating factors (CSF), interferon (IFN), and tumor necrosis factor (TNF)]; natural and synthetic analogs of vitamin A (retinoids) and vitamin D (e.g., $1,25(OH)_2D_3$); steroids (e.g., dexamethasone); prostaglandins; polar-planar compounds [e.g., dimethyl sulfoxide (DMSO), hexamethylene bisacetamide (HMBA), and N-N-dimethyl formamide (DMF)]; short chain fatty acids (e.g., sodium butyrate); dibutyryl cyclic adenosine monophosphate (Bt_2cAMP) and agents that elevate intracellular levels of cAMP [e.g., the phosphodiesterase inhibitor isobutyl-methyl xanthine (IBMX)]; antibiotics and chemotherapeutic agents [e.g., actinomycin D adriamycin and cytosine arabinoside (ara-C)]; and tumor promoting phorbol esters [e.g., 12-O-tetra-decanoylphorbol-13-acetate (TPA)].

Ideally, one would like to find an agent that will be active in vivo and induce all cells within a tumor to undergo complete differentiation and terminal cell division. So far there are only few agents that approach this objective. Many of the above agents have been shown to induce tumor cells to undergo varying degrees of differentiation and to express many of the morphological, biochemical and functional properties of normal mature cells of the tissue in which the tumor originated (69, 85). Since differentiation involves alterations in gene expression the ultimate site for the action of differentiation inducing agents is the cell nucleus. However, many of the early events (triggering) in differentiation induction by exogenous agents occur at the cell surface and some of the markers that are used to indicate the state of differentiation of a cell are surface membrane constituents (e.g., antigens). This short review summarizes the effects that some agents exert on the structure and function of the plasma membrane of malignant cells that are induced to differentiate. A list of some of the membrane components and properties that are affected by differentiation inducers is presented in Table 1.

TABLE 1. <u>Membrane Components and Properties Modulated by Differentiation Inducers</u>

1. Ion pump (Na^+/K^+-ATPase) and ion fluxes (Na^+, Ca^{2+})
2. Enzymes (adenylate cyclase, protein kinases)
3. Protease-sensitive surface component(s)
4. Receptors for growth factors (EGF, PDGF, insulin, transferrin, NGF, IL-2) and other ligands (fibronectin, urokinase, PGE_2)
5. Differentiation antigens (CEA, SSEA-1, SSEA-3)
6. Histocompatibility antigens (HLA-A, B, C; HLA-DR)
7. Adhesion molecules (laminin, fibronectin, I-CAM-1, LFA-1)
8. Proteins, neutral lipids, gangliosides, and glycoproteins
9. Lipid microviscosity and membrane protein lateral diffusion

EFFECTS OF DIFFERENTIATION INDUCING AGENTS ON ION CHANNELS

For the maintenance of an essential ionic gradient between the cell interior and exterior the cell employs a Na^+ pump, the Na^+/K^+-adenosine triphosphatase (ATPase), a membrane-bound enzyme. Monovalent ion fluxes have been implicated in the control of cellular proliferation (92). Ouabain, a specific inhibitor of the enzyme, was found to induce erythroid differentiation in murine erythroleukemia cells (MELC) (67). This observation has led to the suggestion that inhibition of the ATPase is an early event in triggering differentiation (67). Several agents that induce MELC to differentiate (e.g., DMSO, hypoxanthine, and actinomycin D) caused an early (within a few hours) decrease in $^{86}Rb^+$ influx (67). It has been suggested that the decrease in $^{86}Rb^+$-influx after exposure of MELC to DMSO is a secondary event resulting from an inhibition of amino acid uptake, Na^+, K^+, $2Cl^-$ cotransport system, and a lowered Na^+-influx (95). Human promyelocytic leukemia cells (HL-60) are induced to differentiate to granulocytes after treatment with DMSO or β-all-trans retinoic acid (RA). Within a few hours there is an increase in the intracellular concentration of sodium ions and increased activity of the Na^+ pump and, only at a later stage, is there a decrease in the number and turnover of pump molecules on the cell surface (62). It has been proposed that RA stimulates at least one of the sodium transport systems (62). Ouabain accelerated the effect of RA on the increase in intracellular sodium concentration and the activation of the sodium pump and potentiated RA-induced differentiation of the HL-60 cells (62). Under different experimental conditions (depletion of intracellular K^+), DMSO induced in the HL-60 cells an immediate reduction in bidirectional trans- membrane K^+-flux (39). Although amiloride, a passive inhibitor of Na^+-flux across the membrane, was found to block DMSO-induced differentiation of MELC it exhibited a potentiating effect on the induction of myeloid differentiation in HL-60 cells (15). Since amiloride can also inhibit protein synthesis it is not contain whether its effect was limited to the Na^+-pump. The intracellular Na^+ concentration can be increased by monensin (a sodium ionophore), or ouabain. Interestingly, the treatment of pre-B lymphocyte splenic tumor cell line (70Z/3) with these agents induced differentiation similar in magnitude to that induced by lipopolysaccharide (LPS), and LPS itself stimulated sodium ion uptake (89). It is not clear how the differentiating agents modulate ion fluxes and to what extent the changes in ion concentration are related to the process of differentiation. However, the fact that the alterations in ion fluxes are the earliest measurable effects of the agents and that they are caused by different agents in different cell types indicate that they may be important. Obviously, further studies are needed to elucidate the mechanism by which alterations in ion fluxes influence the process of differentiation.

EFFECTS OF DIFFERENTIATION INDUCING AGENTS ON MEMBRANE ENZYMES

The reception and transduction of many signals from extracellular ligands for growth or differentiation induction depends on the activity of specific membrane components. Some of these components are receptors that bind the ligands and others are enzymes (e.g., protein kinases) that form an intricate network for signal transduction. Malignant transformation often abrogates the expression, structure and function of different elements in this system. The induction of differentiation may restore the normal expression of these membrane components. Several studies have demonstrated that granulocytic or monocytic differentiation is accompanied by changes in the ability of the cells to generate cAMP, an established messenger for membrane trans- duction and an endogenous inducer of differentiation of some cell types (1, 30, 42, 46, 93, 106). RA-treated HL-60 cells that differentiate into granulocytes had a higher basal adenylate cyclase (AC) activity (measured in membrane preparations) than undifferentiated cells, however this activity was less stimulated by guanosine triphosphate (GTP) and was not affected by forskolin, which augments AC by activating the catalytic subunit in cooperation with the guanyl regulatory subunit (106). AC activity was not altered in HL-60 cells induced to differentiate with ara-C along the monocytic pathway or in U-937 cells induced with RA to differentiate into monocytes (106). The level of cAMP produced by intact viable cells was lower in the differentiated HL-60 cells under basal conditions and was not increased after histamine treatment (1). Monocytic differentiation of U-937 cells with RA or ara-C did not cause marked changes in AC (106). However, measurement of the cellular cAMP level indicated that the differentiation of the U-937 cells was associated with a lowered ability to generate cAMP under basal conditions, as well as after stimulation of the cells with histamine, isoproterenol, or prostaglandin E_1 (PGE_1) (42). Likewise, the monocytic differentiation of U-937 cells, under the influence of $1,25(OH)_2D_3$ was accompanied by an attenuation of the cAMP response to isoproterenol and forskolin (93). In contrast, the differentiation of murine F9 embryonal carcinoma cells to parietal endoderm, following RA treatment, brought about an increase in the basal, the GTP-stimulated, and the fluoride-stimulated activity of AC (30). The effects on cAMP levels were detected within 1 to 2 days of treatment with the differentiating agents and their relevance to the process of differentiation is not clear. It has been proposed that RA may modulate AC through interacting with the G proteins (GTP-binding proteins) (106, see also the Chapter by Abita et al. in this book).

Changes in cAMP level may have direct effects on the activity of cAMP-dependent protein kinases (pK), which mediate nearly all the actions of cAMP in the cell. These kinases are located in the cytoplasm as well as in the membrane. The activities of cAMP-dependent pK are modulated during differentiation in a pathway-specific fashion. Upon induction of differentiation of HL-60 cells with RA or DMF towards a granulocytic pathway an increased activity of both the cytosolic and the membrane-bound cAMP-dependent pK was observed. An increase in the type I enzyme and the RI regulatory subunit was noted (36). In contrast, monocytic differentiation of these cells, achieved by TPA treatment (91), did not affect the enzyme activity (36). A somewhat similar phenomenon was reported for embryonal carcinoma cells; whereas F9 cells exhibited an increased cAMP-dependent pK activity and higher levels of both RI and RII, following RA-induced differentiation to parietal

endoderm-like cells, the PC13 cells which differentiate to
visceral endoderm by RA treatment, exhibited a decrease in the
enzyme activity, a decrease in the RI level in the membrane and
an increased activity in the cytosol (80).

A cAMP-independent but Ca^{2+}- and phospholipid-dependent pK
(pKC) is considered to be essential for the transduction of
certain signals across the membrane. This enzyme is usually
located in the cytoplasm in an inactive form. However,
diacylglycerol (DAG, a natural metabolite of phosphatidylinositol 4,5-bisphosphate) or TPA, which is structurally similar to
DAG, bind to the enzyme and increase its affinity for Ca^{2+} and
phosphatidylserine, thereby enhancing its translocation from the
cytoplasm to the cell membrane (17). The association with the
membrane activates the enzyme. This activation leads to the
phosphorylation of several membrane and cytoplasmic proteins and
presumably, to alterations of fundamental cellular processes,
including growth, transformation, and differentiation. It is
not surprising, therefore, that the effects of various
differentiation inducers on the activity of pKC have been
analyzed in a number of laboratories (44, 71, 112). TPA
activates pKC purified partially from HL-60 cells as it does in
many other cells (112). In intact HL-60 cells TPA activates pKC
by causing its translocation to the membrane and induces a
monocytic differentiation (44). No translocation to the
membrane was observed with TPA resistant HL-60 cells (55) or
K-562 chronic myelogenous leukemia (CML) cells that do not
undergo differentiation with TPA (44). Although these results
suggest a correlation between activation of pKC and induction of
differentiation there are several experimental findings that
question this contention. For example, U-937 cells can be
induced to differentiate into monocytes either by TPA or by
$1,25(OH)_2D_3$, however, pKC translocation to the membrane only
occurs in the TPA-treated cells (71). These findings suggest
that, either activation of pKC is not an obligatory step in the
monocytic differentiation, or that the vitamin D metabolite can
act along the same pathway as TPA does but at a stage distal to
the membrane events (e.g., in the nucleus).

Tyrosine kinases were implicated in the mechanisms of
oncogene and growth factor action because several proto-
oncogenes that are associated with the cell membrane contain
tyrosine kinase activity. Recently, it has been reported that
when U-937 cells are induced to differentiate with TPA they
express a tyrosine kinase (113). Likewise, when HL-60 cells are
treated with IFN-γ or recombinant TNF-α the cells undergo
monocytic differentiation, and the onset of differentiation (1
or 2 days after exposure to drug) is accompanied by the
appearance of a plasma membrane-associated tyrosine kinase
(45). This enzyme is increased in amount and in activity in
cells induced to differentiate to granulocytes with RA or
DMSO. Thus, it is not limited to cells undergoing monocytic

differentiation. The granulocytic differentiation of HL-60 cells is enhanced synergistically by combining RA and the calcium ionophore A23187 as is the membrane expression of tyrosine kinase in the differentiated cells. Although these experiments tie together RA, Ca^{2+} and tyrosine kinase, the nautre of the interactions among them is unknown. It is possible that the tyrosine kinase plays a role not only in regulation of proliferation but also in the process of differentiation.

Differentiation inudcers have been reported to modulate membrane-bound enzymes that are not related directly to signal transduction. Thus, sodium butyrate treatment of human colon carcinoma cells (line HRT-18) resulted in growth suppression and cell flattening as well as in enhancement of the activities of membrane-associated alkaline phosphatase, γ-glutamyltranspeptidase and sucrase (110). Growth inhibition induced by DMSO or RA in the same cells was not accompanied by increases in the activities of the above enzymes, rather the activities were suppressed (110). Thus, growth inhibition per se is not the cause for changes in these enzymes. Likewise, DMSO inhibited the growth of two human renal carcinoma cell lines but increased the activity of the surface membrane enzyme 5'-nucleotidase in one cell line (Cur) while decreasing the activity in the other (Caki). Butyrate also increase 5'-nucleotidase activity in the Cur cells and induced morphologic changes consistent with increased maturation (84). DMSO induced megakaryotcytic differentiation in K-562 CML cells and induced the expression of surface 5'-nucleotidase (104). RA treatment induced in F9 murine embryonal carcinoma cells differentiation to parietal endoderm and increased the de novo synthesis of cell surface N-acetylglucosaminide β(1--4)galactosyltransferase (75).

EFFECTS OF DIFFERENTIATION INDUCING AGENTS ON MEMBRANE RECEPTORS

The expression of receptors on the cell surface is characteristic of the cell type and the specialized functions that it is "assigned" to perform once it matures. Malignant transformation often involves marked changes in these receptors. Receptors that mediate growth-restricting signals and intercellular interactions may be lost and receptors for mitogenic factors may be overexpressed or expressed ectopically to provide the cancer cell with a greater degree of autonomy. The induction of differentiation and maturation processes by differentiation inducers is usually accompanied by restoration of the membrane receptor repertoire to the one characteristic of the normal counterpart of the cancer cell. Studies with cultured tumor cells revealed that differentation may lead to loss of certain membrane receptors and to an increase in others (Table 2). For example, the differentiation of MELC cells with

TABLE 2.   Modulation of Membrane Receptors and Adhesion-Mediating Molecules by Differentiation Inducers

Cell	Agent	Differentiation Pathway	Change in Membrane Component	Ref.
Human thymic (T) leukemia	TPA	T-cell	loss of transferrin-R	25
HL-60	RA,DMSO	granulocytic	loss of transferrin-R	31
HL-60	butyrate	monocytic	loss of transferrin-R	9
HL-60	RA,DMSO	granulocytic	loss of insulin-R	80
MELC	DMSO	erythroid	loss of insulin-R	43
PC13[a]	RA	visceral endoderm	loss of insulin-R	53
F9,PC13	RA	endoderm	increased PDGF-R	88
PCC.4[a]	RA	parietal endoderm	increased EGF-R	58
NTERA-2[b]	RA	neuronal	decreased EGF-R	13
LA-N-1[c]	RA	neuronal	increased NGF-R	52
JURKAT[d]	TPA	B-cell	increased IL-2-R	47
U-937	$1,25(OH)_2D_3$	monocytic	decreased PGE_2-R	46
MELC	HMBA	erythroid	increased urokinase-R	24
U-937	TPA	monocytic	increased urokinase-R	24
HL-60	TPA	monocytic	increased fibro-nectin-R	83
HL-60	DMSO	granulocytic	increased fibo-nectin-R	83
ML-1[e]	TPA, ara-C	monocytic	increased Fc-R	105
ML-1	DMSO	granulocytic	increased Fc-R	105
HL-60	RA,DMSO	granulocytic	increased C-3b-R	7
JD38[f]	TPA	plasma cell	decreased C3-R	8
U-937	TPA	monocytic	increased I-CAM-1 and LFA-1	90
U-937	TPA, GM-CSF	monocytic	increased Mac-1 and	
HL-60	RA, GM-CSF	granulocytic	p150,95	72

[a]Murine embryonal carcinoma; [b]human embryonal carcinoma; [c]human neuroblastoma; [d]human Burkitt lymphoma; [e]human myeloblastic leukemia; [f]human B lymphoma.

DMSO leads to a loss of insulin receptors (43). Whereas the differentiation of human thymic leukemic cells to mature extrathymic immunocompetent T cells was accompanied by a loss of the transferrin receptor (25). This loss is not restricted to the T maturation process. A similar loss of the trasferrin receptor was observed when HL-60 cells were induced to differentiate either to granulocytes with RA or DMSO (31) or to monocytes with butyrate (9). These cells also lose insulin receptors upon granulocytic differentiation (81). Neuronal differentiation induced in human embryonal carcinoma cells with RA leads to a decrease in EGF receptors whereas the opposite occurs in murine embryonal carcinoma cells (58). Interestingly, murine EC cells also exhibit increases in insulin (53), and PDGF receptors (88) after differentiation into endoderm. Some human neuroblastoma cells (LA-N-1) show an increase in NGF receptors following neuronal differentiation induced by RA (52). The monocytic differentiation of U-937 cells with $1,25(OH)_2D_3$ involves a decrease in PGE_2 (46) and the TPA-induced B-cell maturation of Burkitt's lymphoma cells is accompanied by the increase in IL-2 receptors. Although many of the differentiating cells are losing receptors that are usually present on rapidly proliferating cells (e.g., transferrin and insulin), some cells gain receptors for growth factors. The most plausible explanation is that the expression of these receptors is also under the control of the differentiation program in which the particular cells are engaged, and their loss or gain is a part of the changes in the phenotype of the cells. Receptors for urokinase have been detected on various normal and transformed cells. Their function is still unclear. It is interesting to note that the number of these receptors increases as MELC cells differentiate in response to HMBA (24). The urokinase may actually be involved in the process of commitment to differentiation in these cells becuase when added to the cells together with HMBA it abolishes the time of commitment to terminal differentiation (24).

. Differentiation of several cell types is accompanied by altered interaction with other cells of the same type (homotypic aggregation) or with different cells and the extracellular matrix. The acquisition of adhesive properties is usually the result of expression of specific cell surface constituents (91). HL-60 cells have been shown to express three types of adhesion mediating molecules on their surface after differentiation to either monocytes or granulocytes. These molecules include the fibonectin receptor (83), the Mac-1 and p150,95 adhesive molecules (72) and the C3b receptor (7). The latter receptor is decreased when human B lymphoma cells undergo differentiation to plasma cells (8). The monocytic differentiation of U-937 cells also involves an increased adhesiveness. This property is probably mediated via the I-CAM-1 and LFA-1 complementary adhesion molecules (90). Tumor

cells derived from solid tumors also acquire adhesion mediating
surface molecules during their differentiation. Embryonal
carcinoma cells that are poorly adherent in the undifferentiated
state and often are grown on gelatin-coated dishes to improve
adhesion express both laminin and entactin on their surface upon
differentiation into endodermal cells by RA and dibutyryl cAMP
(14).

EFFECTS OF DIFFERENTIATION INDUCING AGENTS ON SURFACE ANTIGENS

Normal differentiation is accompanied by changes in various
cell surface components. Since some of these components are
immunogenic they can be identified by specific antibodies
(monoclonal or polyclonal). One of the methods used to follow
the differentiation of tumor cells by differentiation inducers
is to determine whether new antigens, characteristic of mature
cells appear and whether antigens characteristic of immature
cells are lost (73). Thus, murine F9 embryonal carcinoma
induced to differentiate with RA lose cell surface expression of
the lactoseries glycolipid SSEA-1 antigen (102) whereas human
embryonal carcinoma TERA-2 induced to differentiate into neurons
with RA, DMSO, HMBA, DMA, or BUdR lose SSEA-3, a globoseries
glycolipid antigen expressed on human EC cells (3). The
RA-induced differentiation of F9 cells to endoderm-like cells
was accompanied by the appearance of i antigen (73) whereas the
differentiation of human NTERA-2 cells involved the appearance
of several lactoseries glycolipid antigens (32). The contents
of carcinoembryonic antigen (CEA) is correlated with the state
of differentiation of colorectal tumors. Butyrate treatment of
HRT-18 colon carcinoma cells increased 20- to 40-fold the
content of CEA (110). Recombinant interferon-γ induced the
expression of 3 differentiation antigens in cultured human
melanoma cell lines (16).

The expression of cell surface antigens related to the
hematopoietic cell differentiation has been particularly well
characterized by a panel of monoclonal antibodies. Antigens
specific for mature T cells (e.g., OKT1, OKT11) appeared on the
surface of several human thymic (T) leukemic cell lines induced
by TPA to differentiate into mature T cells (25). likewise the
TAC antigen (IL-2 receptor) was induced by TPA in select acute
human T lymphocytic leukemia cells (JURKAT and HSB-2) (47).
B-cell lymphoblastic leukemias express common acute
lymphoblastic leukemia antigen (CALLA), surface membrane
immunoglobulin (SMIg) and some express also the Ia antigen.
Induction of differentiation towards plasma cells by DMSO (6) or
TPA (8) resulted in decreased expression of CALLA and Ia antigen
and an increase in SMIg. A distinction has been made between
the effects of TPA and DMSO on an early B-cell lymphoblastoid
cell line. Although both agents inhibited cell proliferation
and caused the accumulation of cells in the G1 phase of the cell

cycle, only DMSO induced maturation to a "late" B-cell phenotype. Thus, the effects of TPA (increased expression of Ia and HLA-A, B, C antigens, and decreased SMIg) could be explained by the increase in G1 phase cells, whereas the effects of DMSO represent expression of mature cell phenotype (6). K-562, CML cells can be induced to differentiate along erythroid, monocytic and megakryocytic lineages by agents such as butyrate, DMSO, RA, and TPA (104). Butyrate induced erythroid differentiation and a marked reduction in the binding of monoclonal antibodies 80H5 and 82H6, which define antigens that are expressed early in hematopoietic differentiation (104). DMSO induced megakaryocytic differentiation and decreased expression of 80H5 antigen. RA also decreased the expression of antigens specific for early hematopoietic differentiation and inhibited the erythroid features of the K-562 cells (104). In contrast, TPA induced a monocytic differentiation and enhanced expression of a monocyte specific antigen defined by monoclonal antibody 82H3 (104).

The monocytic differentiation induced by TPA in the human U-937 premonocytic leukemia or HL-60 promyelocytic leukemia is accompanied by an increased expression of antigen 50,80 (Mo3e determinant), which is characteristic of activated monocytes (108). Interferon (α and β) can induce U-937 monocytic differentiation and increase the expression of an antigen recognized by monoclonal antibody B43.4.1., which is specific for human monocytes (51). Although interferon had no effect on the HL-60 cells (51), the colony stimulating factors G-CSF and GM-CSF induced the differentiation of the HL-60 cells and enhanced the expression of granulocytic and macrophage membrane antigens (10).

The expression of major histocompatibility antigens (MHC) is usually a property of mature differentiated cells. Many agents that induce differentiation increase the expression of these antigens. For example, TPA induced monocytic differentiation of K-562 cells involves an increased expression of · class I (HLA-A, B, C) but not in class II (HLA-DR) MHC antigens (104). Treatment of human B-cell lymphoblastoid cells with either DMSO that induces B-cell differentiation, or with TPA that only inhibits cell growth resulted in increased synthesis of HLA-A, B, C antigens (6). In HL-60 cells TPA induced monocytic differentiation and increased phosphorylation of HLA antigens (33). Interferons (α, β, and γ) are potent inducers of MHC class I and class II expression in various tumors including melanoma (16, 27, 48, 99), breast carcinoma (12, 40, 48), colon carcinoma (48, 81, 99), glioma and cervical cárcinoma (16), HL-60 (61) B-lymphoblastoid cells (27), osteosarcoma (99), and human embryonal carcinoma cells (4). The effects of interferons on MHC expression seem to be unrelated to their effects on cell proliferation or differentiation. In human embryonal carcinoma cells the increase in class I MHC following interferon-γ treatment occurs without induction of differentiation, growth inhibition or resistance to viral infection (4). Likewise, the induction of HLA-DR expression in human breast carcinoma cell lines by interferon-γ was not related to its antiproliferative activity (40). Nonentheless, the increased expression of MHC antigens increases the immunogenicity of the tumor cells (81) and may contribute to the therapeutic potential of interferon in cancer patients.

EFFECTS OF DIFFERENTIATION INDUCING AGENTS ON CELL MEMBRANE PROTEINS AND GLYCOPROTEINS

The antigens described above are proteins, glycoproteins and glycolipids. The changes induced in their expression by various agents have been detected primarily by specific antibodies. Other approaches to the identification of cell surface changes relied on specific radiolabeling of membrane glycoproteins exposed on the cell surface by lactoperoxidase-catalyzed iodination with ^{125}I (20, 31, 64, 110), or by oxidation with periodate or with galactose oxidase (before and after neuraminidase) followed by reduction with sodium borotritiate (20, 38, 64, 65, 109), or on the binding of sugar-binding proteins (lectins) to the cell surface (25, 73, 111). These studies revealed various changes in cell surface proteins and glycoproteins induced by differentiating agents. For example, the differentiation of HL-60 cells along the granulocytic pathway, after treatment with DMSO or RA, was accompanied by a loss of 3 proteins (M_r 95,000; 87,000; and 77,000), and the appearance of 7 new proteins (M_r 270,000; 240,000; 150,000; 135,000; 58,000; 56,000; and 55,000) on the cell surface (31). One of the lost proteins (M_r 95,000) was identified as the transferrin receptor, and one of the new proteins (M_r 55,000) was identified as a major cell surface membrane protein of terminally differentiated myeloid cells (31). Likewise, the induction of monocytic differentiation of HL-60 cells with TPA resulted in increases in surface-iodinated proteins of M_r 150,000; 95,000; 80,000; 60,000; and 50,000 (20). Analyses of cell surface glycoproteins that were based on carbohydrate labeling revealed that granulocytic differentiation induced by DMSO in HL-60 cells resulted in the disappearance of sialoglycoproteins of M_r 155,000 and 130,000 (38). TPA-induced monocytic differentiation of HL-60 cells resulted in a decrease in large glycopeptides (22). A similar differentiation of human myeloid leukemia ML-2 resulted in the labeling of several glycoproteins of M_r 50,000; 95,000; 135,000; and 170,000 and a decreased labeling of glycoproteins with M_r 155,000 (20). Granulocytic differentiation induced by RA in HL-60 cells was characterized by a decrease in chrondroitin sulfate production (85). Increased sialylation of surface glycoproteins was detected in T-cell leukemias induced to differentiate into

mature T cells with TPA (25), in F9 embryonal carcinoma induced
to differentiate to endoderm with RA (23), in K-562 cells
treated with adriamycin (109), in murine melanoma S91 cells
treated with RA (64, 65), and in human squamous carcinoma
treated with RA (66). This increased sialylation was the result
of increased activity of sialyltransferases (25, 26, 28). Other
transferases were also modulated by differentation inducers.
Thus TPA decreased in HL-60 the activities of fucosyl- and
galactosyl-transferases   (28)   whereas   RA   decreased
sialyltransferase and increased fucosyltransferase (63). It is
noteworthy that the glycosyltransferases are membrane-bound
enzymes that are localized primarily in the Golgi apparatus of
the cell. The changes induced in cell surface glycoconjugates
can alter lectin binding. Thus, DMSO-induced erythroid
differentiation of MEL cells resulted and decreased binding of
wheat germ agglutinin (WGA) and decreased agglutination with
this lectin (111). Peanut agglutinin (PNA) binding to T-cell
leukemia induced into mature with TPA diminished due to
increased sialylation (25). Increased sialylation was also the
cause for decreased binding of PNA to embryonal carcinoma
induced with RA to differentiate to endoderm (73). This
differentiation resulted in increased sialylation and decreased
fucosylation of complex glycopeptides (23, 74). Butyrate
treatment of human HRT-18 colon carcinoma cells increased the
amount of a 60 KD membrane glycoprotein with affinity for WGA
and Ricinus communis agglutinin but which binds poorly to PNA
(110). Cytostasis induced by dexamethasone in non-small cell
lung cancer resulted in increased mucin production and increased
incorporation of fucose into glycoproteins (70).

The functions of various proteins and glycoproteins that
are modulated by differentiation inducers are largely unknown.
It is conceivable, though, that at least some of them play a
role in cell surface phenomena that are altered during
differentiation such as cell adhesion, recognition by immune
cells (e.g., natural killer cells), or binding of exogenous
ligands.

Perturbations of the structure of membrane proteins by
exogenously added proteases have been shown to enhance the
erythroid differentiation of MEL and K-562 cells (96, 97,
100). The proteases apparently act at the cell surface since an
immobilized form of protease that cannot penetrate the cells was
capable of inducing MEL cell differentiation with the same
efficiency as a soluble protease (100). Various proteases were
also capable of acting synergistically with DMSO, or other low
molecular weight inducers (96). Similarly, proteases induced
HL-60 cells as well as acute myeloid leukemia cells in priamry
culture to undergo initially a granulocytic differentiation and
subsequently the treated cells acquired properties of mature
macrophages (34). Proteases acted synergistically with DMSO,
RA, butyric acid, or HMBA (34). Treatment of F9 cells with RA

increases the production of plasminogen activator and TPA increase this enzyme in several cell types. It is not clear whether these endogenously produced proteases regulate the differentiated state. The finding of urokinase receptors on the surface of some tumor cells suggests that this enzyme may act also by binding to specific receptors (24).

EFFECTS OF DIFFERENTIATION INDUCING AGENTS ON MEMBRANE LIPIDS AND GLYCOLIPIDS

A variety of changes in cell membrane lipids have been described in various tumor cells induced to differentiate in culture. These changes were both quantitative and qualitative and they affected not only the chemical composition but also the physical properties of the membranes (e.g., microviscosity). Several studies with Friend leukemia cells induced to differentiate with DMSO along the erythroid pathway reported changes in lipid synthesis (50, 87, 114). Suppression of phospholipid synthesis (50), an increase in the molar ratios of phosphatidylcholine (PC) to phosphatidylethanolamine (PE) and PC to sphingomyelin (114), but no change in phospholipid synthesis (87) has been reported by different groups. The reasons for the inconsistent results may be the use of differnt sublines and different periods of exposure to DMSO (87). That the differentiation of the MEL cells is accompanied by changes in lipids is also indicated by the increased microviscosity of the cells (5). Such changes are often the result of an increased cholesterol to phospholipid ratio. The myeloid and monocytic differentiation of HL-60 cells resulted in vastly dissimilar changes in lipid metabolism (11, 21). TPA enhanced phospholipid synthesis within 4 hr after treatment of HL-60 cells and increased the amounts of PC and phosphatidylinositol and enhanced selective incorporation of long-chain fatty acids into triacylglycerols and ether-containing alkylglycerols (11). In contrast, induction of myeloid differentiation of HL-60 cells by DMSO or RA resulted in a rapid suppression of PC synthesis from choline or from the transmethylation of membrane PE and an increase in the ratio of cholesterol to phospholipid (21). These changes were accompanied by an increase in the membrane microviscosity. The modulation of lipid synthesis occurred before the growth inhibitory action of the differntiation inducers could be detected and are presumably related to the sequence of events associated with the onset of commitment to differentiation. Growth inhibition of HL-60 cells by high cell density caused some changes in phospholipid fatty acid composition (41). However, DMSO- or RA-induced myeloid differentiation has led to additional changes such as increased level of arachidonic acid and decreased percentage of monoenoic fatty acids of 16 and 18 carbons. Changes in membrane microviscosity may lead to alterations in the lateral mobility of membrane glycoconjugates. This effect was exemplified in a study of the mobility of fluorescently-labeled WGA bound to surface glycoconjugates on HL-60 or U-937 cells induced with DMSO to differentiate into granulocytes or monocytes, respectively (68). Differentiation along both pathways resulted in a 2-fold reduction in the diffusion of the WGA-glycoconjugate complex in the membrane without a concurrent change in the total number of binding sites (68). It has been proposed that in addition to the changes in lipids one should consider that the reduction in lateral diffusion of the glycoconjugates may result from development of increased transmembrane contact with the cytoskeletal elements of the cells (68). Retinoids have been shown to increase the microviscosity of the membranes of murine embryonal carcinoma cells induced to differentiate into endoderm (59, 98). The diffusion constant obtained for a fluorescent lipid probe in differentiated EC cells was similar to the value measured in endoderm. An increase in free cholesterol to phospholipid ratio observed during the differentiation of the EC cells could account for this effect of differentiation (98).

Gangliosides are sialic acid-containing glycosphingolipids, which are exposed on the surface membrane. The level and type of ganglioside are developmentally regulated and are often modified during the differentiation of normal and tumor cells in vivo and in culture (49). The induction of differentiation of several tumor cell types including human melanoma (56), HL-60 (77, 94), and human T-cell leukemia (60) with TPA was accompanied by an increase in the synthesis of the ganglioside GM3. In HL-60 cells the increase in GM3 occurred only after induction of monocytic differentiation (induced with TPA) whereas granulocytic differentiation (induced with DMSO) resulted in a decrease in GM3 (77, 78). Often a change in globoseries gangliosides is accompanied by an opposite change in lactoseries and ganglioseries glycolipids (77, 78). This phenomenon is also exemplified in the case of human embryonal carcinoma differentiation into a variety of somatic cell types after RA treatment (32). It has been suggested that the changes in glycolipid structures during differentiation result from alterations in the activities of glycosyltransferases that control glycolipid core structure assembly (32). Differentiation of mouse myeloid leukemia M1 cells into macrophages, accomplished by treatment with lymphokine, resulted in the appearance of asialo-GM1 on the cell surface (2). Induction of melanogenesis in mouse S91 melanoma cells by RA resulted in a decreased incorporation of galactose into GM3 and in an increased incorporation into GM1 (64). The cell surface exposure of GM1 was however, reduced in RA-treated cells (64).

The relevance of the changes induced in membrane lipids and glycolipids during the differentiation of tumor cells is not fully understood. Although many of the alterations are probably the result of the acquisition of mature and differentiated phenotype, some changes are rapid and could be important early events in the onset of the differentiation program. An excellent example for the latter contention is the recent report that the addition of exogenous GM3 to cultured HL-60 and U-937 cells and to fresh leukemic cells obtained from patients with acute promyelocytic leukemia resulted in induction of differentiation along the monocytic lineage (79). Thus, the incorporation of this ganglioside into the surface membrane triggers a specific differentiation pathway.

SUMMARY AND CONCLUDING REMARKS

The membrane-associated events described in this Chapter fall under three categories: (i) early events that are related to the induction of differentiation; (ii) events that are the consequence of the expression by tumor cells of a more differentiated phenotype; and (iii) events that are the consequence of exposure to differentiation inducing agents but may not be related directly to differentiation (e.g., changes resulting from growth inhibition).

The cell membrane is the initial target for the action of several differentiation inducers that bind to specific receptors (e.g., CSF, TNF, IL-2, interferon, and TPA) or dissolve in the lipid phase of the membrane [e.g., planar-polar solvents, gangliosides, adriamycin (54), and retinoids]. Binding of some agents to specific receptors is probably followed by switching on signal transduction processes (e.g., phosphorylation of proteins catalyzed by protein kinases) and the biochemical changes that lead eventually to alterations in gene expression and to differentiation. Dissolution of some agents in the membrane may activate signal transduction mechanisms by altering physiochemical properties of the membrane, changing the function of membrane components (e.g., ion channels), or augmenting the response to exogenous ligands present in the serum or growth medium.

Membrane changes that are the consequence of differentiation of tumor cells include alterations in the physicochemical properties of the membrane that may alter membrane receptor functions and adhesive interactions, as well as changes in the expression of cell surface receptors, proteins, glycoconjugates and antigens. There are also changes in cellular properties that follow exposure to differentiation inducers but are related to the suppression of growth and accumulation of cells in the G1 phase of the cell cycle. Cells in G1 may have characteristics that distinguish them from undifferentiated cells as well as from differentiated cells.

Although the mechanism of differentiation induction by various agents is not fully understood the existing knowledge has some implications on differentiation therapy. For example, one way to augment the response to tumor cells to an inducer for which there exist membrane receptors is to increase the number of such receptors. This can be achieved in some cells where treatment with interferon increases the number of TNF receptors. Likewise, interferon increases the level of EGF receptors in some squamous carcinoma cells and the combination of the two agents provides effective suppression of growth. Modulation of ion channels may augment the process of differentiation induction as suggested by the synergism between calcium ionophore and RA. The increased expression of tumor cells membrane MHC antigens by treatment with interferon can render the cells immunogenic and therefore, subject to immune destruction by the host immune response. Similarly, identification of specific changes in cell membrane components resulting from exposure to differentiation inducers can serve as the basis for combination treatment with the agent and monoclonal antibodies against the new membrane component that it induces. Specific changes in membrane components may also serve as markers for the identification of tumor cells responding to the inducers.

The pivotal role that the cell surface membrane plays in the action of many growth factors, differentiation inducers and in the interactions between cells and their environment makes this cell organelle the focus of interest and intensive research. Further studies should clarify the role of membrane components in triggering differentiation and in the maintenance of the differentiated phenotype.

ACKNOWLEDGMENTS

We thank Ms. Susan J. Lyman for manuscript preparation.

REFERENCES

1. Abita, J.P., Gespach, C., Cost, H., Poirier, O., and Saal, F. (1982): IRCS, 10:882-883.
2. Akagawa, K.S, Momoi, T., Nagai, Y., and Tokunaga, T. (1981): FEBS Lett., 130:80-84.
3. Andrews, P.W., Gonczol, E., Plotkin, S.A., Dignazio, M., and Oosterhuis, J.W. (1986): Differentiation, 31:119-126.
4. Andrews, P.W., Trinchieri, G., Perussia, B., and Baglioni, C. (1987): Cancer Res., 47:740-746.
5. Arndt-Jovin, D., Ostertag, W., Eisen, H., Klimek, F., and Jovin, T.M. (1976): J. Histochem. Cytochem., 24:332-347.
6. Ashman, L.K., and Gesche, A.H. (1985): Leukemia Res., 9:157-165.
7. Atkinson, J.P., and Jones, E.A. (1984): J. Clin. Invest., 74:1649-1657.

8. Benjamin, D., Magrath, I.T., Triche, T.J., Schroff, R.W., Jensen, J.P., and Korsmeyer, S.J. (1984): Proc. Natl. Acad. Sci. USA, 81:3547-3551.

9. Boyd, A.W., and Metcalf, D. (1984): Leukemia Res., 8:27-43.

10. Begley, C.G., Metcalf, D., and Nicola, N.A. (1987): Int. J. Cancer, 39:99-105.

11. Cabot, M.C., Welsh, C.J., Callaham, M.F., and Huberman, E. (1980): Cancer Res., 40:3674-3679.

12. Calvo, F., Jabrane, N., Faille, A., Gauville, C., De Cremoux, P., Lagier, G., Abita, J.P., and Lechat, P. (1987): Int. J. Immunopharmac., 9:459-468.

13. Carlin, C.R., and Andrews, P.W. (1985): Exp. Cell Res., 159:17-26.

14. Carlin, B.E., Durkin, M.E., Bender, B., Jaffe, R., and Chung, A.E. (1983): J. Biol. Chem., 258:7729-7737.

15. Carlson, J., Dorey, F., Cragoe, Jr., E., and Koeffler, H.P. (1984): J. Natl. Cancer Institute, 72:13-17.

16. Carrel, S., Schmidt-Kessen, A., and Giuffre, L. (1985): Eur. J. Immunol., 15:118-123.

17. Castagna, M., Rochette-Egly, C., Rosenfeld, C., and Mishal, Z. (1979): FEBS Lett., 100:62-66.

18. Chapekar, M.S., Hartman, K.D., Knode, M.C., and Glazer, R.I. (1986): Mol. Pharmacol., 31:140-145.

19. Cheson, B.D., Jasperse, D.M., Chun, H.G., and Friedman, M.A. (1986): Cancer Treat. Rev., 13:129-145.

20. Chorvath, B., Duraj, J., and Stockbauer, P. (1983): Neoplasma, 30:263-280.

21. Cooper, R.A., Ip, S.H.C., Cassileth, P.A., and Kuo, A.L. (1981): Cancer Res., 41:1847-1852.

22. Cossu, G., Juo, A.L., Pessano, S., Warren, L., and Cooper, R.A. (1982): Cancer Res., 42:484-489.

23. Cossu, G., Cortesi, E., and Warren, L. (1985): Differentiation, 29:63-67.

24. Del Rosso, M., Pucci, M., Fibbi, G., and Dini, G. (1987): Brit. J. Haematol., 66:289-294.

25. Delia, D., Greaves, M.F., Newman, R.A., Sutherland, D.R., Minowada, J., Kung, P., and Goldstein, G. (1982): Int. J. Cancer, 29:23-31.

26. Deutsch, V., and Lotan, R. (1983): Exp. Cell Res., 149:237-245.

27. Dolei, A., Capobianchi, M.R., and Ameglio, F. (1983): Infect. Immun., 40:172-176.

28. Durham, J.P., Ruppert, M., and Fontana, J.A. (1983): Biochem. Biophys. Res. Commun., 110:348-355.

29. Durham, J.P., Emler, C.A., Butcher, F.R., and Fontana, J.A. (1985): FEBS Lett., 185:157-161.

30. Evain, D., Binet, E., and Anderson, W.B. (1981): J. Cell. Physiol., 109:453-459.

31. Felsted, R.L., Gupta, S.K., Glover, C.J., Fischkoff, S.A., and Gallagher, R.E. (1983): Cancer Res., 43:2754-2761.
32. Fenderson, B.A., Andrews, P.W., Nudelman, E., Clausen, H., and Hakomori, S-I. (1987): Develop. Biol., 122:21-34.
33. Feuerstein, N., Monos, D.S., and Cooper, H.L. (1985): Biochem. Biophys. Res. Commun., 126:206-213.
34. Fibach, E., Treves, A., Kidron, M., and Mayer, M. (1985): J. Cell. Physiol., 123:228-234.
35. Fibach, E., Kidron, M., Nachshon, I., and Mayer, M. (1983): Carcinogenesis, 4:1395-1399.
36. Fontana, J.A., Emler, C., Ku, K., McClung, J.K., Butcher, F.R., and Durham, J.P. (1984): J. Cell. Physiol., 120:49-60.
37. Forsbeck, K., Nilsson, K., Hansson, A., Skoglund, G., and Ingelman-Sundberg, M. (1985): Cancer Res., 45:6194-6199.
38. Gahmberg, C.G., Nilsson, K., and Andersson, L.C. (1979): Proc. Natl. Acad. Sci. USA, 76:4087-4091.
39. Gargus, J.J., Adelberg, E.A., and Slayman, C.W. (1984): J. Cell. Physiol., 120:83-90.
40. Gastl, G., Marth, C., Leiter, E., Gattringer, C., Mayer, I., Daxenbichler, G., Flener, R., and Huber, C. (1985): Cancer Res., 45:2957-2961.
41. Geny, B., Lagarde, M., Ladoux, A., and Abita, J.P. (1987): Submitted.
42. Gespach, C., Cost, H., and Abita, J.P. (1985): FEBS Lett., 184:207-213.
43. Ginsberg, B.H., Brown, T.J., and Raizada, M.K. (1979): Diabetes, 28:823-828.
44. Girard, P.R., Stevens, V.L., Blackshear, P.J., Merrill, Jr., A.H., Wood, J.G., and Kuo, J.F. (1987): Cancer Res., 47:2892-2898.
45. Glazer, R.I., Chapekar, M.S., Hartman, K.D., and Knode, M.C. (1986): 140:908-915.
46. Goldring, S.R., Amento, E.P., Roelke, MS., and Krane, S.M. (1986): J. Immunol., 136:3461-3466.
47. Greene, W.C., Robb, R.J., Depper, J.M., Leonard, W.J., Drogula, C., Svetlik, P.B., Wong-Staal, F., Gallo, R.C., and Waldmann, T.A. (1984): J. Immunol., 133:1042-1047.
48. Greiner, J.W., Horan Hand, P., Colcher, D., Weeks, M., Thor, A., Noguchi, P., Pestka, S., and Schlom, J. (1987): J. Lab. Clin. Med., 109:244-261.
49. Hakomori, S.J. (1985): Cancer Res., 45:2405-2414.
50. Harel, L., Lacour, F., Friend, C., Durbin, P., and Semmel, M. (1979): J. Cell Physiol., 101:25-32.
51. Hattori, T., Pack, M., Bougnoux, P., Chang, Z.L., and Hoffman, T. (1983): J. Clin. Invest., 72:237-244.
52. Haskell, B.E., Stach, R.W., Werrbach-Perez, K., and Perez-Polo, J.R. (1987): Cell Tissue Res., 247:67-73.

53. Heath, J., Bell, S., and Rees, A.R. (1981): J. Cell Biol., 91:293-297.
54. Hickman, J.A., Chahwala, S.B., and Thompson, M.G. (1986): Adv. Enzy. Reg., 24:263-274.
55. Homma, Y., Chubb, C.B.H., and Huberman, E. (1986): Proc. Natl. Acad. Sci. USA, 83:7316-7319.
56. Huberman, E., Heckman, C., and Langenbach, R. (1979): Cancer Res., 39;2618-2624.
57. Ishimura, K., Hiragun, A., and Mitsui, H. (1980): Biochem. Biophys. Res. Commun., 93:293-300.
58. Jetten, A.M. (1980): Nature, 284:626-629.
59. Jetten, A.M., De Luca, L.M., and Meeks, R.G. (1982): Exp. Cell Res., 130:494-498.
60. Kiguchi, K., Henning-Chubb, C., and Huberman, E. (1986). Cancer Res., 46:3027-3033.
61. Koeffler, H.P., Ranyard, J., Yelton, L., Billing, R., and Bohman, R. (1984): Proc. Natl. Acad. Sci. USA, 81:4080-4084.
62. Ladoux, A., Abita, J.P., and Geny, B. (1986): Differentiation, 33:142-147.
63. Liu, C.K., Schmeid, R., Schreiber, C., Rosen, A., Qian, G.X., and Waxman, S. 91983): Exp. Hematol., 11:738-746.
64. Lotan, R., Neumann, G., and Deutsch, V. (1983): Cancer Res., 43:303-312.
65. Lotan, R., Lotan, D., and Meromsky, L. (1984): Cancer Res., 44:5805-5812.
66. Lotan, R., Lotan, D., Sacks, P.G., and Hong, W.K. (1987): Int. J. Cancer, 40:224-229.
67. Mager, D., and Bernstein, A. (1978): J. Supramol. Struct., 8:431-438.
68. Magnusson, K.E., Wojcieszyn, J., Dahlgren, C., Stendahl, O., Sundqvist, T., and Jacobson, K. (1983): Cell Biophys., 5:119-128.
69. Marks, P.A., Sheffery, M., and Rifkinol, R.A. (1987): Cancer Res., 47:659-666.
70. McLean, J.S., Frame, M.C., Freshney, R.I., Vaughan, P.F.T., and Mackie, A.E. (1986): Anticancer Res., 6:1101-1106.
71. Mezzetti, G., Bagnara, G.P., Monti, M.G., Pernecco Casolo, L., Bonsi, L., and Brunelli, M.A. (1987): Life Sci., 40:2111-2117.
72. Miller, L.J., Schwarting, R., and Springer, T.A. (1986): J. Immunol., 137:2891-2900.
73. Muramatsu, T. (1984): Cell Diff., 15:101-108.
74. Muramatsu, H., and Muramatsu, T. (1982): Develop. Biol., 90:441-444.
75. Nakhasi, H.L., Nagarajan, L., and Anderson, W.B. (1984): FEBS Lett., 168:222-226.
76. Nicolson, G.L. (1976): Biochem. Biophys. Acta, 458:1-72.

77. Nojiri, H., Takaku, F., Tetsuka, T., Motoyoshi, K., Miura, Y., and Saito, M. (1984): Blood, 64:534-541.
78. Nojiri, H., Takaku, F., Ohta, M., Miura, Y., and Saito, M. (1985): Cancer Res., 45:6100-6106.
79. Nojiri, H., Takaku, F., Terui, Y., Miura, Y., and Saito, M. (1986): Proc. Natl. Acad. Sci. USA, 83:782-786.
80. Palumbo, A., Brossa, C., Turco, G., and Pegoraro, P. (1983): Endocrinol., 112:964-970.
81. Pfizenmaier, K., Bartsch, H., Scheurich, P., Seliger, B., Ucer, U., Vehmeyer, K., and Nagel, G.A. (1985): Cancer Res., 45:3503-3509.
82. Plet, A., Gerbaud, P., Anderson, W.B., and Evain Brion, D. (1985): Differentiation, 30:159-164.
83. Pommier, C.G., O'Shea, J., Chused, T., Takahashi, T., Ochoa, M., Nutman, T.B., Bianco, C., and Brown, E.J. (1984): Blood, 64:858-866.
84. Prager, M.D., and Kanar, M.C. (1984) Cancer Lett., 24:81-88.
85. Reiss, M., Magnilia, C.A., and Sartorelli, A.C. (1985): Cancer Res., 45:2092-2097.
86. Reiss, M., Gamba-Vitalo, C., and Sartorelli, A.C. (1986): Cancer Treat. Rep., 70:201-218.
87. Rittmann, L.S., Jelsema, C.L., Schwartz, E.L., Tsiftsoglou, A.S., and Sartorelli, A.C. (1982): J. Cell. Physiol., 110:50-55.
88. Rizzino, A., and Bowen-Pope, D.F. (1985): Develop. Biol., 110:15-22.
89. Rosoff, P.M., and Cantley, L.C. (1983): Proc. Natl. Acad. Sci. USA, 80:7547-7550.
90. Rothlein, R., Dustin, M.L., Marlin, S.D., and Springer, T.A. (1986): J. Immunol., 137:1270-1274.
91. Rovera, G., Santoli, D., and Damsky, C. (1979): Proc. Natl. Acad. Sci. USA, 76:2779-2783.
92. Rozengurt, E., and Mendoza, S. (1980): Ann. N.Y. Acad. Sci., 339:175-189.
93. Rubin, J.E., and Catherwood, B.D. (1984): Biochem. Biophys. Res. Commun., 123:210-215.
94. Ryan, J.L., Yohe, H.C., and Malech, H.L. (1985): Yale J. Biol. Med., 58:125-131.
95. Schaefer, A., Munter, K.H., Geck, P., and Koch, G. (1984): J. Cell. Physiol., 119:335-340.
96. Scher, W., Scher, B.M., and Waxman, S. (1982): Biochem. Biophys. Res. Commun., 109:348-354.
97. Scher, W., Hellinger, N., and Waxman, S. (1985): Exp. Hematol., 13:36-43.
98. Searls, D.B., and Edidin, M. (1981): Cell, 24:511-517.
99. Shaw, A.R.E., Chan, J.K.W., Reid, S., and Seehafer, J. (1985): J. Natl. Cancer Inst., 74:1261-1268.
100. Slosberg, E.A., Scher, B.M., Scher, W., Josephson, S., and Waxman, S. (1986): Exp. Hematol., 14:442, Abst. #171.

101. Smets, L.A., and Van Beek, W.P. 91984): Biochim. Biophys. Acta, 738:237-249.
102. Solter, D., Shevinski, L., Knowles, B.B., and Strickland, S. (1979): Dev. Biol., 70:515-521.
103. Subtelny, S., and Wessells, N.K. (1980): The Cell Surface: Mediator of Developmental Process. Academic Press, New York.
104. Sutherland, J.A., Turner, A.R., Mannoni, P., McGann, L.E., and Turc, J-M. (1986): J. Biol. Res. Mod., 5:250-262.
105. Takeda, K., Minowada, J., and Bloch, A. (1982): Cancer Res., 42:5152-5158.
106. Thomas, G., Chomienne, C., Balitrand, N., Schaison, G., Abita, J.P., and Baulieu, E.E. (1986): Anticancer Res., 6:725-728.
107. Todd, R.F., Griffin, J.D., Ritz, J., Nadler, L.M., Abrams, T., and Schlossman, S.F. (1981): Leukemia Res., 5:491-495.
108. Todd, III, R.F., and Liu, D.Y. (1986): Fed. Proc., 45:2829-2836.
109. Trentesaux, C., Laplace, B., Madoulet, C., Rebel, G., and Jardillier, J.C. (1987): Anticancer Res., 7:187-192.
110. Tsao, D., Morita, A., Bella, Jr., A., Luu, P., and Kim, Y.S. (1982): Cancer Res., 42:1052-1058.
111. Tsiftsoglou, A.S., and Sartorelli, A.C. (1981): Biochim. Biophys. Acta, 649:105-112.
112. Vandenbark, G.R., Kuhn, L.J., and Niedel, J.E. (1984): J. Clin. Invest., 73:448-457.
113. Zick, Y., Grunberger, G., Rees-Jones, R.W., and Comi, R.J. (1985): Eur. J. Biochem., 148:177-182.
114. Zwingelstein, G., Tapiero, H., Portoukalian, J., and Fourcade, A. (1982): Biochem. Biophys. Res. Commun., 108:437-446.

Some Membrane Events Linked to the Differentiation of Human Myeloid Leukemic Cells

J.P. Abita, B. Geny, C. Chomienne and A. Ladoux

Inserm U 204, Centre Hayem, Hôpital St. Louis
75475 Paris Cedex 10, France

INTRODUCTION

HL-60 cells are promyelocytic leukemia cells that can be induced to differentiate either into granulocyte or to monocyte-like cells depending on the inducer used. For example, granulocytic differentiation can be achieved by retinoic acid (RA) or by dimethyl sulfoxide (DMSO) (8,4), while the acquisition of the monocytic properties can be induced by phorbol esters or butyrate (3,41). U-937 cells have monoblast-like characters and are induced to differentiate exclusively into cells having many morphological and functional properties of mature monocytes-macrophages when cultured in the presence of all the agents cited above (36, 33,34). Both cell lines thus constitute ideal models to study the intracellular signals as well as the molecular changes triggered by the different inducers.

In this report we focus on changes involving systems localized in the plasma membrane.

METHODS

HL-60 and U-937 cells were grown in suspension in RPMI 1640 medium containing 2mM L-Glutamine, antibiotics and supplemented with 15% heat inactivated fetal bovine serum. Differentiation was assessed by many criteria including morphology, NBT reduction test non-specific esterases and monoclonal antibodies staining.

Intracellular pH (pHi) measurements were performed using either the distribution of the weak acid (^{14}C)-benzoic acid, or the fluorescent probe 2',7'-biscarboxyethyl-5(6)-carboxyfluorescein acetoxymethylester (BCECF). In this latter case fluorescence was recorded using either a spectrofluorimeter (excitation wave length: 500 nm; emission wave length: 530 nm) or an Ortho cytofluorograph 50 H equipped with a model 2150 computer and an argon laser tuned at 488 nm. Fluorescence emission of BCECF was detected at two different wavelenths: 520 nm (10 nm band pass) and 640 nm (highpass filter).

Na^+-K^+-ATPase activity was determined as the ouabain-inhibitable $^{86}Rb^+$ uptake according to (24).

Adenylate cyclase activity of membrane preparations was measured essentialy according to Salomon et al.(44).

RESULTS

Intracellular pH

The pHi value of undifferentiated U-937 cells was found to be 7.03+0.02 (n=51). Eukaryotic cells regulate their pHi through a number of systems located in the plasma membrane. They are best studied by following how cells recover their normal pHi after an intracellular acidosis. Such an experiment, using the fluorescent probe BCECF, is presented in Fig.1. U-937 cells were acidified to a pHi of about 6.3 by use of the K^+/H^+ ionophore nigericin, in a Na^+ and bicarbonate free medium. Nigericin was then quenched with BSA.

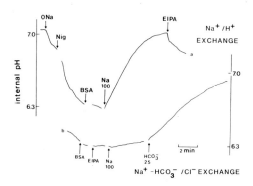

FIG.1. Two pHi regulating mechanisms cohexist in U-937 cells. The experiment was performed at 20°.

Trace a shows that the addition of 100 mM Na^+ promoted the rapid recovery to the initial pHi value. In the presence of 100 µM ethylisopropyl amiloride (EIPA), a known specific inhibitor of the Na^+/H^+ exchange system (48,49), no recovery could be induced by raising the external Na^+ concentration (first part of trace b). Last part of trace a shows also that the addition of EIPA to U-937 cells that had recovered their pHi, produced a cell acidification to pHi=6.8, a value close to that found after incubation of the cells in a Na^+ free medium (first part of trace a). These simple experiments identify the Na^+/H^+ exchanger as a major mechanism allowing U-937 cells to recover their pHi after a cellular acidifi-

cation. The second part of trace b shows that pHi recovery occurs
also, even in the presence of EIPA, upon addition of 25 mM bicarbonate to the incubation medium. Further experiments have indicated that in this latter case pHi recovery was due to the operation
of a Na⁺ dependent HCO_3^-/Cl^- exchange system (27). Flow cytometric
measurements presented in Fig.2 confirmed the existence of these
two regulating mechanisms in U-937 cells.

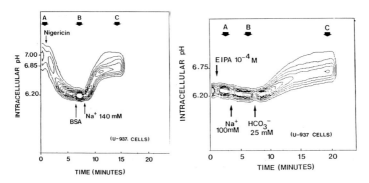

FIG.2. Flow cytometric measurements of pHi variations in U-937
cells. Left: cells, loaded with BCECF, were equilibrated in a Na⁺
free, 5 mM K⁺ modified Earle's salt solution (MESS). At times indicated by the small arrows, nigericin (1 μM), BSA and Na⁺ (140mM)
were added to the cells. Right: U-937 cells were incubated in the
medium described above. At times indicated by the arrows, EIPA
(0.1 mM), Na⁺ (100 mM) and bicarbonate (25 mM) were added to the
cells. Fluorescence was recorded as described in METHODS. These
experiments are based on the analysis of about 700,000 cells using
the list mode of the computer. Contour lines enclose different per
centiles of the cell population.

Fig.3 (main panel) shows that 1 μM RA induces a time-dependent
differentiation of U-937 cells which was preceded , by about 24 h,
by an increase in pHi. After 4 days, 75±5% of the cells had acquired the characters of monocytes and had a mean pHi of 7.23±0.03
(n=35). Both increase in pHi and differentiation occured in the
same range of RA concentrations with an ED_{50} = 300 nM (Fig.3inset).
   We had already demonstrated that the same two systems regulate
also the pHi of HL-60 cells (26). Fig.4 shows that the RA-induced
differentiation of HL-60 cells is also preceded by an increase of
the cell pHi. Undifferentiated cells have a mean pHi of 7.00±0.03
(n=27). After 5 days of culture in the presence of 1 uM RA, 90+5%
of the cells had acquired the characters of granulocytes and had
a mean pHi of 7.37±0.02 (n=21). In this case too the dose response
curves for RA-induced differentiation and increase in pHi were su-
perposable (26).
   We have demonstrated using BCECF that, in both HL-60 and U-937
cells, the increase in pHi seen during differentiation was due essentially to the activation of the Na⁺/H⁺ exchange system.

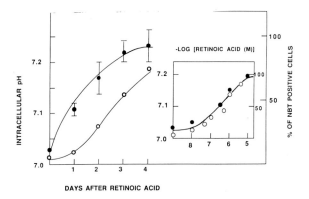

FIG.3. Effect of retinoic acid on the pHi and on
the differentiation of U-937 cells. Main panel:
time courses of pHi changes (●) and of appearance
of NBT positive cells (O) induced by 1 µM RA. pHi
measurements were performed using the distribution
of benzoic acid. Each bar represents the mean±sdm
from 18-51 experimental values. Inset: dose response
curves for RA action on the pHi (●) and on the differentiation (O) of U-937 cells.

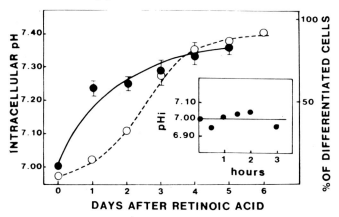

FIG.4. Time course of pHi changes during the differentiation of HL-60 cells. Main panel: pHi measurements (●) and differentiation (O). RA was used
at 1 µM. Each bar represent the mean±sdm of 9-13
experiments.
Inset: pHi measurements in HL-60 cells during the
first 3 hours following RA addition.

[22]Na^+uptake experiments (26) indicated that the rate of EIPA-sensitive [22]Na^+uptake by undifferentiated HL-60 cells was 1.95 ± 0.4 mmol/min/10^6 cells (n=7) compared to 3.99 ± 0.4 mmol/min/10^6 cells (n=7) for RA-differentiated cells. On the contrary, the rate of the HCO_3^-/Cl^-exchanger was about the same for both types of cells: 0.5 ± 0.11 mmol/min/10^6 cells and 0.34 ± 0.1 mmol/min/10^6cells. The same findings were made with U-937 cells: the rate of [22]Na^+uptake mediated by the Na^+/H^+exchanger was twice higher in differentiated than in undifferentiated cells (3.3 ± 0.6 mmol/min/10^6cells versus 1.43 ± 0.33 mmol/min/10^6 cells); whereas the rate of EIPA-insensitive, HCO_3^- activated [22]Na^+uptake did not change after differentiation: 0.56 ± 0.11 mmol/min/10^6cells compared to 0.54 ± 0.14 mmol/min/10^6 cells .

$Na^+K^+ATPase.$

The activity of the plasma membrane $Na^+K^+ATPase$ of HL-60 cells was measured by the difference between [86]Rb^+ uptake with and without 1 mM ouabain. Under physiological conditions, this activity was found to be 1.05 fmol/cell/min in undifferentiated cells. As shown in Fig.5, 1 μM RA induced a stimulation of the sodium pump activity which reached a maximum (170% of the initial value) after 7-8 hours. The pump activity returned to normal at about 12h.

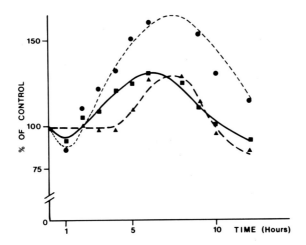

FIG.5. Na-K-ATPase activity (●) and intracellular Na (■) and K (▲) concentrations measured in HL-60 cells after addition of 1 uM RA.

During this period the number of enzyme molecules, measured by the specific binding of ^{3}H-ouabain, remained constant (25). Fig.5 shows also that following RA addition to HL-60 cells, there was a transient increase in the intracellular concentrations of Na^+ and K^+. The maximum in $(K^+)i$ coincided with the maximum obser-

ved in the sodium pump activity whereas the maximum in $(Na^+)i$ preceded it.

Ouabain, the specific inhibitor of the $Na^+K^+ATPase$, was found
to be without effect on the differentiation of HL-60 cells at concentrations below 0.05 µM and was cytotoxic at higher concentrations. When ouabain was added at 0.025µM, 16 hours before addition
of 0.1 µM RA, (a concentration which by itself induced the differentiation of 30-40% of the cells in 4 days), there was an acce-
leration and a potentialization of the RA-induced differentiation
(see Fig. 6). We have verified that not only the percentage, but
also the absolute number of NBT positive cells increased concomitantly (25). Under these conditions there was an early increase
in the activity of the sodium pump which peaked at 145% of the initial value after only 3 hours.

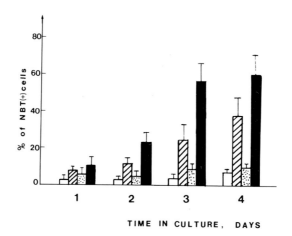

TIME IN CULTURE, DAYS

FIG.6. Percentage of NBT positivecells in
HL-60 cells cultured during 4 days in the
presence or absence of drugs.
Open columns: control cells; cross-hetched
columns: cells cultured in the in the presence of 0.1 µM RA; dotted columns: cells
cultured with 0.025 µM ouabain; dark columns:
cells cultured during 16 hours with ouabain
and then with 0.1 µM RA. Columns and bars
represent the means±sdm of 4 experiments
made in triplicate.

Adenylate cyclase.

Adenylate cyclase (AC) activity was measured on crude membrane
preparations of HL-60 cells. The effects of the differentiation
induced by 1 µM RA are shown in Fig.7. Basal activity was significantly higher in differentiated than in undifferentiated cells
($p<0.01$). In untreated cells GTP and forskolin (Fsk) stimulated

AC activity 2.7 and 2.1 fold respectively, whereas in RA-differen
tiated cells only GTP stimulated AC activity 1.6 fold (p<0.05)
and Fsk had no effect. In untreated cells, enzyme activity in the
presence of both GTP and Fsk was not different from the activity
seen in the presence of GTP alone. In RA-differentiated cells,
activity in the presence of both compounds was 50% less than that
with GTP alone. Dose response curves for AC activity in the presence of GTP and/or Fsk are shown in Fig.8. In both types of cells, GTP exhibited a biphasic effect with a maximum at 1 μM. In either case the effects of GTP and Fsk were not additive. We have
verified that when RA (0.01 to 100 μM) was added to membrane preparations of undifferentiated cells, it had no significant effect
on AC activity (47).

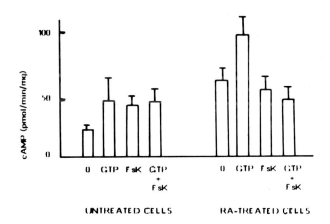

FIG. 7. Effects of RA-induced differentiation on
HL-60 cells adenylate cyclase activity.
Enzyme activity was measured in the absence (**O**)
or the presence of GTP (100 μM), Fsk (100 μM) or
both. Results are mean±sdm of 4 independent experiments performed in triplicate.

DISCUSSION

Our experiments have shown that two pharmacologically distinct
pHi regulating mechanisms are present in the plasma membrane of
U-937 and HL-60 leukemic cell lines. One is the amiloride sensitive Na^+/H^+ exchanger. This system is present in most animal cells,
including rat and human lymphocytes (14) and neutrophils (16,17,
45). However the exchanger of the leukemic cells differs from that

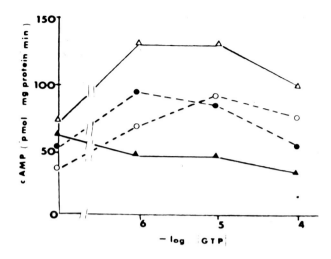

FIG.8 . Effect of GTP and Forskolin on AC activity
in HL-60 cells. Enzyme activity was measured in
undifferentiated (circles) and RA-differentiated
(triangles) cells with increasing concentrations
of GTP in the presence (●▲) or in the absence (O△)
of 100 μM Fsk. Results shown are means of one series of 5 experiments performed in triplicate.
Within assay standard deviations are less than
7% of the means graphed.

of other cells in its high affinities for amiloride and its derivatives and by relatively low affinities for Na^+ and Li^+ (26,14).
For instance the IC_{50} value for amiloride inhibition of the Na^+/H^+
exchanger of human mature granulocytes, measured at 140 mM external Na^+, is 75 μM (46); in U-937 and HL-60 cells it is equal to
2-5 μM. Another distinct property of leukemic cells is that the
Na^+/H^+ exchanger of normal lymphocytes and granulocytes can be activated by osmotic shocks (15,18) whereas the antiport of U-937 and
HL-60 cells cannot.

An additional pHi regulating system that allows U-937 and HL-60
cells to recover from an intracellular acidification is a Na^+ dependent HCO_3^- / Cl^- exchange system. The properties of this exchanger have been extensively studied and will be reported elsewere
(27). One important point is that normal human granulocytes lack
a Na^+ dependent HCO_3^-/Cl^- exchanger. They possess a Na^+ independent
HCO_3^- /Cl^- exchange system (45).

Whether the unique properties of the Na^+/H^+ antiport found in
both Hl-60 and U-937 cells and the presence of a Na^+ dependent
HCO_3^- /Cl^- exchange system are linked in some way to their transformed state is not yet known. In a recent study the existence of fundamental differences in the electrical properties of U-937 cells

and human monocyte-derived macrophages have been reported (28).

In both leukemic cell lines, RA produced a cell alkalinization which developped over 48 hours, which clearly preceded the appearance of the differentiated phenotype and which was due to a 2 fold increase in the activity of the Na^+/H^+ exchanger. Previous studies on the regulation of the activity of this exchanger in various cell types have shown that it is very sensitive to a variety of stimuli. Mitogens or phorbol esters elicit activations that are observed within seconds to minutes (11,19), whereas others such as metabolic acidosis (21), glucocorticoids (23) or thyroxine (22) induce responses that take hours or days to develop. Our data indicate that RA-induced activation of the Na^+/H^+ exchanger in U-937 and HL-60 cells belongs to the category of slow responses.

Activators of the Na^+/H^+ exchanger differ also in their effects on the kinetic properties of the system. Phorbol myristate acetate produces a shift in the pHi dependence of the exchanger into the alkaline range without modifying its maximal velocity measured at acidic pHi values (50,31); however epidermal growth factor produces an activation of the exchanger at all pHi values, suggesting a "Vmax" effect (50). We have shown, in both HL-60 (26) and U-937 cells (unpublished results), that the long term activation of the Na^+/H^+ exchanger does not involve a change in its internal pHi dependence. It remains to be determined whether this activation is the result of an increased expression of the exchanger at the cell surface or whether it results from the increased turnover rate of already existing exchangers as reported recently for rabbit kidneys undergoing hypertrophy (51).

Although RA induced the same changes in HL-60 and in U-937 cells, the two lines entered a distinct differentiation pathway. One difference between the two cell types is that a 2 fold increase in the activity of the Na^+/H^+ exchanger resulted in a >0.35 pH unit increase in HL-60 and only a 0.2 pH unit increase in U-937 cells. This could suggest a possible role of the pHi for the cell commitment to one or the other pathway. All the more that we have found that DMSO triggers also a 0.37 pHi unit increase in HL-60 cells (26) whereas recombinant human gamma interferon (rHu-IFN-γ RU 42 369) and 1,25 dihydroxyvitamin D_3 which differentiate HL-60 cells into monocyte-like cells produce a 0.13 and 0.23 pH unit increase respectively. On the other hand, Etretinate, a synthetic retinoid which differentiates neither HL-60 nor U-937 cells (7), does not change the pHi of either cell line even at 10 µM.

Our data have also shown that intracellular concentrations of Na^+ and K^+ as well as the activity of the sodium pump are also increased in the first few hours following RA addition to HL-60 cells They suggest that the early stimulation of the sodium pump may be due to the increase in $(Na^+)i$ and would in turn lead to the increase in $(K^+)i$. This suggest that RA stimulates one (or many) of the Na^+ transport systems known to exist in the cell plasma membrane. Our experiments on the Na^+/H^+ exchanger have indicated however that this system is not activated in the first 3 h following RA addition (Fig.5, inset).

Another point that arises from our studies is that ouabain, at a concentration which binds to and inhibits about 70% of the sodium pump molecules, which is not cytotoxic and which has no differentiating effect by itself, accelerates and potentiates RA-induced differentiation of HL-60 cells. When RA and ouabain are both present stimulation of the $Na^+K^+ATPase$ is detected earlier than when RA only is present. These results, and the fact that they ha-been found also with DMSO and butyrate suggest that intracellular concentrations of monovalent cations may play a role in the cascade of events leading to the differentiation of leukemic cells.Similar findings have been reported for the differentiation of the murine pre-B cell line 70Z/3 (39) and also, as suggested by our results, that both $(Na^+)i$ and pHi have to be increased to get succesful differentiation (40).

Differentiation of HL-60 and U-937 cells is known to be accompanied by an arrest of cell proliferation and by a decreased expression of the cellular proto-oncogene c-myc (52,37). It is interesting to note that the very same events described here: increase in $(Na^+)i$ and $(K^+)i$, activation of the sodium pump, activation of the Na^+/H^+ exchanger, increase in pHi; occur also as early events in the mitogens-induced proliferation of a variety of cell lines (30,35,42). This proliferation is accompanied by an increase in the expression of c-myc (20,29). How the same intracellular signals can lead to opposite effects remains an unresolved question.

While RA added directly to HL-60 cells membrane preparations had no effect on adenylate cyclase activity, incubation of these cells with 1 µM RA led concomitantly to differentiation and to changes in AC activity. In differentiated cells basal AC activity was significantly higher than in control cells. Similar findings were reported by Roberts et al.(38) and Fontana et al.(10). However this increased activity was not reflected in cAMP production measured in intact HL-60 (1) or in U-937 cells (12), even after total inhibition of cAMP phosphodiesterase activity. On the other hand, in differentiated cells AC activity was less succeptible to stimulation by GTP, was not affected by Fsk and, in the presence of Fsk, GTP inhibited enzyme activity at lower concentration and to a greater extent than in untreated cells. Studies of cAMP production in whole cell have shown comparable results: RA-differentiated cells have a decreased capacity to generate cAMP upon hormonal stimulation of AC (1,12); and 1,25 dihydroxyvitamin D_3 differentiated U-937 cells produce twice less cAMP, compared to control cells, when stimulated by isoproterenol or Fsk (43). Whilst in the case of the hormonal ligands the decreased cAMP production may be explained either by a lower number of membrane receptors or by a defective coupling between the receptors and the enzyme, with Fsk this decreased production implies an alteration in the regulatory G proteins (13). Recent experiments using the ADP-ribosilation of G_s by cholera toxin and of G_i by pertussis toxin have shown a 3 to 4 fold decrease in the amount of G_s after differentia tion. (unpublished). On the other hand, Didsburry et al.(9) have shown that differentiation of U-937 cells by dibutyryl cAMP resulted in a 3.6 fold increase in the $G_i\alpha$, 41kDa, protein.

This decreased capacity of AC to be hormonally stimulated after granulocytic or monocytic differentiation could be explained if one considers the role played by intracellular cAMP levels in leukemic versus normal mature myeloid cells: increased cAMP levels favor the differentiation of leukemic cells (33,32), whereas increased cAMP levels inhibit the functions of normal mature cells (6,2,5).

In summary, the results presented indicate that some of the early events triggered by the differentiation inducers, especially retinoic acid, are comparable to that induced by mitogens, although the final results are quite opposite. They suggest also that retinoic acid might act, at least on leukemic cells, directly on the plasma membrane.

REFERENCES

1. Abita, J.P., Gespach, C., Cost, H., Poirier, O., and Saal, F. (1982): IRCS Medical Science 10:882-883.
2. Anderson, R.A., Glover, A., and Rabson, A.R. (1977):J. Immunol. 118:1690-1696.
3. Boyd, A.W., and Metcalf, D. (1984): Leuk. Res. 8:27-43.
4. Breitman, T.R., Selonick, S.E., and Collins, S.J. (1980): Proc. Natl. Acad. Sci. USA 77:2936-2940.
5. Bryant, R.E., and Sutcliffe, M.C. (1974): J. Clin. Invest. 54: 1241-1244.
6. Busse, W.W., and Sosman, J. (1976): Science 194: 737-738.
7. Chomienne, C., Balitrand, N., Cost, H., Degos, L., and Abita, J.P. (1986): Leuk. Res. 11: 1301-1305.
8. Collins, S.J., Ruscetti, F.W., Gallagher, R.E., and Gallo, R.C. (1978): Proc. Natl. Acad. Sci. USA 75: 2458-2462.
9. Didsburry, J.R., Ho, Y.S., and Snyderman, R. (1987): FEBS Letters 211: 160-164.
10. Fontana, J., Miksis, G., and Durham, J. (1987): Exp. Cell Res. 168: 487-493.
11. Frelin, C., Vigne, P., and Lazdunski, M. (1985): In: Hormones and cell regulation, edited by J.E. Dumont, B. Hamprecht, and J. Nunez, Vol.9, pp. 259-268.Elsevier, Amsterdam.
12. Gespach, C., Cost, H., and Abita, J.P. (1985): FEBS Letters 184: 207-213.
13. Gilman, A.G. (1984): J. Clin. Invest.73: 1-4.
14. Grinstein, S., Cohen, S., Lederman, H.M., and Gelfand, E.W. (1984): J. Cell. Physiol. 121: 87-95.
15. Grinstein, S., Rothstein, A., and Cohen, S. (1985): J. Gen. Physiol. 85: 765-787.
16. Grinstein, S., and Furuya, W. (1986): Am. J. Physiol. 250: C283-C291.
17. Grinstein, S., Furuya, W., and Biggar, W.D. (1986): J. Biol. Chem. 261: 512-514.

18. Grinstein, S., Furuya, W., and Cragoe, E.J. (1986): J. Cell. Physiol. 128: 33-40.
19. Grinstein, S., and Rothstein, A. (1986): J. Membr. Biol. 90: 1-12.
20. Kelly, K., Cochran, B.H., Stiles, C.D., and Leder, P. (1983): Cell 35: 603-610.
21. Kinsella, J., Cujdik, T., and Sacktor, B. (1984): J. Biol. Chem. 259: 13224-13227.
22. Kinsella, J., and Sacktor, B. (1985): Proc. Natl. Acad. Sci. USA 82: 3606-3610.
23. Kinsella, J., Freiberg, J., and Sacktor, B. (1985): Am. J. Physiol. 248: F233-F239.
24. Ladoux, A., Geny, B., Marrec, N., and Abita, J.P. (1984): FEBS Letters 176: 467-472.
25. Ladoux, A., Abita, J.P., and Geny, B. (1986): Differentiation 33: 142-147.
26. Ladoux, A., Cragoe, E.J., Geny, B., Abita, J.P., and Frelin,C. (1987): J. Biol. Chem. 262: 811-816.
27. Ladoux, A., Krawice, I., Cragoe, E.J., Abita, J.P. and Frelin C. (1987) Eur. J. Biochem. in press.
28. McCann, F.V., Keller, T.M., and Guyer, P.M. (1987): J. Membr. Biol. 96: 57-64.
29. Makino, R., Hayashi, K., and Sugimura, T. (1984): Nature Lon. 310: 697-698.
30. Moolenaar, W.H., De Laat, S.W., Mummery, C.L., and Van der Saag, P.T. (1982): In: Ions, Cell proliferation, and Cancer, edited by A.L. Boyton, W.L. McKeehan, and J.F. Whitfield, pp. 151-174. Academic Press, Inc. New York.
31. Moolenaar, W.H., Tertoolen, L.G.H., and De Laat, S.W. (1984) Nature Lon. 312: 371-374.
32. Olsson, I.L., and Breitman, T.R. (1982): Cancer Res. 42: 3924-3927.
33. Olsson, I.L., Breitman, T.R., and Gallo, R.C. (1982): Cancer Res. 42: 3928-3933.
34. Olsson, I.L., Gulberg, U., Ivhed, I., and Nilsson, K. (1983) Cancer Res. 43: 5862-5867.
35. Pouyssegur, J., Paris, S., and Chambard, J.C. (1982):In: Ions, Cell proliferation, and Cancer, edited by A.L. Boyton, W.L. McKeehan, and J.F. Whitfield, pp. 205-218. Academic Press, Inc. New York.
36. Radzun, H.J., Parwaresh, M.R., Sundström, C., Nilsson, K., and Eissner, M. (1983): Int. J. Cancer 31: 181-186.
37. Reitsma, P.H., Rothberg, P.G., Astrin, S.M., Trial, J., Bar-Shavit, Z., Hall, A., Teitelbaum, S.L., and Kahn, A.J. (1983): Nature Lon. 306: 492-494.
38. Roberts, P.J., Venge, P., and Segal, A.W. (1985): 19th Annual Meeting of the European Society for Clinical Investigation, 24-27 April, Toulouse, France, p.A47, Abs. 280.
39. Rosoff, P.M., and Cantley, L.C. (1983): Proc. Natl. Acad. Sci. USA 80: 7547-7550.
40. Rosoff, P.M., Stein, L.F., and Cantley, L.C. (1984): J. Biol.

    Chem. 259: 773-780.
41. Rovera, G., Santoli, D., and Damsky, C. (1979): Proc. Natl.
    Acad. Sci. USA 76: 2779-2783.
42. Rozengurt, E., and Mendoza, S.A. (1986): In: The role of Mem-
    branes in Cell Growth and Differentiation, edited by L.J.
    Mandel, and D.J. Benos, pp. 163-191. Academic Press, Inc.
    New York.
43. Rubin, J.E., and Catherwood, B.D. (1984): Biochem. Biophys.
    Res. Commun. 123: 210-215.
44. Salomon, Y., Londos, C., and Rodbell, M. (1974): Anal. Biochem
    58: 541-548.
45. Simchowitz, L., and Roos, A. (1985): J. Gen. Physiol. 85:
    443-470.
46. Simchowitz, L., and Cragoe, E.J. (1986): Mol. Pharmac. 30:
    122-130.
47. Thomas, G., Chomienne, C., Balitrand, N., Schaison, G., Abita,
    J.P., and Baulieu, E.E. (1986): Anticancer Res. 6: 857-860.
48. Vigne, P., Frelin, C., Cragoe, E.J., and Lazdunski, M. (1983):
    Biochem. Biophys. Res. Commun. 116: 86-90.
49. Vigne, P., Frelin, C., Cragoe, E.J., and Lazdunski, M. (1984):
    Mol. Pharmac. 25: 131-136.
50. Vigne, P., Frelin, C., and Lazdunski, M. (1985): Eur. J. Bio-
    chem. 65: 293-306.
51. Vigne, P., Jean, T., Barbry, P., Frelin, C., Fine, L., and
    Lazdunski, M. (1985): J. Biol. Chem. 260: 14120-14125.
52. Westin, E.H., Wong-Staal, F., Gelman, E.P., Dalla-Favera, R.,
    Papas, T.S., Lautenberger, J.A., Eva, A., Reddy, E.P., Tro-
    nick, S.R., Aaronson, S.A., and Gallo, R.C. (1982): Proc.
    Natl. Acad. Sci. USA 79: 2490-2494.

BIOLOGICAL MODIFICATIONS AS AN APPROACH TO DIFFERENTIATION THERAPY

Control of Growth and Differentiation: Possible Control Mechanisms, Mutations Producing Neoplasia and Therapeutic Implications

J. Paul[1] and P.T. Rowley[2]

[1]Beatson Institute for Cancer Research, Garscube Estate,
Switchback Road, Bearsden Glasgow G61 1BO, Scotland;
[2]Department of Medicine and Division of Genetics
University of Rochester School of Medicine
Rochester NY 14642, USA

SUMMARY

In this report theoretical models for mechanisms of growth and differentiation, their relevance to neoplasia, implications for replacement therapy, and in vitro models for investigating these ideas are discussed. The simplest model systems involve a single factor with a single action and are limited to four components, viz. a growth or differentiation–inducing factor, a receptor, a mediator across the nuclear membrane, and a target chromatin. It is concluded that a defect in any component may give rise to similar phenotypes and some of the defects may give rise to constitutive growth. If single cell systems are considered, defects in a negative control system are more likely to be amenable to treatment by replacement than those of a positive growth system. However, although negative feedback is an important aspect of control, most current findings point to the existence of positive controls. Reasons for the paradox are discussed: it is likely that the target cells which have been investigated form only part of a loop involving at least two cell-types. In practice, therefore, more complex models have to be considered. Stem cells have the option of entering a symmetrical self-renewal mitosis or an asymmetrical mitosis in which one daughter becomes committed to terminal differentiation. Promotion of the latter alternative may reduce the growth fraction of a tumor cell-line. This strategy may also enable cells blocked in a replicating transit population to proceed to non-dividing mature cells. The usefulness of cell culture models to investigate these models particularly in relation to research by Working Group VI is discussed.

I. INTRODUCTION

Tumors vary in phenotype from those which appear undifferentiated to those which are highly differentiated. Features of differentiation generally vary inversely with the fraction of mitotic cells and, since most terminally differentiated cells have no further capacity for cell division, it is argued that, if tumour cells could be caused to proceed to terminal differentiation, the clinical course of a tumour could be improved. In theory, if pushed far enough, the stem-cell-like pool of tumour cells might become exhausted.

Since very little is known about the regulation of cell differentiation, to investigate this hypothesis, empirical approaches have to be adopted. These include attempts to develop models, both theoretical and practical.

Model building is an activity that provides the scientist with two major benefits. The first is making explicit the assumptions required to generalize from the specific case to the general case. The second is the identification of gaps in fundamental knowledge and the recognition that certain experiments may permit a choice between alternative assumptions. The value of a model lies in the thought process involved in its construction and its ability to be tested experimentally.

II. THEORETICAL MODELS

A. Assumptions of Proposed Models

The assumptions underlying the models to be proposed are as follows:

1. A neoplasm arises by the accumulation of mutations, which may be genetic or epigenetic (23).
2. The multistage process by which a cell of normal phenotype becomes a cell with a neoplastic phenotype involves one critical mutation which disrupts the normal pattern of growth constraints.
3. This critical mutation involves a component of the normal growth control mechanism. (Of all such mutations, many have no effect and others will be lethal to the cell in which they occur).
4. Most mutations reduce or eliminate a capability rather than creating a new capability, and thus represent a deficiency or loss.

The models to be proposed initially represent simplest cases. In particular, they utilize the smallest likely number of elements in a growth control system. Nevertheless, this small number yields a large number of possible alterations. It is recognized that actual control systems are likely to have many additional components and even multiple systems per target cell type.

The models have been greatly influenced by recent studies, e.g. of epidermal growth factor for which it has been shown that a mutation in the structural gene for its receptor gives rise to unregulated growth of the target cell. This discovery was provocative because it combines two essential ingredients of a model for the mutational basis of neoplasia, (1) the phenotype of unregulated growth and (2) its arising from the loss of a function, in this case giving rise to the ability of the receptor to institute a positive growth signal in the absence of its ligand. Although this is a "new" function, it is nevertheless a loss, not only of a portion of the protein product, but also of susceptibility to regulation. Many of the proto-oncogenes which can be activated by mutation are components of a cascade concerned with initiation of DNA synthesis (24).

B. Model System Components

Several model system components are proposed. The first is the growth factor itself, whose ultimate effect on growth may be stimulatory or inhibitory. It will be assumed to vary normally only in availability due to changes in synthesis or release by its cell of origin. The second is the receptor, which is assumed to be a component of the cytoplasmic membrane of the target cell and responds to the binding of the growth factor by generating an intra-cytoplasmic signal. The third is a mediator, a signaling component which crosses the nuclear membrane. It is activated when the growth factor binds to the receptor. The mediator acts on the fourth component, a target in chromatin which stimulates or inhibits expression of particular genes assumed to control DNA synthesis and cell division.

C. Positive Growth Control Model

A positive growth control model is one in which the components form a cascade in which increase of any element leads to an increase in subsequent elements (Figure 1).

Simple mutations leading to defects, in the growth stimulator, receptor, mediator or target in this model, will lead to deficiency of growth, not growth excess. Only special types of mutations in the structural gene for each component will lead to constitutive growth. These are illustrated in Figure 2.

In most in vitro experimental systems, we select for growth and, in studying tumours, we are studying colonies in which selection for growth is an important factor. As a result, in most of the mutations which have been identified the functions of the components of the system are altered in a special way rather than destroyed. The v-sis gene product provides an example of an altered agonist, the v-erbB and v-fms products examples of altered receptors, the v-ras gene products examples of altered mediators and v-fos and v-myc gene products are possible examples of modified chromatin targets. In all cases these mutations give rise, not to cessation of growth, but to defective control of growth.

D. Negative Growth Control Model

An alternative type of model is a negative control model in which one or more components are inhibitors of DNA synthesis or mitosis. The simplest form of such a model is one in which a growth inhibitor interacts with a receptor in a manner similar to a growth factor with its receptor and this in turn stimulates a cascade which results in interaction with a chromatin target to cause inhibition of DNA synthesis and cell division (Figure 3).

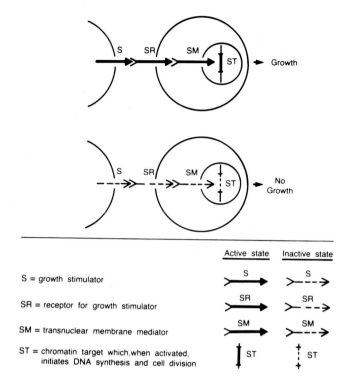

Figure 1. Model illustrating positive control of growth.

This model has theoretical attractions because it permits the postulation of growth control by feedback inhibition which is the simplest and most stable way of regulating a reaction and this model, therefore, formed the basis of the chalone hypothesis. However, little reliable direct evidence has been found to support these proposals. The interest in these models for cancer is that mutations of genes for growth inhibitors or repressors are likely to result in uncontrolled constitutive growth (Figure 4).

E. Combined Models

(1) Multicellular models

The fact that most of the evidence currently available implicates positive controls, whereas theory would require a negative control model, is a paradox. The explanation may simply be that individual cells are only part of a system in which we have one cell-type producing growth factors which stimulate a target cell-type. Target cells, in turn, may produce metabolites or factors which inhibit growth factor production. Provided the two components are kept separate they provide a fail-safe system because mutations in a positive control system result in non-growth, the equivalent of genetic death of a cell. However, there are two ways in which this mixed cell system can be circumvented. If the production of growth factor is increased (for example, interleukin-2

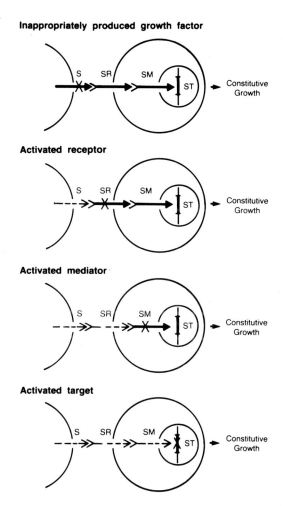

Figure 2. Mutations of positive growth control system which may cause constitutive growth.

in T-cell leukaemias), or growth factor is produced by cells carrying a receptor (autocrine stimulation), excessive growth of target cells may result.

(2) Intracellular combined models

There is ample evidence that most genes are responsive to both positive and negative regulatory factors; real control circuits may, therefore, be quite complex. The most relevant model here is that which proposes a competition between differentiation and growth. This is a longstanding idea in embryology and there are numerous examples where it seems to hold. It has been particularly analysed in relation to haemopoietic stem cells and is a model of great relevance to

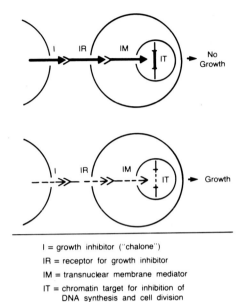

I = growth inhibitor ("chalone")
IR = receptor for growth inhibitor
IM = transnuclear membrane mediator
IT = chromatin target for inhibition of
     DNA synthesis and cell division

Figure 3. Model illustrating negative control of growth.

differentiation therapy, as described by Lajtha. It is discussed in more
detail below but, in essence, postulates that stem cells may either
replicate to give identical daughters or divide asymmetrically to give a
daughter identical to the original cell and one which goes on to terminal
differentiation.   The decision may be influenced by metabolites in the
environment released by differentiated cells. Such factors may operate
through the types of mechanisms described in sections A and B.

     This type of model, which is typical of haemopoietic cells, is
illustrated in Figure 5. When stem cells have divided asymmetrically the
committed daughter cell then may undergo a series of amplifying
divisions in a "transit compartment" before responding to further signals
and entering terminal differentiation (Figure 5).

III. IN VITRO MODELS

     In the early mammalian embryo, cells in the inner cell mass are
pluripotent; they give rise to all cell types found in the adult animal.
With successive cell divisions the developmental fate of each generation
becomes progressively restricted, the process of determination or
commitment. The early divisions result in different kinds of stem cells,
many of which persist throughout the life of the animal. Some retain an
ability to differentiate along diverging pathways, but their progeny have
progressively limited potential and indeed may only be able to proceed
down a single pathway. The committed stem cells respond to demand
with a series of amplifying divisions and eventually this transit
population enters into a terminal differentiation or maturation pathway

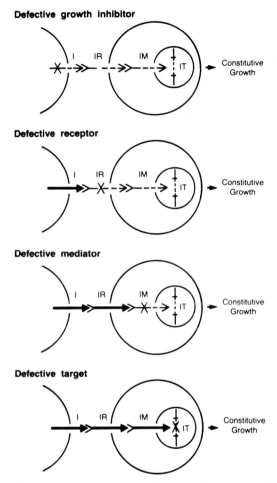

Figure 4. Mutations of negative growth control system which may cause constitutive growth.

yielding fully differentiated cells which are incapable of further differentiating and commonly also incapable of further dividing.

An ideal tissue culture model for the study of cell differentiation would mimic this behaviour. It would be a culture of pluripotent cells with different developmental potentials maintained in defined medium and capable of direction into required pathways by the addition of defined factors. It should have characteristic quantifiable features and it should be possible to grow colonies from single cells.

How near can we come to this ideal? It is possible to grow pluripotent cells from mammalian blastocysts but only small amounts can be obtained and we do not know how to direct their developmental fates. However, in recent years there has been great interest in established cultures of teratocarcinoma cells which are thought in many respects to be the equivalent of blastocyst cells (16, 26). In <u>vivo</u> they

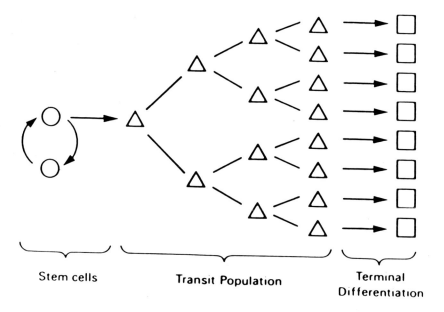

Stem cells   **Transit Population**   Terminal
Differentiation

Figure 5. Transit cell population separating stem cells from terminally differentiated cells.

give tumours with a variety of tissue types and they can be maintained in vitro indefinitely. They tend not to differentiate if grown in sparse inocula but, if allowed to pile up and form 3-dimensional structures, some differentiation may occur. They also show some response to treatment with factors such as DMSO or retinoic acid. Since these cells can replicate indefinitely, colonies can be grown from individual cells and the cultures can be reinjected into syngenic animals in which they will usually form tumours containing differentiating elements. They have been regarded as a very promising model for early cell differentiation but so far there has been only limited success in directing differentiation into well-defined pathways.

Experience with this and other systems, including observations on cell differentiation in the developing embryo, has raised the question as to whether differentiation can, in fact, be directed by extraneous factors. Three main theories have been proposed.

1. Directive theories. According to these theories the decision to develop along a specific pathway is directly influenced by factors in the environment which trigger a "developmental switch" of the kind referred to earlier.

2. The stochastic theory. According to this theory, the developmental pathways followed by daughters of a cell division are determined solely by random endogenous events. Hence, diverging cells arise randomly and the predominance of one cell type over another depends solely on selective factors in the environment.

3. Modified stochastic theories. According to theories of this type an endogenous stochastic mechanism determines whether a cell will diverge

into one pathway or another but the probability of any course can be influenced by factors in the environment.

The experience with very early stem cell lines and teratocarcinoma lines has given little encouragement for directive theories. This could be because endogenous factors are predominant in the early stages of cell differentiation but it might also simply mean that extraneous directing factors have not so far been identified. However, in cells at later stages of development, i.e., committed stem cells, there is clear evidence of effects of environmental factors. This has formed the basis of many studies in model tissue culture systems.

Tissue culture models for cell differentiation have had three different but related objectives:

1. Culture of differentiated cells, for example, to study the synthesis of specialised products such as haemoglobin.
2. Study of stages and mechanisms of differentiation. This calls for differentiating cell systems.
3. Attempts to reverse blocks to differentiation, usually in tumour cells.

A. Culture of Differentiated Cells.

It is relatively easy to maintain any differentiated tissue in organ culture for limited periods (usually a few days) and this classical technique has been in use for at least 80 years.

In more recent years much effort has gone into establishing cell lines with differentiated characteristics. The problem is that most normal differentiated cells senesce more or less rapidly but it has been found that cells from differentiated tumours can often be established in vitro. This technique was exploited particularly by Sato and his colleagues (30) to obtain cell lines which perform differentiated functions such as the synthesis of peptide or steroid hormones. Other important examples are erythroid cell lines and myeloma and lymphoma cell lines, synthesizing immunoglobulins. Cell lines of this type have two interesting features. First, they offer a system in which details of specialized function can be studied. Secondly, they offer models for the investigation of strategies based on the concept of Differentiation Therapy.

B. In Vitro Differentiating Systems

The most intensively studied systems have been concerned with haematopoiesis. These have involved the primary culture of colonies from haemopoietic tissue, such as bone marrow, and have led to the identification of different haemopoietic colony-forming cells (e.g. CFU-E and CFU-C) and associated factors including G-CSF, M-CSF, GM-CSF and erythropoietin. These are well-established, highly quantifiable and standardizable systems. The main disadvantages in their use are that it is not easy to obtain large amounts of material for study and primary cultures have to be established for each experiment. Moreover, reproducible neoplastic transformation has not been achieved in vitro in mammalian systems although avian haemopoietic cells can be transformed by retroviruses (2).

However, some established haemopoietic cell lines established from tumours have some desirable properties. The Murine Erythroleukaemia lines (MEL) such as Friend cell lines are good examples (8). In standard culture conditions these have the morphology of blast cells but, on treatment with dimethylsulfoxide (DMSO) or other inducers (notably HMBA), they undergo maturation to normoblast- or reticulocyte-like cells. Moreover, these cells will grow as tumours in mice and hence in vivo and in vitro conditions can be alternated.

Epithelial cells are also of particular interest in that they can be maintained in culture through many passages in low Ca^{++} medium but differentiate into keratinized squamous cells when the Ca^{++} concentration is raised (15). Transformed cells, if present, do not respond to high calcium treatment (18). They apparently are blocked at an immature stage.

The situation regarding fibroblasts is less clearcut mainly because the relationship of stem cells to mature cells is not well established. It might be argued that all fibroblasts behave as stem cells or, on the contrary, that the synthesis of collagen and other connective-tissue matrices is a criterion of cell differentiation. The relationship is simply not so clearly defined as it is for haemopoietic and epithelial cells.

Other primary cell lines exhibit differentiation in vitro, for example myoblasts, which differentiated into myotubes, but few of them have been exploited in the investigation of Differentiation Therapy.

C. Reversal of Block to Differentiation

One of the most prevalent interpretations of the behaviour of tumor cell lines, such as the Friend cell or K562 cell, is that they represent cells blocked at an early stage of maturation, in these examples in the transit population state (Figure 5).

This hypothesis can be extended to almost all tumour cells with the corollary that treatment with factors which release the block will lead to amelioration of the tumour. It follows that any established tumour cell line in which a block to cell differentiation may exist, provides an experimental system for the investigation of Differentiation Therapy.

The idea that in many tumours a block to differentiation occurs so that the cells continue to replicate without differentiation, or at least the balance between differentiation and replication is in favour of replication, raises three questions. First, at which stage during cell differentiation does the lesion occur which results in the block? Second, what is the mechanism of the block? Third, can it be influenced by environmental factors?

The first question is complex because there is strong evidence that carcinogenesis is a multistage process in which tumour initiation can only be recognised after several stages have occurred. Examples are retinoblastoma and Wilm's tumour in which the tendency to tumour formation is represented by a recessive mutation in the genome, as previously noted. For this to give rise to a tumour, two further events are needed. One is that the lesion should become homozygous, and the other that this should occur in the target tissue in which presumably the correct epigenetic conditions are present to permit tumourigenesis. Only when these conditions have been fulfilled (and possibly others) is a tumour initiated.

When then does initiation occur in common human tumours? There are numerous arguments that early initiation events involve stem cells. This is particularly exemplified in chronic granulocytic leukaemia in which the marker Philadelphia chromosome almost certainly arises in a pluripotential stem cell population in bone marrow. However, although the initiating lesions may occur at this early stage, the block to differentiation may be expressed much later. For example, the Friend cell is thought almost certainly to represent an erythroid cell blocked at the CFU-E stage. Indeed it resembles most closely an early pro-erythroblast. The question which arises is, how much earlier in the maturation pathway did the lesion occur which resulted in the block? We have no satisfactory answer.

What of the nature of the block itself? Insufficient information is available but one suggestion, derived from the modified stochastic theory, proposes that the balance between a decision to continue division and a decision to enter terminal differentiation is biased towards the former by an enhanced stimulus to mitosis, which is a common consequence of activation of many oncogenes (24).

IV. IMPLICATIONS FOR THERAPY WITH BIOLOGICAL MODULATORS

With the above schema for possible mutations underlying the neoplastic phenotype, we may now consider the degree to which replacement of deficient factors may revert the cellular phenotype towards the normal state. Obviously many components other than "differentiation factors" would be needed.

First, let us consider models which invoke factors controlling growth. In the positive growth control systems, only a special type of mutation in a receptor, mediator, or target causes constitutive growth. Since such mutations presumably have dominant phenotypes, replacement of the normal gene might be ineffectual. However, in the case of a negative growth control system, replacement may be more promising. Since these mutations presumably have somatic recessive phenotypes, replacement of the normal factor would be expected to be ameliorative.

Finally, let us consider the models which involve factors controlling differentiation. Substances which may reverse a differentiation block fall into two categories. In view of the evidence, such as studies on the effects of hormones on cultures of plant tumour callus (3) and the normal differentiation of cells derived from teratocarcinoma when transplanted to the early embryo (21), one strongly-held conviction is that exposure of tissue to very strong normal morphogenetic signals may rectify anomalous behaviour. Hence, attempts have been made to remove differentiation blocks with hormones and other growth and differentiation factors.

Experience with endocrine hormones has provided little encouragement for their use as therapeutic agents in cancer. On the contrary, in hormone-dependent tumours, deprivation of hormones has proved helpful. This has been studied in vitro by the isolation and investigation of the behaviour of hormone-dependent cell lines, mostly derived from tumours. In the treatment of breast cancer, oophorectomy and drugs such as Tamoxifen have been practical applications. In a similar way, growth factors such as EGF serve to maintain the growth of cells carrying receptors rather than to rectify differentiation blocks but to date these observations have not been exploited in therapy.

Many of the normal factors identified in haemopoietic systems , such as erythropoietin, probably function as growth factors as well as differentiation-inducing factors and may not, therefore, have a place in Differentiation Therapy. However, certain factors may have different kinds of effects. For example, Sachs (28) has maintained that his factor MGI, which is the same as G-CSF, can reverse a differentiation block in myeloid leukaemic cell lines in vitro. Also nerve growth factor may reverse a block in a phaeochromocytoma cell line (12). It is possible that TGF beta and interferon may behave in a similar fashion.

On the whole, however, the use of physiological differentiation factors in cancer therapy has so far proved disappointing - perhaps because we know too little about them. More success has attended the use of substances without a clearly defined physiological function in differentiation but which have been found quite empirically to reverse differentiation blocks. Best known among those are dimethysulphoxide and related polar-planar compounds, retinoic acid, hexamethylene bisacetamide, gamma-interferon, butyrate and dihydroxyvitamin D_3.

V. PRACTICAL ASPECTS OF IN VITRO MODELS

The most important requirement for a model system is reproducibility. It is not too important whether the plating efficiency of a cell line is 0.1% or 100% provided the same cells are always cloned with the same efficiency in different laboratories at different times. The two main sources of variability are the cells and the medium in which they are grown.

A. Variation Among Cells.

Little can be done about this in primary cultures, e.g. growth of Colony Forming Cells from bone marrow, but it is essential to know what the normal variation is in order to be able to attribute significance to observations outside the normal range. In inbred mice, variation is low and even within non-inbred populations (e.g. humans) there is not great variation among normal individuals.

In contrast, in continuous culture systems, a high level of reproducibility requires meticulous technique because cells in culture can diverge very rapidly. The mutation rate of most genes is on the order of 10^{-6} per cell per mitosis and, since most bulk cultures consist of some millions of cells, it is obvious that several mutations of nearly every gene may be present in a standard cell culture. Whereas, in the intact animal, selection might not be expected to favour them, in the artificial conditions of tissue culture some of them may enjoy a selective advantage. Hence, it is a matter of common observation that cell cultures in continuous passage may diverge rapidly from the original culture. Even if the progeny of a colony derived from a single-cell are cloned, the resulting colonies are already found to exhibit considerable variation.

To minimize variation, it is therefore desirable to work from frozen stock derived from as uniform a population as possible. To achieve uniformity, early passage primary cells may be used or, in the case of continuous lines, cells derived from single-cell cloning at as low a post-cloning passage number as possible. Common practice is to thaw out a fresh ampoule each month, grow it up during one month and then use it in experiments during the next month. In this way no cells used in experiments have had more than ten or so passages from the original stock.

B. Variation Due to Medium

This is much more difficult to control, especially as most differentiated or differentiating cells have a high serum requirement and the properties of serum vary enormously from batch to batch. We have often observed that nominally identical batches of serum behave quite differently towards Friend cells and K562 cells. Even among those which support high plating efficiencies some will show high levels of spontaneous induction of haemoglobin synthesis while others will give low levels. Moreover, some will display a good response to inducers while some will display a poor or no response. The reasons for this behaviour are not known but, since serum contains a variety of growth factors which can be influenced by methods of preparation and storage, it is not too surprising. To minimize the effect of this kind of variation, we routinely obtain sample batches of new serum supplies before the current batch runs out, check them for suitability against the current batch and then order a replacement supply of a batch which closely matches that in current use.

The failure of some laboratories to reproduce the results in others is almost always due to failure to conform to good housekeeping practice of the kind outlined. Unfortunately, this also leads to much confusion in the literature and to apparently conflicting claims.

VI. RESULTS FROM WORKING GROUP VI

Dr. Paul Fisher (New York) conducted studies on the effects of various recombinant human interferons on growth, differentiation, and tumor-associated antigen expression and shedding by melanoma, breast carcinoma and colon carcinoma cells (7, 11, 13, 14). If one assumes that altered tumor-associated antigen expression may relate to the state of differentiation of the treated cell, then interferon may prove useful in enhancing the targeting and therefore increasing the therapeutic potential of monoclonal antibodies (a form of differentiation therapy).

Drs. Yoshihiro Fujii and Noritoshi Takeichi (Sapporo, Japan) have tested differentiation therapy in a rat myelomonocytic leukemia model. C-WRT-7 cells were induced to differentiate to macrophage-like cells after a short-term incubation with lipopolysaccharide (LPS) and to lose their leukemogenicity in syngeneic rats (9). Administration of LPS alone or together with daunorubicin induced the in vivo differentiation of leukemia cells. This method proved to be effective in curing as well as prolonging survival. Long-term incubation of these cells with LPS resulted in the establishment of an LPS-resistant subline, probably by selection of minor populations, which displayed enhanced expression of Ia antigens and less IL3-like activity and were less leukemogenic than the parental cells.

One of us (Rowley, Rochester) has explored the utility of the human leukemic cell line K562, both as a model of erythroid differentiation (5, 22) and as a model of a multipotent hematopoetic cell which can be induced into different pathways of differentiation (20). Phorbol esters were shown to induce striking megakaryocytic characteristics including increased cell size, reduced growth rate, polyploidy, platelet glycoprotein antigens, expression of the sis proto-oncogene (which is the structural gene for the B chain of platelet-derived growth factor), and the release of mitogenic activity into the medium (19). GM-CSF was shown to reduce, not only growth, but also the expression of the abl oncogene (27).

Dr. Blanche Alter (New York) has shown that hemin stimulates erythropoiesis and hemoglobin synthesis by peripheral blood progenitors from normal adults and from patients with sickle cell anemia cultured in methycellulose with erythropoietin (17). Erythropoietin also increases hemoglobin F if added during the last three to seven days of culture, implying that it acts on CFU-E or early erythroblasts. Dr. Shigeru Sassa (New York) has studied the mechanism of induction of heme synthesis in murine hepatoma cells (10, 29). DMSO increased delta-amino laevulinate dehydratase and decreased growth rate. The regulation of the heme synthesis was found to differ from that in erythroid marrow cells.

Dr. Anders Rosen (Stockholm) has described a new lymphokine (MP-6 BSF) (25). Produced by a T-helper cell x MOLT4 human hybridoma, it influences the differentiation of normal B lymphocytes. It induces differentiation in B-cell CLL and modifies T-cells by up-regulating IL2 receptors. This B-cell growth factor activity can be modified by two monoclonal antibodies.

Many of the participating laboratories have been investigating interferons. Dr. Ferdinando Dianzani's group (Rome) has obtained evidence that a diffusible signal for lymphocyte production of gamma-interferon is induced by oxidation of terminal galactose residues on the surface of macrophages (1). His group has used a short-term (72 hrs) in vitro culture system to study the effect of alpha-interferon on mononuclear cells from peripheral blood of hairy cell leukaemia patients and have shown effects on both membrane and cytoplasmic features, particularly the density of surface immunoglobulin accompanied by dramatic reduction of cytoplasmic acid phosphatases (6).

Dr. Felice Gavosto's laboratory (Turin) has shown that gamma-interferon is a potent inducer of HLA class II antigens. CFU-GM from CML are less sensitive than normal CFU-GM to the inhibitory action of prostaglandin E (PGE), possibly because of abnormal expression of HLA class II antigens. However, gamma-interferon in liquid culture does not significantly affect expression of HLA class II antigens by progenitor cells, although it may increase their sensitivity to PGE.

Dr. Fabien Calvo's group (Paris) have found that MHC class I and II antigens in H466-BT47-D breast carcinoma cell lines respond to treatment with gamma-interferon.

Dr. Antonia Dolei's group (Sassari) has shown that peripheral blood mononuclear cells, when treated with growth inhibitors, yield an interferon-like molecule which is not alpha-, beta-, or gamma-interferon (4).

Dr. Charles Chany's group (Paris) (31) have made the very remarkable observation that BALB/c embryonic fibroblasts transformed by Moloney sarcoma virus and then cultivated for over 600 generations in the presence of mouse alpha-beta interferon revert to a normal phenotype and fail to produce tumours in nude mice, although they retain integrated Moloney sarcoma virus. DNA from these cells can still give rise to foci in transfected cells and hybridisation with a v-mos probe can be demonstrated. Even after withdrawal of the interferon, the cells did not revert for 100 generations, although mos transcripts were present. The cells produced no mos-containing virions.

In two review articles, one of us (23, 24) has discussed some of the theoretical problems encountered in analysing carcinogenesis.

REFERENCES

1. Antonelli, G., Blalock, J.E., and Dianzani, F. (1985): Cellular Immunology, 94:440-446.
2. Beug, H., von Kirchback, A., Doderlein, G., Conscience, J.F., and Graf, T. (1979): Cell, 18:375-390.
3. Braun, A.C. (1969): The Cancer Problem: A Critical Analysis and Modern Synthesis. Columbia University Press, New York.
4. Dianzani, F., Dolei, A. and Di Marco, P. (1986): J. Interferon Res., 6:43-50.
5. Farley, B.A., Ohlsson-Wilhelm B.M., and Rowley, P.T. (1987): Int J Cell Cloning, 5:27-34.
6. Fattorossi, A., Dolei, A., Pizzolo, J.G., Cafolla, A., Mandelli, F. and Dianzani, F. (1987): J. Biol. Regul. Homeo. Agents, 1:17-22.
7. Fisher, P.B., Hermo, H., Jr., Solowey, W.E., Dietrich, M.C., Edwalds, G.M., Weinstein, I.B., Langer, J.A., Pestka, S., Giacomini, P., Kusama, M., and Ferrone, S. (1986): Anticancer Research, 6:765-774.
8. Friend, C., Scher, W., Holland, J.G. and Sato, T. (1971): Proc. Natl. Acad. Sci. USA, 68:378-382.
9. Fujii, Y., Yuki, N., Takeichi, N., Kobayashi, H. and Miyazaki, T. (1987): Cancer Research, 47:1668-1673.
10. Galbraith, R.A., Sassa, S., and Kappas, A. (1986): Biochem. J., 237:597-600.
11. Giacomini, P., Gambari, R., Barbieri, R., Nistico, P., Tecce, R., Pestka, S., Gustafsson, K., Natali, P.G., and Fisher, P.B. (1986): Anticancer Research, 6:877-884.
12. Greene, I.A. and Tischler, A.S. (1976): Proc. Natl. Acad. Sci. USA, 73:2424-2428.
13. Greiner, J.W., Guadagni, F., Noguchi, P., Pestka, S., Colcher, D., Fisher, P.B., and Schlom, J. (1987): Science, 235:895-898.
14. Greiner, J.W., Schlom, J., Pestka, S., Langer, J.A., Giacomini, P., Kusama, M., Ferrone, S., and Fisher, P.B. (1987): Pharmac. Ther. In press.
15. Hennings, H., Michael, D., Cheng, C., Steinert, P., Holbrook, K. and Yuspa, S.H. (1980): Cell, 19:245-254.
16. Kahan, B.W., Ephrussi, B. (1970): J. Natl. Cancer Inst., 44:1015-1036.

17. Kaye, F.J., Weinberg, R.S., Schofield, M.J., and Alter, B.P. (1986): Int. J. Cell Cloning, 4:432–446.
18. Kulesz-Martin, M.F., Koehler, B., Hennings, H. and Yuspa, S.H. (1980): Carcinogenesis (Lond.) 1:995–1006.
19. Leary, J.F., Farley, B.A., Giuliano, R., Kosciolek, B.A., LaBella, S., and Rowley, P.T. (1987): J. Biol. Regul. Homeo. Agents, 1:73–80.
20. Leary, J.F., Ohlsson-Wilhelm B.M., Giuliano R., LaBella S., Farley, B.A., and Rowley, P.T. (1987): Leuk. Res. In press.
21. Mintz, B. and Illmensee, K. (1975): Proc. Natl. Acad. Sci. USA, 72:3585–3589.
22. Ohlsson-Wilhelm, B.M., Farley, B.A., and Rowley, P.T. (1987): Exp. Hematol. 15:817–821.
23. Paul, J. (1987): In: Oncogenesis: Recent Advances in Histopathology, edited by P.P. Anthony and R.N.M. MacSween, pp.13–31. Churchill Livingstone, Edinburgh.
24. Paul, J. (1987): In: Theories of Carcinogenesis: Proceedings from the 1986 International Conference on Cancer Research, edited by O.H. Iversen. Hemisphere Publishing Corp., New York.
25. Rosen, A., Uggla, C., Szigeti, R., Kallin, B., Lindqvist, C. and Zeuthen, J. (1986): Lymphokine Res., 5:185.
26. Rosenthal, M.D., Wishnow, R.M., and Sato, G.H. (1970): J. Natl. Cancer Inst., 44:1001–1014.
27. Rowley, P.T., Leary, J.F., Skuse, G.R., Farley, B., Giuliano, R., and LaBella, S. Blood. In press.
28. Sachs, L. (1978): In: Differentiation of Normal and Neoplastic Hemopoietic Cells, edited by B. Clarkson, P.A. Marks and J.A. Till. Cold Spring Harbor Laboratory.
29. Sassa, S., Sugita, O., Galbraith, R.A., and Kappas, A. (1987): Biochem. Biophys. Res. Commun., 143, 1:52–57.
30. Sato, G., Augusti-Tocco, G., Posner, M., and Kelly, P., (1970). Recent Prog. Hormone Res., 26:539.
31. Sergiescu, D., Gerfaux, J., Joret, A.M., and Chany, C. (1986): Proc. Natl. Acad. Sci. USA, 83:5764–5768.

Interferons Modulation of Growth and Differentiation of Friend Erythroleukemia Cells

G.B. Rossi[1], E.M. Coccia[1], M. Federico[1], F. Titti[1], N. Mechti[2], B. Lebleu[2], G. Romeo[3] and E. Affabris[3]

[1]Laboratory of Virology, Istituto Superiore di Sanità,
Viale Regina Elena 299, 00161 Rome;
[2]Department of Protein Biochemistry, ERA CNRS 482;
University of Montpellier II, Montpellier, France
[3]Department of Cellular and Developmental Biology,
University "La Sapienza", Via degli Apuli 1, 00185 Rome, Italy

The possibility that differentiation inducers may turn out to be useful in the treatment of some malignancies is being considered lately. This concept is predicated on the belief that neoplasia originates from a block of cell differentiation which, if relieved, would result in a more differentiated or in a terminally differentiatied phenotype with the possible loss of malignant potential. As a concept for therapy this approach holds the further promise that induction of differentiation could increase the number of functional (differentiated) vs neoplastic (undifferentiated) cells, somehow remedying unbalanced pathological situations which certainly characterize some malignancies.

Interferons (IFNs), once identified for their antiviral activity, do indeed induce several additional effects such as inhibition of tumor cell growth, both in vitro and in vivo, modulation of various immunological properties including enhancement of natural killer cell activity, enhanced expression of histocompatibility antigens and of tumor associated antigens. Finally, indications that IFNs play a role in the process of cell differentiation originate from observations in many differentiating and differentiated cell systems (for an extensive review see 18). Whether differentiation is induced or inhibited may depend on the target cell.

The mechanisms by which IFNs induce their antitumor effect are not known. However, their ability to modulate cell differentiation and expression of oncogene(s) may play a role. Tumor cell populations differentiating upon exposure to IFNs may undergo a partial or complete suppression of their growth potential. In this respect a good example is provided by the observation of the strikingly favorable effect of IFN-alpha administration in patients with hairy cell leukemia (2, 13). In fact, IFN-alpha or -beta (but not -gamma) may act as differentiating agents on hairy cells that represent B lymphocyte precursors blocked at a pre-terminal stage of development. It appears that the cellular marker of these precursors in patients with hairy cell leukemia is their strict requirement for the continuous exposure to IFNs (14).

With respect to IFNs effects on the oncogene expression, it has been reported that IFNs may in certain cell systems selectively either induce or reduce the accumulation of some mRNAs. In particular IFNs reduce c-myc mRNA levels in Daudi Burkitt lymphoma cells (5, 9). The analysis of a Daudi variant line resistant to growth inhibition by IFNs and of several other resistant leukemic cell lines suggests a close link between the IFNs-mediated c-myc inhibition and the accompanying G_o/G_1 arrest of cells exposed to IFNs and exhibiting this effect (5). On the other hand, terminally differentiated cells such as HL60, U937 and Friend Erythroleukemia cells (FLC), that become arrested in the G_o/G_1 phase of the cell cycle, show a parallel sharp decline in the amount of c-myc mRNA (5). Recently, it has also been found that the constitutive expression of an exogenous c-myc is able to block DMSO-induced differentiation (4, 12).

Several FLC clones exhibiting resistance to one or more IFNs effects have been studied to define the molecular mechanism by which IFNs induce their differentiation-modulating and tumor growth-suppressing effects. This system appears amenable to genetically controlled analysis and dissociation of IFN effects, briefly summarized herebelow:

a)   the bell-shaped dose-response curve of IFN-alphabeta on FLC differentiation is due to opposite effects of IFN-alpha and IFN-beta.

It had been observed that doses of murine fibroblast IFN (a mixture of the alpha and beta species) below 500 U/ml enhance DMSO-induced differentiation of FLC whereas doses above 10,000 units consistently decrease it (3, 6, 15-17). Experiments with recently available recombinant mu-IFN-alpha$_1$ and -beta preparations indicate a more precise attribution of the reported effects to the different IFN species. In wild-type (w.t.) cells IFN-beta inhibits cellular growth but stimulates erythroid differentiation. FLC variants that are either alpha,beta-resistant (α, β-R) or alpha,beta,gamma-resistant (α, β, γ-R) are unresponsive to both the inhibitory effect on cell growth and the stimulatory effect on erythroid differentiation of IFN-beta. In w.t. cells treated with dimethylsulfoxide (DMSO) differentiation is not enhanced by exposure to low doses of mu-IFN-α_1, whereas is inhibited upon exposure to >1,000 U/ml of this IFN species. This is even more pronounced in cells of both resistant clo-

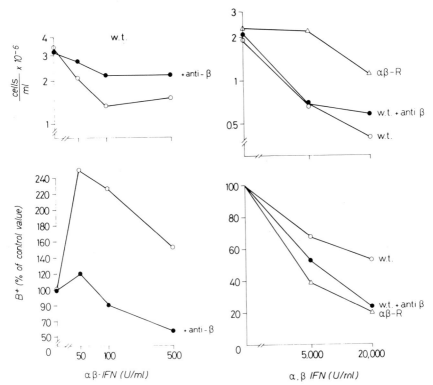

Fig.1 —   Neutralization of the effects of low (left) and high
(right) doses of murine fibroblast IFN on growth and
differentiation of DMSO-treated wt (○–○) and α, β-R
(△–△) FLC by preincubation with anti-IFN-beta monoclonal antibodies generous gift of Drs Y. Watanabe and Y.
Kawade, Kyoto University, Japan. Briefly, IFN and the
neutralizing monoclonal antibody were incubated overnight at +4°C in 50 μl of RPMI 1640 supplemented with
5% foetal calf serum (ratio between neutralizing units
and IFN units: 2). A 96-well microtiter plate, washed
once with supplemented culture medium, was used. Then
each well was added with 25 ul of DMSO (4x the concentration used in supplemented culture medium) and 25 μl
of a cell suspension at 4×10^5 cells/ml. Cultures were
grown for three days, then cells were counted and the
percentage of benzidine-positive (B^+) cells evaluated
according to the wet benzidine staining method (11).
Cell mortality, evaluated by the trypan blue dye exclusion method, never exceeded 2%. Each condition was
performed in duplicate. Fibroblast IFN: Sp. act. 3×10^7
IU/mg protein. Anti-mouse IFN-beta (7F.D3) purified
IgG, 4,4 A_{280} units/ml PBS. 10 U/ml of L cell fibroblast IFN were neutralized up to an antibody dilution
of $1:4\times10^5$. Empty symbols: without monoclonal antibodies; full symbols: with monoclonal antibodies. 100%
values of B+ cells: left panel, 0,6% DMSO 21 (○), 22
(●); right panel, 1,5% DMSO 68 (○), 65 (●), 60 (△).

nes, as observed previously with fibroblast IFN preparations
(1), where the inhibition of differentiation is not accompanied by any significant inhibition of cellular growth. In
FLC exposed to fibroblast IFN preparation the inhibitory
effect of the less abundant alpha type is obviously oversha-
dowed by the simultaneous presence of a majority of IFN-beta
molecules exerting the opposite effect. We show in fact
that when fibroblast IFN is incubated with excess amounts of
a monoclonal antibody neutralizing IFN-beta (Fig. 1, left)
FLC differentiation is obviously not enhanced; in fact, when
high dosages of fibroblast IFN are employed, differentiation
is inhibited by the exposure to the non neutralized IFN-alpha species (Fig. 1, right). The reverse experiment, i.e.
incubation of fibroblast IFN with a monoclonal antibody neutralizing one IFN-alpha subspecies, yields less satisfactory
results because the antibodies may not neutralize all the
other IFN-alpha subspecies.

b) Effects of different IFN species on FLC commitment to terminal differentiation.

Full FLC commitment to terminal differentiation (i.e.
all progeny cells are hemoglobinized) is known to occurs
14-20 hrs after cell seeding in the presence of DMSO as no
further commitment takes place later (8,10). We investigated
whether the opposite effects of IFN-alpha$_1$ and IFN-beta on
differentiation are mediated by different pathways influenc-
ing the commitment event. Cells were treated with DMSO plus
either recombinant IFN-alpha$_1$ or IFN-beta, were then washed
out of all compounds and plated in soft-agar. Differentiation was evaluated by scoring colonies stained with Benzidine after three days of culture. Colonies were scored as
blue if all the cells are stained, white if none of the
cells are stained, and mixed if only some of the cells are
stained. Hence, white colonies represent the progeny of
fully uncommitted progenitor cells, blue colonies that of
fully committed cells, and mixed colonies represent the progeny of progenitor cells partially committed at plating time
(8). Treatment with IFN-beta does not modify the percentage
of committed (mixed + blue colonies) vs uncommitted (white
colonies) precursor cells. It merely accelerates the rate of
full hemoglobinization (relative ratio of blue vs mixed colo
nies) as blue colonies are more numerous than in DMSO-treated cells. Conversely, treatment with IFN-alpha$_1$ blocks commitment as it markedly increases the percentage of white
colonies vs that of blue+mixed colonies (submitted for publi
cation). It may be concluded that the mechanisms underlying
the stimulatory (IFN-beta) vs the inhibitory (IFN-alpha)
effect on FLC differentiation are different.

c) Modulation of FLC tumorigenity by treatment with IFN-alpha-
beta.

FLC retain malignancy: they are able to induce subcutaneous tumors (reticular cell sarcoma) by subcutaneous in-

jection or ascitic tumors when injected intraperitoneally in syngeneic mice. In vitro DMSO treatment of FLC causes cessation of cell proliferation (after 4-5 days) and terminal differentiation. When Friend cells are injected in DBA/2 mice after in vitro DMSO treatment, a 2-log reduction of TCID$_{50}$ is observed (7). Parenthetically, DMSO administration to mice injected with FLC does not give the same result as it simultaneously induces a wave of production of Friend virus that will in turn induce the typical leukemic picture. On the other hand, when FLC are treated with DMSO and high doses of fibroblast IFN, the observed 2-log TCID$_{50}$ reduction does not take place. In the opposite experiment, i.e. DBA/2 mice given FLC treated in vitro with DMSO and low doses of fibroblast IFN, mice were observed for three months during which time the size of the developing tumor and the ensuing mortality were assessed to evaluate the possible reduction of tumorigenity due to the stimulatory effect of differentiation of IFN-beta. The data of a large, but still preliminary experiment do not convincingly point to a protective effect of IFN-beta with respect to the tumorigenicity of FLC pre-exposed in vitro to subliminal doses of DMSO and to low doses of IFN-beta. This appears to be consistent with the previous results discussed with respect to the effects of IFN-alpha-beta on the commitment decision of FLC to undergo terminal differentiation. In fact, we have reported that FLC exposure to low doses of fibroblast IFN merely accelerates the process of full hemoglobinization of DMSO-treated FLC but does not modify the percentage of committed cells.

d) c-myc expression during IFN modulation of FLC growth and differentiation.

We have investigated by Northern blot analysis the effects of fibroblast IFN administered at low doses on c-myc expression in the FLC. Briefly:

- mu fibroblast IFN causes a significant but rather transient reduction of c-myc mRNA levels while not affecting those of Galactose Phosphodehydrogenase mRNA (Fig. 2, upper panel). This treatment does not induce any evident increase of B$^+$ cells.

- low doses (0.5%) of DMSO induce a moderate level of FLC differentiation (20% of B$^+$ cells after 4 days of culture) and cause a transient depletion of c-myc RNA level. The addition of fibroblast IFN (low doses) does not result in any dramatic changes of c-myc mRNA expression while it potentiates DMSO-induced differentiation (up to 48% of B$^+$ cells). When looking carefully to the figure, (2-hr time point), however, IFN appears to somehow expand DMSO-induced down-regulation of c-myc expression (Fig. 2, lower panel).

Once again, this is not inconsistent with previous data indicating that a sustained depletion of c-myc mRNA expression is required for efficient FLC differentiation.

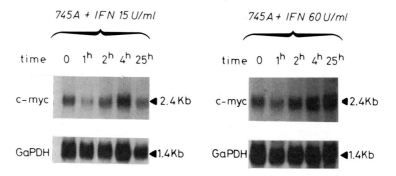

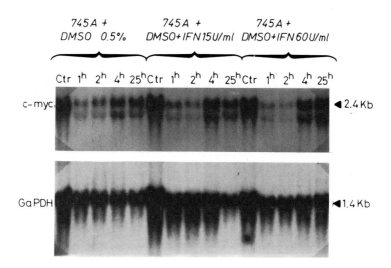

Fig.2.   Blot hybridization analysis of RNA from wt FLC treated
or not with DMSO and the indicated doses of fibroblast
IFN. Cells seeded at 10^5/ml were treated with or
without the indicated doses of DMSO and fibroblast IFN.
At different times cells were collected and RNA extracted by the guanidine/cesium chloride method. 30 μg of
RNA was run on denaturing 1,2% agarose gel containing
formaldehyde, transferred onto nylon filter and hybridized to the nick-translated murine c-myc cDNA (19).
Hybridization with rat GaPDH cDNA was also performed.

ACKNOWLEDGEMENTS

This work was supported in part by grants from Consiglio Nazionale delle Ricerche, Rome, Italy, Progetti Finalizzati "Oncologia" No. 87.01151.44 and No. 86.02683.44, and from the Associazione Italiana per la Ricerca contro il Cancro, Milan, Italy. The skillful secretarial assistance of Ms. L. Leone and Mr. G. Caricati is gratefully acknowledged.

REFERENCES

1. Affabris, E., Jemma, C., and Rossi, G.B. (1982): Virology, 120:441-452.

2. Bottomley, J.M., Cawley, J.C., Catovsky, D., Bevan, P.C., Worman, P.C., Nethershell, A.B.W., and Finter, N.B. (1985): In: The interferon System, edited by F. Dianzani and G.B. Rossi, vol. 24, Raven Press.

3. Cioè, L., Dolei, A., Rossi, G.B., Belardelli, F., Affabris, E., Gambari, E., and Fantoni, A. (1978): In: In vitro Aspects of erythropoiesis, edited by M. Murphi, pp. 159-171, Springer Verlag, Heidelberg.

4. Coppola, J.A., and Cole, M.D. (1986): Nature, 320:760-763.

5. Einat, M., Resnitzky, D., and Kimchi, A. (1985): Nature, 313:597-600.

6. Dolei, A., Colletta, G., Capobianchi, M.R., Rossi, G.B., and Vecchio, G. (1980): J. Gen. Virol., 46:227-236.

7. Friend, C., Scher, W., Holland, J.C., et al. (1971): PNAS USA, 68:378-382.

8. Gusella, J., Geller, R., Clarke, B., Weecs, V., and Housman, D. (1976): Cell, 9:221-230.

9. Jonak, G.J., and Knight, E.J. (1984): Proc. Natl. Acad. Sci. USA, 81:1747-1750.

10. Marks, P.A., Sheffery, M., and Rifkind, R.A. (1987): Cancer Res., 47:659-666.

11. Orkin, S.M., Harosi, F., and Leder, P. (1975): Proc. Natl. Acad. Sci. USA, 72:98-102.

12. Prochownik, E.V., and Kukowska, J. (1986): Nature, 322:848-850.

13. Quesada, J.R., Reuben, J., Manning, J.T., Hersh, E.M., and Gutterman, J.U. (1984): New Eng. J. Med., 310-1:15-18.

14. Michaleviez, R., and Revel, M. (1987): Proc. Natl. Acad. Sci. USA, 84:2307-2311.

15. Rossi, G.B., Dolei, A., Cioé, L., Benedetto, A., Matarese, G., and Belardelli, F. (1977): Proc. Natl. Acad. Sci. USA, 74:1655-.....

16. Rossi, G.B., Dolei, A., Cioé, L., Benedetto, A., Matarese, G.P., F. Belardelli, and Rita, G. (1977): Tex. Rep. Biol. Med. 35:420-428.

17. Rossi, G.B., Matarese, G.B., Grappelli, C., Belardelli, F., and Benedetto, A. (1977): Nature, 267:50-52.

18. Rossi, G.B., Affabris, E., Romeo, G., Federico, M., and Coccia, E.M. (1987): In: The Interferon System: A current review to 1987, edited by S. Baron, F. Dianzani, G.J. Staton, and W.R. Fleischman, Jr., pp. 285-297, University of Texas Press, Austin.

19. Stanton, L.W., Farlander, P.D., Tesser, P.M., and Marcu, K.B. (1984): Nature, 319:423-425.

Direct Effects of IFN-α on the Malignant Cells in Hairy-Cell Leukemia

F. Sigaux[1], S. Castaigne[2], G. Flandrin[1] and L. Degos

*From the [1]Institut National de la Santé et de la Recherche Medicale U301
and Laboratoire Central d'Hématologie,
[2]Inserm U93 and Department d'Hématologie, Hopital Saint Louis, 75475 Paris,
Cedex 10*

INTRODUCTION

Hairy cell leukemia (HCL) is a rare chronic lymphoid neoplasm associated with splenomegaly, pancytopenia and an increased incidence of severe infections (10). As shown by studies of cell phenotype and gene rearrangements (1,19), this disease is a clonal proliferation of B cells arrested at a late stage of cell differentiation. In the past, splenectomy was the only treatment with proven efficacy (16). More recently, it was shown by a number of groups (6,18,22,23,25,29-31), including our own, that IFN-α is a highly effective therapy in most patients with HCL. While the efficacy of IFN-α is now well established, the mechanism of the therapeutic effect is currently poorly understood. In the present review, we summarize data which show that IFN-α is able to directly interact with hairy cells. We suggest that the efficacy of IFN-α is due to an inhibition of an autocrine proliferative loop.

IFN-α IS A HIGLY EFFECTIVE THERAPY IN HCL

A number of trials have shown that low dose continuous IFN-α therapy can induce remissions in the majority of HCL. During the first months of treatment, a decrease in circulating hairy cells (in most cases, disappearance) and granulocytes are usually observed in the peripheral blood. During the same period, the neoplastic infiltration of bone marrow decreases, while a rise in the volume of myeloid cells is usually found by stereological methods (11). Complete or partial remissions are observed in most patients after 7-12 months of therapy. In our experience based on 51 HCL patients, complete remission was observed in 23 cases and partial remission in 19. Treatments by Roferon A ® or Intron A ®   give similar results, with few patients failing to respond to this treatment.

In the search for the mechanism of the therapeutic effect, three clinical findings should be emphasized. First, in patients treated by IFN-α, the decrease of circulating hairy cells is often dramatic, leading, in a few weeks, to virtual disappearance of these neoplastic cells. Similary, splenomegaly if present, has usually resolved after the first month of treatment. The same pattern is observed in bone marrow, where the decrease in hairy cell infiltration starts before the increase in myeloid cells. This suggests that the decrease in the total number of neoplastic cells may induce a restoration of normal haematopoiesis and is consistent with recent data showing that either serum from hairy cell patients or supernatants of cultured hairy cells produce a clear inhibitory effect on the growth of haematopoietic precursors (20). It is thus probable that IFN-α primarily affects the hairy cell and not the myeloid cells. The second important clinical finding is the high frequency of relapses observed after cessation of therapy (26). Our experience is based on 44 patients with a median follow-up (from cessation of treatment) of either 18 months after 7 month therapy or 12 months after 12 month therapy. The actuarial probability of relapses at 18 months after cessation of treatment is 65%. Interestingly, re-treatment by IFN-α usually induces the same therapeutic effects. The last point worth noting is the probable inefficacy of IFN-γ in this disease.

IFN-α INTERACTS WITH HAIRY CELLS

Is IFN involved in indirect cytotoxicity?

IFN-α could act indirectly on hairy cells via a cytotoxic cell. So far, no studies analysing the generation of cytotoxic T cells have been published. This would be interesting as it has been shown that IFN-α is able to induce, both T-cell receptor alpha chain gene rearrangement and cytotoxicity in T-cell clones (7). Numerous studies have been performed on natural killer (NK) cell activity. IFN-α is a potent activator of natural killer (NK) cells. It is well established that the NK activity of blood is decreased in patients with hairy cell leukemia. Sequential studies of NK activity after INF-α therapy have demonstrated a return to normal function after a few months in some patients (27). It was thus necessary to demonstrated that NK cells can kill hairy cells. Negative results were obtained by two independant studies (14,28). Although it is possible that a low level of cytotoxicity would be missed in the standard ^{51}Cr release assay used in these experiments, these results do not support the view that the efficiency of IFN-α treatment in HCL is mediated by NK cells.

Direct effects on hairy cells

If IFN-α exerts a direct effect on hairy cells then these cells must express high affinity IFN-α receptors . It was demonstrated that puri fied peripheral blood hairy cells express IFN-α receptors but with a quite variable density (3,8). Moreover in vitro or in vivo treatment by IFN-α induces a down regulation of these receptors. In one of two patients resistant to therapy, no receptor was detected on the cell surface even after in vitro culture (4). All these data show that IFN-α may directly interact with hairy cells, in the majority of cases.

After binding to receptors IFN-α can induce many events, including 2'5' oligoadenylate (2-5 A) synthetase induction, enhanced MHC expression (2) and antiproliferative effects. 2-5 A synthetase is an enzyme which appears to be involved in many physiological mechanisms, including the control of cell division and differentiation. In vivo treatment by IFN-α induces a 2 to 7 fold stimulation of 2-5 A synthetase activity in the hairy cells of most patients with similar kinetics to that observed for the IFN-α receptor down regulation (5,9). It does not however affect the 2-5 A synthetase activity of resistant receptor negative hairy cells. In addition, IFN-γ, which is ineffective in HCL, is unable to enhance the 2-5 A synthetase activity despite the presence of specific receptors.

Numerous oncogenes are involved in cell proliferation and differentiation. The c-myc proto-oncogene is one of the members of a family of genes composed of c-myc, n-myc and l-myc which are assumed to play a crucial role in the control of cell proliferation. On the other hand, the c-fos proto-oncogene encodes a protein whose expression seems to be largely restricted to differentiated cells. We have therefore studied the effects of IFN-α on oncogene transcription in HCL. Seven patients, including two cases resistant to the treatment, were studied by Northern analysis and probes recognizing v-fos and c-myc oncogenes (21). C-myc transcripts were only detectable (using total RNA) in the cells from the two resistant cases. This transcription was not modified by IFN-α therapy. In constrast, c-fos transcripts were detected in all patients and in-vivo treatement by IFN-α was able to modulate this transcription. Although the significance of these findings remain unclear, it is possible that the modulation of c-fos oncogene transcription might indicate an alteration of the differentiation status of hairy-cells.

B cell growth factor (BCGF) has recently been shown to induce in vitro proliferation of hairy cells (12). To further investigate the interaction between IFN-α and hairy cells proliferation, the effects of IFN-α on the proliferative response of hairy cells to human BCGF were investigated. In vitro treatment of hairy cells with 1000 IU IFN-α, but not IFN-γ, resulted in an inhibition of this response (24). Since in-vivo treatment (around $3\ 10^6$ IU/day) induces lower serum concentration of IFN-α, it was necessary to analyse the effects of in vivo treatment and to compare those with the results obtained in vitro using low IFN concentrations. It was observed (15) that a marked inhibition of the BCGF-dependant proliferation, was obtained with concentrations of 100 IU/ml similar to those obtained after in vivo treatment. Similar results were observed using IFN-β but not IFN-γ. Moreover, it was shown that a single dose of $3\ 10^6$ IU was able within 6-12 hr after administration to induce the same effects.

It is known that extracts from Ebstein Barr virus transformed B cells, as well as B cell tumours or activated B cells contain a BCGF-like activity. Moreover, cytosolic extracts of hairy cells also contain a factor similar to the high molecular weight precursor form of the BCGF produced by T cells. This factor acts as an autostimulary factor on hairy cells (13). It might be hypothesized that IFN-α exerts its action on HCL through inhibition of an autocrine loop involving a BCGF-like molecule (15). The steps involved in this process might be inhibition of BCGF receptor expression on hairy cells or impairment of transduction both resulting for example from cell differentiation. Work is in progress to analyse the involvement of some molecules such as CD23 which may serve as the receptor for low molecular weight BCGF (17).

REFERENCES

1. ANDERSON, K., BOYD, A.W., FISHER, D.C., LESLIE, D., SCHLOSSMAN, S.F. and NADLER, L. (1985) Hairy cell leukemia: a tumor of pre-plasma cells. Blood, **65**, 620-629

2. BALDINI, L., CORTELEZZI, A., POLLI, N., NENI, A., NOBILI, L., MAIOLO, A.T., LAMBERTENGHI-DELILIERS, G. and POLLI, E.E. (1986) Human recombinant interferon alpha-2-C enhances the expression of classe II HLA antigens on hairy cells. Blood, **67**, 458-464

3. BILLARD, C., SIGAUX, F., CASTAIGNE, S., VALENSI, F., FLANDRIN, G., DEGOS, L., FALCOFF, E. and AGUET, M. (1986) Treatment of hairy cell leukemia with recombinant alpha interferon. II. In vivo down regulation of alpha interferon receptors on tumor cells. Blood, **67**, 821-826

4. BILLARD, C., FALCOFF, E., SIGAUX, F., CASTAIGNE, S., FLANDRIN, G., DEGOS, L., FERBUS, D. and AGUET, M. (1987) Absence of interferon alpha receptor on hairy cells from a patient resistant to interferon-alpha therapy. Cancer J., **1**, 231-232

5. BILLARD, C., FERBUS, D., SIGAUX, F., CASTAIGNE, S., FLANDRIN, G., DEGOS, L., FLANDRIN, G. and FALCOFF, E. Action of interferon alpha on hairy cell leukemia: expression of specific receptors and (2'-5') oligo (A) synthetase in tumor cells from sensitive and resistant patients. Leuk. Res. (in press)

6. CASTAIGNE, S., SIGAUX, F., CANTELL, K., FALCOFF, E., BOIRON, M., FLANDRIN, G. and DEGOS, L. (1986) Interferon alpha in the treatment of hairy cell leukemia. Cancer, **57**, 1681-1684

7. CHEN, L.K., MATHIEU-MAHUL, D., SASPORTES, M., DEGOS, L. and BENSUSSAN, A. (1986) What is a T-cell clone ?: effect

of rIFN on T cell clone function and T-cell receptor gene rearrangement. Human Immunol., **17**, 214-223

8. FALTYNEK, C.R., PRINCLER, G.L., ROSSIO, J.L., RUSCETTI, F.N., MALUISH, A.E., ABRAMS, P.G., and FOON, K.A. (1986) Relationship of the clinical response and binding of recombinant interferon alpha in patients with lymphoproliferative diseases. Blood, **67**, 1077-1082

9. FERBUS, D., BILLARD, C., SIGAUX, F., THANG, and FALCOFF, E. (1987) In vivo and in vitro induction of (2'-5') oligoadenylate synthetase by human interferons in leukocytes from heathly donors and patients with renal cancer and hairy cell leukemia. J. Biol. Reg. Homeo. Ag., **1**, 9-15

10. FLANDRIN, G., SIGAUX, F., SEBAHOUN, G. and BOUFFETTE, P. (1984) Hairy cell leukemia: clinical presentation and follow-up of 211 patients. Semin Oncol, **11**, 458-471

11. FLANDRIN, G., SIGAUX, F., CASTAIGNE, S., BILLARD, C., AGUET, M., BOIRON, M. FALCOFF, E. and DEGOS, L. (1986) Treatment of hairy cell leukemia with recombinant alpha interferon. I. Quantitative study of bone marrow changes during the first months of treatment. Blood, **67**, 817-820

12. FORD, R., YOSHIMURA, J., MORGAN, J., QUESADA, R., MONTANA, A.D., and MAIZEL, A.L. (1985). Growth factor mediated tumor cell proliferation in hairy cell leukemia. J. Exp. Med., **162**, 1093-1098

13. FORD, R., KWOK, D., QUESADA, J. and SAHASRABUDDHE, C.G. (1986) Production of B cell growth factor(s) by neoplastic B cells from hairy cell leukemia patients. Blood, **67**, 573-577

14. GASTL, G., AULITZKY, W., LEITER, E., FLENER, R., and HUBER, C. (1986) Alpha interferon induces remission in hairy cell leukemia without enhancement of natural killing. Blut, **52**, 273-277

15. GENOT, E., BILLARD, C., MATHIOT, C., FALCOFF, E., SIGAUX, F., and KOLB, J.P. (1987) Proliferative response of hairy cells to B cell growth factor (BCGF): in vivo inhibition by interferon-α and in vitro effects of interféron-α, -β, and -γ. Leukemia, 1, 590-596

16. GOLOMB, H.M. and VARDIMAN, J. (1983) Response to splenectomy in sixty five patients with hairy cell leukemia: an evaluation of spleen weight and bone marrow involvement. Blood, 61, 349-352

17. GORDON, J., WEBB, A.J., WALKER, L., GUY, G.R., and ROWE, M. (1986) Evidence for an association between CD23 and the receptor for a low molecular weight B cell growth factor. Eur. J. Immunol., 16, 1627-1630

18. JACOBS, A.D., CHANILIN, R.E., and GOLDE, D.W. (1985). Recombinant alpha-2 interferon for hairy cell leukemia. Blood, 65, 1017-1020

19. KORSMEYER, F.J., GREENE, W.C., COSSMAN, J., HSU, S.M., NECKERS, L., DEPPER, J.M., LEONARD, W.J., JAFFE, E.S.,AND WALDMANN, T.A. (1983). Rearrangement and expression of immunoglobulin genes and expression of Tac antigen in hary cell leukemia. Proc. Natl. Acad. Sci. USA., 80, 4522-4526

20. LAURIA, F., GUARINI, A., BAGNARA, G.P., CATANI, L., GAGGIOLI, L, GUGLIOTTA, L., RASPADORI, D., BUZZI, M., ZAULI, G., and TURA, S. (1987) Inhibitory effect of hairy cell leukemia (HCL) serum on the "in vitro" growth of haematopoietic precursors. 4th Intern. Symposium on Therapy of acute Leu. Rome 7-12 Feb. 1987, 264a

21. LEHN, P., SIGAUX, F., GRAUSZ, D., LOISEAU, P., CASTAIGNE, S., DEGOS, L., FLANDRIN, G. and DAUTRY, F. (1987) C-myc and c-fos expression during interferon-alpha therapy for hairy cell leukemia. Blood, 68, 967-970

22. QUESADA, J.R., REUBEN, J., MANNING, J.T., HERSH, E.M. and GUTTERMAN, (1984) J. Alpha interferon for induction of

remission in hairy cell leukemia. N. Eng. J. Med., **310**, 15-18

23. QUESADA, J.R., GUTTERMAN, J.U., and HIRSH, E.M. (1987) Treatment of hairy cell leukemia with alpha interferon. Cancer, **57**, 1678-1688

24. PAGANELLI, K.A, EVANS, S.S., HAN, T. and OZER, H. (1986) B cell growth factor induced proliferation of hairy cell lymphocytes and inhibition by type I interferon in vitro. Blood, **67**, 937-942

25. RATAIN, M.J., GOLOMB, H.M., VARDIMAN, J.W., VOKES, E.E., JACOBS, R.H., and DALY, K. (1985) Treatment of hairy cell leukemia with recombinant alpha-2 interferon. Blood, **65**, 644-648

26. RATAIN, M.J., GOLOMB, H.M., BARDAWIE, R.G., VARDIMAN, J.W., WESTHROOK, C.A., KAMINER, L.S., LEMBERSKY, B.C., BITTER, M.A., and DALY, K. (1987) Durability of responses to interferon alpha-2b in advanced hairy cell leukemia. Blood, **69**, 872-877

27. SEMENZATO, G., PIZZOLO, G., AGOSTINI, A., AMBROSETTI, R., ZAMBELLO, L., TRENTIN, M., LUCA, M., MASCIARELLI, M., CHILOSI, M., VIVANTE, F., PERONA, G. and CETTO, G.(1986) Alpha interferon activates the natural killer system in patients with hairy cell leukemia. Blood, **68**, 293-296

28. SIGAUX, F., CHAPUIS, F., CASTAIGNE, S., DEGOS, L., FLANDRIN, G. and GLUCKMAN, J.P. (1987) hairy cells are not lysed by NK cells. Blut, **54**, 319-320

29. THOMSON, J.A., BRADY, J., KIDD, P., and FEFER, A. (1985) Recombinant alpha-2 interferon in the treatment of hairy cell leukemia. Cancer Treat. Rep. , **69**, 791-793

30. THOMSON, J.A., and FEFER, A. (1987) Interferon in the treatment of hairy cell leukemia. Cancer, **59**, 605-609

31. WORMAN, C.P., CATOVSKY, D., BEVAN, P.C., CAMBA, J., JOYNER, M., GREEN, P.J., WILLIAMS, H.J.H., BOTTOMLEY, J.M., GORDON-SMITH, E.C., and CAWLEY, J.C. (1985) Interferon is effective in hairy cell leukemia. Br. J. Haemat., **60**, 759-763

GROWTH FACTORS
AND DIFFERENTIATION THERAPY

The Role of Hematopoietic Growth Factors in Normal and Leukemic Cell Differentiation

M.A.S. Moore and T.M. Dexter*

*Laboratory of Developmental Hematopoiesis, Memorial Sloan
Kettering Cancer Center, NY 10021;
*Department of Experimental Haematology, Paterson Institute for Cancer Research,
Christie Hospital, Manchester*

INTRODUCTION

The extent of proliferative activity required to maintain circulating myeloid cells at their normal levels can be gauged from the finding that about 3.7×10^{11} cells need to be produced each day of adult life. Occasional mistakes are made during replication, resulting in the emergence of leukemic cells. What is surprising, is that leukemias occur so infrequently: obviously many controls are built into the system to maintain its integrity. These controls are both intrinsic to the cells ('genetic house-keeping') and extrinsic in the form of environ-ental influences.

These external influences are many and diverse, encompassing interactions of developing hemato-poietic cells with extracellular matrix molecules, with a variety of stromal cell types and with growth factors. The area of hematopoietic growth factor (HGF) research has expanded dramatically in the last 2-3 years with the availability of recombinant materials in quantities allowing direct in vivo testing in both pre-clinical and clinical systems. HGFs, variously characterized as colony stimulating factors (CSF's) and Interleukins (IL's), comprise a family of glycosylated polypeptides with biological specificity defined by their ability to support proliferation and differentiation of hematopoietic cells of various lineages, usually in a semi-solid clonal assay system. The biological specificities of

activation of mature end cells. The original family
of CSF's comprised CSF-1 (M-CSF), with macrophage
specificity, G-CSF with neutrophil granulocyte
specificity and GM-CSF with capacity to induce
differentiation in both lineages, (and in human
marrow culture the additional capacity to stimulate,
eosinophil megakaryocyte and erythroid,
progenitors). Interleukin-3 (Multi-CSF) is capable
of stimulating proliferation of all classes of
myeloid progenitors including a subset of pluripotential stem cells at one extreme, and highly
differentiated mast cells at another (for review see
3,10,14). Four additional lymphokines with highly
specialized functions are now considered part of the
family of HGFs. IL-4 is a lymphokine that is
intimately involved in the allergic response,
stimulating mast cell growth and differentiation
acting synergistically with IL-3, promoting B cell
proliferation, Ig secretion and inducing IgE
receptors and also acting as a T cell growth factor
(8). IL-5, formerly known as eosinophil
differentiating factor or BCGF-II is a lymphokine
functioning as a CSF for eosinophil-restricted
progenitors and as a functional activator of the
mature eosinophil (20). In additon it is a growth
factor for preactivated B cell and is a T-cell
replacing factor in certain antibody responses. IL-6
has interferon-like activity (IFN Beta 2) and is a B
cell growth and differentiation factor (30) and a
recently reported Pre-B cell growth factor is under
preliminary consideration as IL-7.

    The CSF's and Interleukins are heavily N-
glycosylated, or in the case of G-CSF, O-glycosylated
in their secreted state, although all are active in
vitro in a non-glycosylated form. In every case,
both murine and human gene products are available
which is important in the case of factors whose
action is species restricted (IL-3, IL-4, GM-CSF).
No significant sequence homology exists between the
different factors (with the exception of G-CSF and
IL-6) arguing against their evolution from a common
primordial gene. Between species, considerable con-
servation is seen at the nucleotide and amino acid
level with amino acid homologies between mouse and
man of 70-80% for G-CSF, CSF-1 and IL-5, 50-55% for
GM-CSF and IL-4 and 29% for IL-3. With the exception
of CSF-1 which is a dimeric structure with identical
14,500Mr subunits, the factors are comprised of
single polypeptide chains of 120-178 amino acids.
Recent chromosomal localization studies have

identified single copy genes for M-CSF, GM-CSF and IL-3 clustered on the distal portion of the long arm of human chromosome 5 at a site frequently involved in deletions or translocations associated with myeloid leukemia and myelodysplastic syndromes. The G-CSF gene is on chromosome 17 near a site involved in translocations associated with acute promyelocytic leukemia. Differentiation or lineage commitment has been explained by several models ranging from a purely stochastic to a deterministic hematopoietic inductive microenvironment. It is likely that the actual situation is a compromise between these hypotheses with stochastic events occurring with a probability that can be modulated by external growth factors.

Hematopoietic cell development in association with marrow stromal cells occurs only if the developing hematopoietic cells and the stroma are in intimate cell contact. It has also been shown that the marrow stroma contains phenotypically diverse cell types and that distinctive interactions occur between, e.g. developing granulocytes and stromal cells undergoing lipid accumulation, and between developing erythroid cells and macrophages (1). It is unlikely that these associations are trivial; rather, they are almost certainly important at the mechanistic level of cell development.

A clue to the processes involved in stromal cell-hematopoietic cell interaction has emerged from two recent observations. First, using purified (FACS-enriched) multipotential cells (CFU-S) it was shown that marrow stromal cells in vitro do not secrete growth or developmental factors to which the multipotential cells could respond in soft-gel assays in vitro, but if the population enriched for CFU-S was allowed to attach to the stroma the cells underwent proliferation and development to produce mature myeloid cells (24). A similar result was found with some IL-3-dependent multipotential stem cell lines (24,19). Other IL-3-dependent cell lines, however, were unable to attach to the marrow stroma and they rapidly died in the absence of added growth factor. Thus it was concluded that the attachment per se was a critical event in the subsequent response of the stem cells to whatever is the 'growth factor' that is being produced by the stromal cells. Furthermore, the inability to detect the growth factor as secreted material implies that it must be bound to the surface of the stromal cells and is effective only when the stroma and stem cells are in intimate contact. Perhaps more significantly, it was shown that stem cells could attach to metabolically dead stromal cells (fixed in glutaraldehyde) and proliferate and develop into mature progeny, i.e. sufficient amounts of growth promoter were present on the surface of the stromal cells to facilitate proliferation and development of the stem cells (19).

What is the nature of this stromal cell-associated growth promoter? A recent observation offers a possible explanation. It has been thought for some time that molecules of the extracellular matrix may play an important cell/tissue-specific role in development. It has now been shown that an extracellular matrix, which incorporates glycosaminoglycans, can bind growth factors such as GM-CSF and present these growth factors to the appropriate hematopoietic target cells (6). It has also been shown that hematopoiesis can be modulated by agents that interfere with proteoglycan synthesis (3,24), and that the different types of marrow stromal cells show major differences in their expression of the various extracellular matrix components. It is possible that the various 'hematopoietic microenvironments' represent complexes of stromal cell/extracellular matrix molecules/growth factors. To what extent these growth factors are produced by the stromal cells or merely sequestered from circulating molecules has not yet been determined. Nonetheless, this represents a reasonable working model for investigating developmental processes at the mechanistic level.

CLINICAL UTILIZATION OF RECOMBINANT HEMATOPOIETIC GROWTH FACTORS

HGFs, including G, GM, M-CSFs and Interleukin-3 have potent effects on stimulating recovery of bone marrow following intensive chemotherapy or irradiation (11,12,13). The stimulation of production of differentiated hematopoietic cells following growth factor therapy is paralleled by augmented regeneration of early bone marrow stem cells and committed progenitor cells. Preclinical evaluation of HGFs has indicated that combination biotherapy using CSFs and Interleukins is more efficacious than single agent treatment in stimulating recovery of normal immunohematopoiesis.

It has been demonstrated that IL-1 synergistically interacted both in vitro and in vivo in potentiating the action of G-, GM-CSF and IL-3 and IL-5 (11,12,13,14,27). IL-1 possesses the ability to stimulate primitive pluripotent stem cells to express receptors for other hematopoietic growth factors and at the same time is able to induce growth factor production by a direct action on T cells, endothelial cells and bone marrow stromal fibroblasts (9,22). A phase I-II clinical trial has been completed using G-CSF to counteract the myelosuppression associated with a high-dose chemotherapy regimen in patients with bladder cancer (9,22). The results of this trial point to the relative non-toxicity of this growth factor and indicate a future role in combatting significant side effects of conventional chemotherapy and irradiation therapy. Preclinical studies in murine and primate autologous and allogenic bone marrow transplantation point to a potential application of these growth factors in stimulating hematopoietic reconstitution in humans in similar transplant situations (5).

CSF DEPENDENCE OF MYELOID LEUKEMIC PROGENITOR CELLS

The early in vitro studies indicated that leukemic cells from patients with AML, CML or pre-leukemic states were absolutely dependent upon a source of stimulatory factors for their clonal proliferation in culture at low plating densities. As with normal progenitor assays "spontaneous" leukemic cloning is observed as the marrow cell or peripheral blood leukocyte plating density is increased. This may be due to endogenous production of CSF's by accessory populations which may be residual normal cells of T cell lineage or leukemic cell sub-populations.

The autocrine concept of malignant transformation proposes that cells become malignant by the endogenous production of polypeptide growth factors that act upon their producer cells via functional external receptors. Support for the concept has been obtained by studies on oncogene action since oncogenes may confer growth factor autonomy on cancer cells by coding directly for autocrine polypeptide growth factors or their receptors, or by amplifying the mitogenic signals generated as a consequence of growth-factor-receptor interaction.

Normal hematopoiesis is most generally considered to be regulated by a paracrine mechanism whereby cells within the responding tissue produce growth factors acting locally on adjacent hemato-poietic targets. More classic endocrine mechanisms have been shown in the case of erythropoietin action, but even here, paracrine mechanisms may operate. Autocrine-type mechanisms have been implicated in the case of macrophages where the mature macrophage is responsive to stimulatory growth factors that it, itself can produce (such as CSF-1), as well as inhibitory factors such as prostaglandin E. In contrast to neoplastic cell populations, autocrine control of hematopoiesis is tightly regulated by a balance between stimulating and inhibiting factors which may become uncoupled following leukemic transformation. In this context, growth factor production in a system such as granulocyte-macrophage regulation involves inducibility for factor produc-tion by exogenous agents such as endotoxin, whereas in many leukemic situations, growth factor production is both autonomous and constitutive. The possible phenotypes in leukemia range from autonomy with factor production still inducible; to constitutive but factor dependent; to fully autonomous with pro-liferation in the absence of detectable exogenous growth factor, and where investigated, absence of growth factor gene activation and mRNA production. This latter state is more frequently achieved after prolonged in vitro selection and culture adaption of leukemic cell lines and is rarely a phenotypic manifestation of the natural evolution of leukemia in vivo. Support for the autocrine model has been developed by studies of myeloid leukemia in a number of species.

Strong evidence for an autocrine role for GM-CSF has been provided in a study of 22 cases of primary human acute myeloid leukemia in which Northern blot analysis revealed expression of the GM-CSF gene in 11 cases (32). GM-CSF expression was not found in normal hematopoietic tissue with the exception of activated T cells, strongly indicating that the GM-CSF gene activation was intimately associated with the transformation event. Furthermore, in 6 cases, GM-CSF was secreted by leukemic cells of both early and late stages of differentiation, and activity was specifically neutralized by antiserum to GM-CSF. The paradox of CSF-dependence of primary human myeloid leukemias in clonal assay, and autocrine production of GM-CSF can be answered in part by the concentra-

tion at which the cells are plated. At high concentration "spontaneous" leukemic colony or cluster
formation is the norm. In the study of Young et al
(32) 9/22 cases showed autonomous growth of leukemic
clusters when cells were plated at 5×10^4 per ml yet
exogeneous GM-CSF increased cloning number and clone
size in 15/22 cases. It is possible that in some
cases, GM-CSF is not actually secreted by the
leukemic cells but is present in active form as a
membrane-bound moiety. In this regard, Nara and
McCulloch (15) showed purified cell membranes from
cells of some AML patients, but not normal bone
marrow, or ALL cells could promote proliferation of
AML cells in short term suspension culture, enhancing
self-renewal. A direct link between constitutive GM-
CSF expression and leukemic transformation was
provided by Lang et al (7) who transfected the murine
GM-CSF gene into CSF-dependent, non-leukemic myeloid
cell lines and produced leukemic cell lines that
constitutively secreted GM-CSF. To date, no example
of human myeloid leukemia constitutively producing
and responding to IL-3 has been reported but in the
mouse system, the well characterized spontaneous
murine myelomonocytic leukemia WEHI-3 constitutively
secretes IL-3, apparently due to insertion of retroviral sequences adjacent to the IL-3 gene.

Inappropriate production of CSF can not be the
only mechanism leading to transformation since the
normal action of CSF is to sustain proliferation
leading to terminal differentiation. Thus, uncoupl-
ing of the proliferative from the differentiative
action of CSF must accompany the transformation
event. Some insight into this is provided by the NFS
60 murine cell line which was derived from a primary
retrovirus induced myeloid leukemia. These leukemic
cells are IL-3 dependent, and also proliferate in
response to G-CSF but fail to differentiate. The
line is characterized by a rearranged c-myb locus
associated with production of truncated RNA and the
introduction of a terminator condon at the junction
of the long terminal repeat and the c-myb locus
(23). Clearly this rearrangement is not associated
with abrogation of factor-dependence, in contrast to
the action of myc and abl which abrogate IL-3 requirements. This intriguing observation suggests
that the myb protooncogene may be intimately involved
in factor-dependent myeloid differentiation and the
truncated c-myb gene product may transmit proliferative signals induced by G-CSF and IL-3 but
uncouple these from the granulocyte differentiation

program.

Therapeutic strategy in the face of GM-CSF or IL-3-dependent leukemogenesis, either autocrine or paracrine, would require intervention to block CSF production or action. High affinity antibodies to the factor or its receptor, in the latter case coupled to some form of toxin, may be one possible strategy which is under active consideration as a therapy in the case of IL-2 dependent T cell lymphoma (anti-IL-2 receptor antibody and IL-2 toxin conjugates). A second strategy envisages the use of GM-CSF to recruit resting leukemic stem cells into cell cycle and synchronize the population in S phase in conjunction with cycle specific chemotherapy.

CSF INDUCTION OF LEUKEMIA CELL DIFFERENTIATION

The original characterization of mouse G-CSF (16) as a hematopoietic growth factor distinct from other CSF species and the purification and cloning of the human homolog (29,17) was facilitated by its unique ability to induce differentiation of the murine myelomonocytic leukemic cell line WEHI-3 and the HL-60 leukemia. In both instances G-CSF induced neutrophil differentiation together with macrophage. This was quantitated in suspension culture of the cell lines where 4-6 days was required to obtain maximum maturation, or was measured in clonal assay where differentiation was associated with conversion of compact undifferentiated leukemic colonies to diffuse, differentiated. HL-60 cells required approximately 5 times more G-CSF than did WEHI-3 cells for comparable effect and morphological and cytochemical analysis of the colonies revealed that up to 75% were induced to contain significant numbers (10%) of polymorphonuclear neutrophils and there was increased intensity of alphanapthyl acetate esterase staining (17,18). Many endogenous cytokines and lymphokines appear capable of inducing both neutrophil and monocytoid maturation changes in HL-60 cells and of mature monocyte and macrophage functional features in the U937 monocytic leukemic cell line. Since functional neutrophil and macrophage maturation involves changes in lysosomal enzyme activity, in cytoskeletal protein, glycolipid profiles and altered expression of cell surface receptors in a coordinated, temporal sequence, no single criterion of differentiation can establish the exact developmental state of induced cells. For this reason, we elected to characterize HL-60 and U937 leukemic cell differentiation, using a panel of markers characteristic of mature granulocytes and macrophages and applied to leukemic cells cultured for 2-6 days in simple suspension culture in the presence of G-CSF sources of cytokine/lymphokine differentiation inducers (17,18). G-CSF is also a potent inducer of macrophage differentiation of the murine MI myeloid leukemic cell lines with 1/2 maximum response as measured by induced phagocytic activity and lysozyme secretion induced with 10ng/ml hG-CSF (25). MI cells when synchronized in early G_1 by density inhibition in the absence of serum, when stimulated by G-CSF showed enhanced expression of FcR and lysozyme within 18 hrs. (26). Exponentially growing cells or cells arrested in late G_1 by addition of aphidicolin did not show enhanced expression of differentiation markers until 72 hrs. after addition of G-CSF. These observations suggest that the G_1 phase can be separated into an early permissive and a late non-permissive phase with respect to G-CSF induced differentiation.

    If differentiation-induction is to have therapeutic potential it is necessary to establish that it translates into extinction of the self renewal potential of the leukemic cells. In the case of WEHI-3, G-CSF suppression of clonogenic cells, as measured by decline in recloning capacity, usually requires 14-28 days because of the asynchronous nature of events influencing self-renewal versus differentiation. Eventually however, physiological concentrations of G-CSF in vitro extinguish leukemic self-renewal and upon subsequent transfer to syngeneic Balb/c mice no leukemias develop. Both G- and GM-CSF can enhance proliferation of HL-60 cells in short term suspension and clonogenic assay but ultimately, and particularly with G-CSF, enhanced differentiation leads to complete suppression of HL-60 recloning (2). These observations are of value in guiding analysis of responsiveness of primary human myeloid leukemia to growth factors. Without question, in short-term suspension culture and primary leukemic clonogenic assay, G-CSF, like GM-CSF, is a growth stimulating factor in the majority of cases and can synergize with GM-CSF to increase leukemic colony numbeer and size. Indeed, in some cases it may increase the recloning capacity of primary leukemic colonies. However in long-term suspension cultures or upon more rigorous serial recloning the differentiation-inducing action of G-CSF ultimately outweighs its proliferation-inducing action and final extinction of leukemic cloning is observed.

At the present time there is insufficient information available concerning the biology of human myeloid leukemia or preleukemic syndrome to state unequivocally that G-CSF "maturation" therapy would prove clinically effective. Caution must be exercised in view of the potential for emergence of leukemic clones that are totally uncoupled, where G-CSF provides a proliferative but not a differentiative signal (e.g. phenotypiclly like the murine NFS-60 leukemic cell line). It is possible that G-CSF receptor negative clones could be selected in the face of chronic G-CSF therapy. Information is accumulating on the distribution of G-CSF receptors on leukemic cells. Competitive binding studies with ^{125}I-labelled hG-CSF has revealed high affinity receptors, with a frequency comparable to their distribution on normal cells (50-500 per cell), on fresh human leukemic marrow cells classified as M2,3 and 4, as well as on murine WEHI-3, NSF-60 and M1 myeloid leukemic cell lines, and on human HL-60 and U937 lines (23,14). In all cases but NFS-60, a close correlation was found between G-CSF receptor display and the ability of the leukemic cells to differentiate in response to G-CSF. We have combined receptor analysis with suspension culture of primary human leukemic marrow to document the responsiveness of primary human leukemias to G-CSF differentiation. Approximately 1/3 of all cases of ANLL showed enhanced terminal differentiation to segmented neutrophils and/or macrophages following 4-6 days of suspension culture in the presence of G-CSF (1).

Preliminary in vivo studies in mice bearing the WEHI-3 myelomonocytic leukemia have indicated the feasibility of G-CSF maturation therapy in this model system. An indirect approach was used by Schlick and Ruscetti (21) who used a biological response modifying agent, maleic anhydride divinyl ether copolymer (MVE-2) in conjunction with cyclophosphamide to increase survival and produce up to 50% disease free survivors in mice transplanted with WEHI-3 cells. The MVE-2 was a potent inducer of macrophage production of G-CSF and caused elevated serum levels of this CSF species, suggesting that its efficacy was indirectly due to G-CSF induction of leukemic cell differentiation. Less specific effects on host defence function were probably not primarily involved in this anti-leukemic effect since G-CSF receptor negative WEHI-3 D-Variant cell lines were equally leukemogenic when transplanted into mice treated or not treated with MVE-2 and the survival promoting action was only seen with the G-CSF receptor positive D+ WEHI-3 line. In more direct studies we have shown (1) that daily rhG-CSF give intraperitonealy or subcutaneously to Balb/c mice bearing intraperitoneal WEHI-3 leukemic cells resulted in significant prolongation of survival, and with lower numbers of leukemic cells injected, up to 80% long-term disease free survivors. The response was seen only with leukemic cell lines that were G-CSF receptor positive and not with G-CSF receptor negative, differentiation non-inducible variant lines, or with a G-CSF non-responsive but vitamin D_3 macrophage differentiation inducible subline.

Since the major treatment modalities for leukemia and lymphoma involve chemotherapy and/or radiotherapy with severe depression of hematopoiesis and immune function, treatment with G-CSF may be advantageous in terms of 1). boosting host natural immunity (neutrophil ADCC, macrophage effector), 2). inducing an increased proportion of leukemic stem cels to undergo differentiation and lose self-renewal potential, and 3). stimulate recovery of normal hematopoietic progenitor cell populations.

<u>REFERENCES</u>

1. Allen, T.D. and Dexter, T.M. (1983): Scan. Elec. Microsc., 4:1851-1858.
2. Begley, C., Metcalf, D. and Nicola, N. (1987): Int. J. Cancer, 39:99-104.
3. Dexter, T.M. (1987): J. Cell Science, 88:1-6.
4. Gabrilove, J., Jakubowski, A., Fain, K., Scher, H., Grous, J., Sternberg, C., Yagoda, A., Clarkson, B., Moore, M.A.S., Bonilla, H. F., Oetggen, H.F., Alton, M., Downing, M., Welte, K., and Souza, L.M. (1987): Blood, 70:394a.
5. Gillio, A.P., Bonilla, M.A., O'Reilly, R.J., Potter, G.K., Boone, T., Souza, L. and Welte, K. (1986): Blood, 68:283a.
6. Gordon, M.Y., Riley, G.P., Watt, S.M. and Greaves, M.F. (1987): Nature, 326:403-406.
7. Lang, R., Metcalf, D. and Gough, N. (1985): Cell, 43:531-536.
8. Lee, F., Yokota, T., and Otsuka, T. (1986): Proc. Natl. Acad. Sci. USA., 83:2061-2064.

9.   Lovhaug, D., Pelus, L.M., Nordlie, E.M., Botum, A. and Moore M.A.S. (1987): Exp. Hematol., 14:1037-1042.
10. Metcalf, D. (1986): Blood, 67:257-267.
11. Moore, M.A.S., Welte, K., Gabrilove, J. and Souza, L. (1987): Blut, (in press).
12. Moore, M.A.S. and Warren, D.J. (1987): Proc. Natl. Acad. Sci. USA, 84:7134-7138.
13. Moore, M.A.S., Warren, D.J. & Souza, L. (1987): In: Leukemia: Recent Advances in Leukemia and Lymphoma, edited by R. P. Gale and D. W. Golde, (in press), Alan R. Liss, New York.
14. Moore, M.A.S. (1987): In: Important Advances n Oncology 1988, edited by V. DeVita, S. Rosenberg and S. J. Hellman, (in press). J. P. Lippencott Co., Philadelphia.
15. Nara, N. and McCulloch, E. (1985): J. Exp. Med., 162:1435-1440.
16. Nicola, N., Metcalf, D., and Matsumoto, M. (1983): J. Biol. Chem., 258:9017-9027.
17. Platzer, E., Welte, K., Gabrilove, J., Lu, L., Harris, P., Mertelsmann, R., and Moore, M.A.S. (1985): J. Exp. Med., 162:1788-1801.
18. Platzer, E., Oez, S., Welte, K., Sandler, A., Gabrilove, J., Mertelsmann, R., Moore, M.A.S. and Kalden, J. (1986): Immunobiol., 172:185-190.
19. Roberts, R.A., Spooncer, E., Parkinson, E.K., Lord, B.I., Allen, T.D. and Dexter, T.M. (1987): J. Cell Physiol., 132:203-209.
20. Sanderson, C., O'Garra, A., and Warren D. (1986): Proc. Natl. Acad. Sci. USA, 83:437-443.
21. Schlick, E. and Ruscetti, F.W. (1986): Blood, 67:980-988.
22. Sieff, C.A., Tsai, S. and Faller, D.V. (1987): J. Clin Invest., 79:48-54.
23. Souza, L., Boone, T., Gabrilove, J., Lai, P.H., Zsebo, K.M., Murdock, D.C., Chazin, V.R., Platzer, E., Moore, M.A.S., Mertelsmann, R., and Welte, K. (1986): Science, 232:61-65.
24. Spooncer, E., Heyworth, C.M., Dunn, A. and Dexter, T.M. (1986): Differentiation, 31:111-118.
25. Tomida, M., Yamamoto-Yamaguchi, Y., Hozumi, M., Okabe, T., and Takaku, K. (1986): FEBS Lett., 207:271-275.
26. Tsuda, H., Necker, L. and Pluznik, D. (1986): Proc. Natl. Acad. Sci. USA., 83:4317-4321.
27. Warren, D.J. and Moore M.A.S. (1987): J. Immunol., (in press).

28. Weinstein, Y., Ihle, J., Lavu, S., et al. (1986): Proc. Natl. Acad. Sci. USA, 83:5010-5014.
29. Welte, K., Platzer, E., Lu, L., Gabrilove, J., Levi, E., Polivka, A., Mertelsmann, R., and Moore, M.A.S. (1985): Proc. Natl. Acad. Sci. USA, 82:1526-1530.
30. Yasukawa , K., Hirano, T., Watanabe, Y., Muratani, K., Matsuda, T., Nakai, S. and Kishmoto, T. (1987): EMBO Journal 6:2939-
31. Ymer, S., Tucker, Q., Sanderson, C., et al. (1985): Nature, 317:255-261.
32. Young, D., Wagner, K. and Griffin, J. (1987): J. Clin. Invest., 79:100-108.

Intracellular Factors Involved in Erythroid Differentiation of Mouse Erythroleukemia (MEL) Cells

T. Watanabe, S. Nomura, T. Kaneko, S. Yamagoe,
T. Kamiya and M. Oishi

*Institute of Applied Microbiology, University of Tokyo,
Bunkyo-ku, Tokyo 113, Japan*

SUMMARY

In order to investigate intracellular factors involved in mouse erythroleukemia (MEL) cells (Friend cells) differentiation, we first analyzed the differentiation process by cell fusion and cytoplast fusion experiments. From these experiments, we obtained basic information regarding the differentiation process as summarized below. (1) The process is a synergistic result of two different inducible intracellular reactions. (2) One reaction is induced following disturbance of DNA metabolism or replication and is not specific to MEL cells. (3) The other reaction is induced by dimethylsulfoxide (DMSO) or hexamethylenebisacetamide (HMBA) even at suboptimal concentrations of these agents and is specific to MEL cells. This reaction is inhibited by tumor-promoting phorbol esters and cycloheximide. The induced activity remains transiently in the cells and located in cytoplasts.

Based upon these findings, two factors (DIF-I and DIF-II) corresponding to these reactions were detected and partially purified from the cytosol. When these factors were introduced in undifferentiated MEL cells, they triggered erythroid induction, provided that the cells had been potentiated by the induction of either one of the two reactions. Both of the factors are proteinaceous.

INTRODUCTION

Mouse erythroleukemia (MEL) cells, which were established by Friend (1), have been studied extensively as a model for not only terminal erythroid differentiation but for in vitro differentiation in general. Following exposure to agents such as DMSO (2), HMBA (10) or butyric acid (5, 15), MEL cells are redifferentiated in vitro to express a variety of cellular functions characteristics observed in normal erythropoiesis. Despite a number of studies, however, the nature of the reaction leading to the differentiation is not well understood and none of the intracellular factors involved in the process has been identified.

In the last several years, we have been studying the mechanism of the in vitro erythroid differentiation and attempting to identify intracellular molecules involved in the differentiation (4, 6, 8, 17, 18). In this article, we present our experimental results regarding such intracellular factors involved in erythroid differentiation of MEL cells.

Nature of the differentiation process revealed by cell and cytoplast fusion experiments

In order to characterize the complex process leading to erythroid differntiation, we attempted to dissect the process by separating it into two different entities. For this, a series of cell fusion and cytoplast fusion experiments were designed. First, we employed two different mutant MEL cells (Tk$^-$ and Hprt$^-$). Neither of them was able to grow in HAT medium but when they were fused each other they became able to grow in the medium. We treated one of the mutant cells with a suboptimal concentration (or dose) of a known inducing agent, the concentration at which no erythroid differentiation was observed, and fused them with the other mutant cells which had been treated with a different inducing agent also at a suboptimal level. The fused cells were then incubated in HAT medium and among the survived cells hemoglobin-accumulated cells were scored.

We tested a number of combinations with different known inducing agents and concluded that the MEL cell differentiation is a synergistic result of at least two different intracellular reactions (6). One reaction is induced by agents which affect DNA replication (or cell division as a consequence) such as ultraviolet light (UV) irradiation, mitomycin C (MMC) or araC treatment and the other reaction is induced by typical inducing agents such as DMSO or HMBA even at suboptimal concentrations. A typical result of such a synergistic effect by UV irradiation and DMSO treatment is shown in Table 1. The result is consistant with the previous observations made by Sachs (11), Scher and Friend (13) and Terada et al. (16). One of the important conclusions drawn by the cell fusion experiment, employing cells with different origins, was that the UV inducible reaction is not specific to MEL cells but can be induced among various mammalian cells including cells of human origin.

The DMSO (HMBA) inducible second reaction was studied more extensively (4). When assayed by cell (cytoplast) fusion, the reaction, which is specific to MEL cells, was fully induced by the brief exposure to DMSO, for example, 2 hr at 2%, a condition which normally does not induce erythroid differentiation. In a typical experiment, DMSO-pulsed cells were fused with UV irradiated

Table 1. Erythroid differentiation of fused MEL cells

Treatment		Benzidine-positive
DS19(Tk⁻)	DS19(Hprt⁻)	cells, %
—	—	0.1
—	UV	3.8
UV	—	4.0
UV	UV	4.5
—	DMSO	1.7
DMSO	—	1.5
DMSO	DMSO	2.6
UV	DMSO	33.7
DMSO	UV	35.8

DS19(Tk⁻) and DS19(Hprt⁻) MEL cells were grown in fetal calf serum-supplemented minimal essential medium to a cell density of 2×10^6 cells/ml. One of the cell preparations (Tk⁻ or Hprt⁻) was exposed to 1.8% (v/v) DMSO for 16 hr and the other was irradiated by UV light (20 J/m^2) and incubated for 24 hr. Cell fusion was then performed, followed by incubation in fetal calf serum-supplemented minimal essential medium for 20 hr. The cells were then collected, washed once with phosphate- buffered saline (PBS), and incubated in fetal calf serum-supplemented HAT medium. Benzidine-positive cells were scored on the 5th day. Data from reference (6).

partner MEL cells at different time intervals after removal of DMSO and the erythroid differentiation was assayed five days later. As shown in Fig. 1, the DMSO pulse induced an erythroid inducing potential which was detected only after cell fusion with UV irradiated MEL cells. As seen in the figure, we found that the induction process was transient the activity declining to the pretreatment level at 30 hrs after pulse. The induction was inhibited by cycloheximide suggesting de novo protein synthesis to be involved in the process and also by tumor-promoting phorbol esters such as TPA (12-0-tetradecanoylphorbol 13-acetate).

By use of cytoplast fusion the induction process was further characterized. For this, chloramphenicol resistant MEL cells were incubated with DMSO and cytoplasts were prepared at different time intervals. The cytoplasts were then fused with UV irradiated MEL cells and cybrids were selected in the presence of chloram- phenicol, ouabain and oligomycin (17). An activity similar to the

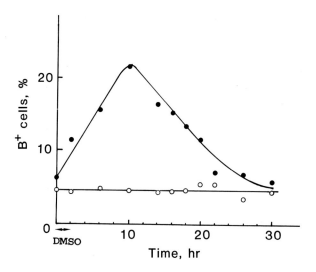

Fig. 1. Induction of the activity leading to erythroid differentiation as revealed by cell fusion with UV-irradiated cells. MEL cells, DS19(Tk$^-$Hprt$^-$) , were grown in MEM supplemented with fetal calf serum (12%) to a cell density of 2 x 10^6 cells/ml. The cells were then diluted 1:1 with the same medium, and DMSO was added to a final concentration of 1.8% (v/v). After 2 hr incubation, the cells were centrifuged (1,200 x g, 5 min), washed twice with PBS, resuspended in medium (1 x10^6 cells/ml), and further incubated at 37°C. At different time intervals as shown, 1.0 ml samples were withdrawn and mixed with 1 x 10^6 cells which had been UV irradiated 24 hr before cell fusion (see below).

For UV-irradiated cells, MEL cells [DS19(Tk$^+$Hprt$^-$)] were grown in fetal calf serum (12%) supplemented MEM to a cell density of 1 x 10^6 cells/ml. The cells were then centrifuged, resuspended in PBS to a cell density of 5 x 10^6 cells/ml, and irradiated with UV light (25 J/m^2) in a Petri dish (60 mm diameter) with constant rotary shaking at 13 rpm. The cells were then centrifuged (1,200 x g, 5 min), resuspended in fetal calf serum (12%) supplemented MEM at a cell density of 7 x 10^5 cells/ml, and further incubated for 24 hr at 37°C. As a control (non UV irradiated cells), cells were treated in the same way except for UV irradiation. These cells were then used for cell fusion with DMSO-treated cells. DMSO-treated cells fused with UV irradiated cells (●); DMSO-treated cells fused with control cells (O). After cell fusion, the cells were incubated in HAT medium for 5 days, and benzidine-positive (B$^+$) (9) cells were scored. Data from reference (4).

one found in the intact cells also appeared in the cytoplasts with
essentially the same kinetics as appeared in the intact cells
(Fig. 2A) and the induction of the activity was inhibited by TPA
or cycloheximide. No activity was induced, however, when
cytoplasts were first prepared and treated with DMSO (Fig. 2B),
suggesting that the induction of the activity requires nuclei,
although the activity is located in cytoplasts.

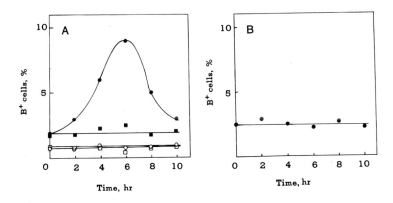

Fig. 2. (A) Induction of intracellular erythroid-inducing
activity in cytoplasts by DMSO. MEL cells, IAM111 (Oua^S Cm^r), were
grown in MEM supplemented with fetal calf serum (12%) at 37°C to a
cell density of 2 x 10^6 cells/ml. The cells were then diluted
(1:1) with the same medium and DMSO was added to a final
concentration of 1.8% (v/v). At different time intervals, the
cells were enucleated and cytoplasts were fused with IAM101 (Oua^r
Cm^s) cells which had been irradiated by UV light (20 J/m^2) 24 hr
before. After 4 days incubation with chloramphenicol (80 µg/ml)
and ouabain (3 mM), oligomycin (10 ng/ml) was added to the medium
and the cells were incubated for one more day. Benzidine-positive
(B$^+$) cells were then scored. Cytoplasts from DMSO-treated cells;
fused with (●), UV irradiated cells; (○), control (-UV) cells.
Cytoplasts from control cells; fused with (■), UV-irradiated cells;
(□), control (-UV) cells. A total of approximately 3 x 10^3 cells
were scored for each sample.
    (B) Absence of erythroid-inducing activity in cytoplasts

directly treated with DMSO. MEL cells, IAM111 (Oua^s Cm^r), were grown in MEM supplemented with fetal calf serum (12%) at 37°C to a cell density of 2 x 10^6 cells/ml. The cells were then enucleated. The cytoplasts were suspended in the same medium (1 x 10^6 cytoplasts/ml) and exposed to 1.8% (v/v) DMSO for various length of periods. At different intervals as shown in the figure, the cytoplasts were withdrawn, washed once with MEM and mixed with IAM101 cells (Oua^{r}Cm^s, 1 x 10^{6}cells) which had been irradiated by UV light (20 J/m^2) at 24 hr before. After cytoplast fusion, the samples were incubated with chloramphenicol (80 µg/ml) and ouabain (3 mM) for 4 days. Oligomycin (10 ng/ml) was then added to the medium and the cells were incubated for one more day. Benzidine-positive (B$^+$) cells (9) were then scored. A total of approx. 3 x 10^3 cells were scored for each sample. Data from reference (17).

The results of these cells and cytoplast fusion experiments summarized as follows. (1) The erythroid induction is a synergistic result of two distinctive cellular reactions. (2) The first reaction originates from inhibition or cessation of DNA replication (or cell division as a consequence). The reaction is not specific to MEL cells. (3) The second reaction is specific to MEL cells and involves, a transmembrane signal which is triggered by DMSO and HMBA. The induction process accompanies de novo protein synthesis and the induced activity is transiently located in cytoplasts. Based upon these results, at least two different kinds of trans-acting factors were implicated in the differentiation process. We designated these putative factors as differentiation inducing factor I (DIF-I) for the one induced by UV and other DNA damaging agents and differentiation inducing factor II (DIF-II) for the one induced by DMSO or HMBA.

Detection of DIF-I in cell-free extracts

Based upon the information described above, we searched for these putative intracellular factors in the extracts prepared from MEL cells. For DIF-I, we prepared cell-free extracts from UV or MMC treated MEL cells and introduced them into MEL cells which had been briefly exposed to DMSO. When such cells were cultured for several days, the number of cells that accumulated hemoglobin increased several fold over the untreated control cells. To introduce proteins into MEL cells, a procedure to permeabilize cells to proteins was devised (7). The procedure involved exposure of cells to a hypertonic condition followed by L-α-lyso-phosphatidylcholine treatment. The activity was also detected in the extracts from non-erythroid cells. Fig. 3 shows a typical pattern of the appearance of the erythroid inducing activity in the cell-free extracts prepared from non-erythroid FM3A cells established from a mouse mammary gland tumor cells at different time intervals after treatment of the cells with UV or MMC. As seen in the figure, the erythroid inducing activity in the extracts started to appear at 15 hr after the treatment and reached a maximal level at approximately 24 hr incubation. Although the inducing activity was low, this experiment indicated the presence of an erythroid inducing activity in the extracts which appeared in an inducible manner after the treatment. As also seen in the figure, the induction process was inhibited by cycloheximide, suggesting de novo protein synthesis to be involved in the induction process. The activity was not detected when the recipient MEL cells were not treated with DMSO prior to the exposure to the extracts or were not permeabilized to proteins. A similar activity was also induced in UV (or MMC) treated cells from other speices such as HeLa cells (Yamagoe et al., manuscript in preparation). Although recent experiments suggest a minor portion is present in nuclei, most of the active factor was located in the cytoplasm. These characteristics coincided well with the nature of the putative trans-acting factor (DIF-I) implicated by the previous cell fusion experiments.

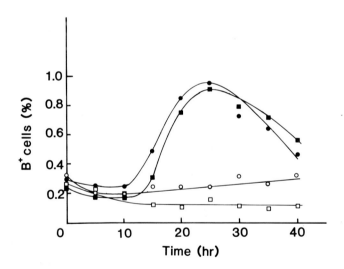

Fig. 3. Erythroid inducing activity in the extract from FM3A cells as a function of time of incubation after treatment of the cells with MMC or UV irradiation. Mouse FM3A cells were cultured in ES (2% calf serum). The cultures were treated with MMC (1μg /ml), MMC (1 μ g/ml) plus cycloheximide (1 μ g/ml) or subjected to UV irradiation (each 30 liter). For UV irradiation, the cells were centrifuged, resuspended in PBS (5 x 10^6 cells/ml) and irradiated under germicidal lamps at an intensity of 20 J/m^2. After centrifugation, the irradiated cells were resuspended in 10

vol of ES (2% calf serum) and incubated under the same condition as the other samples. At the time indicated in the abscissa, the cells from each 1 liter of the culture were harvested by centrifugation and cell-free extracts (cytosol fractions) were prepared and the erythroid-inducing activities (B^+ cells) of the fractions (20 μl, 10 μg protein) were assayed after introduction into DMSO pulsed MEL cells (7). (O); control, (●); MMC treatment, (■); UV irradiation and (□); MMC plus cycloheximide.

By employing a series of column chromatographies the active factor was partially purified from the cell-free extracts (8). The factor was non-dialyzable, sensitive to proteases (trypsin and proteinase K) and the activity was lost after heat treatment (60 C 15 min), suggesting it to be a protein. The molecular weight of the factor was in the range of 80,000 to 100,000 daltons. The partially purified factor induced erythroid differentiation at a level almost equivalent to the one induced with DMSO or HMBA. The induced cells contained a high concentration of hemoglobin and lost their proliferation capacity as observed with the cells induced with DMSO or HMBA (2, 3). We are currently purifying the factor, hopefully to a homogeneity, to elucidate molecular structure of the protein, to detect a possible enzymatic activity associated with it and to clone the gene.

Detection of DIF-II in cell-free extracts

By use of the same strategy employed for DIF-I, we tried to detect the second factor (DIF-II) which also had been implicated by cell and cytoplast fusion experiments. Since the maximal level of putative second factor was obtained at 6 hrs after DMSO (HMBA) treatment from the results obtained from cytoplast fusion experiments (17), cell-free extracts were prepared from MEL cells which had been exposed to DMSO (1.8%) for 6 hr. The extracts were then introduced into MEL cells which had been exposed to UV light, thereby maximizing the production of DIF-I which should act synergistically with DMSO inducible DIF-II. Whereas no erythroid inducing activity was detected in the crude extracts, an activity was detected in the eluate after DEAE chromatography of the extract (Fig. 4B) (18). The activity was eluted from the column at 50 mM NaCl but no such activity was detected in the same eluate from the control cells (Fig. 4A). The activity was not detected without the UV pretreatment or without permeabilization of the recipient cells, suggesting that the induction of DIF-I (by UV treatment) in the recipient cells and incorporation of the factor into the cells are prerequisite for detecting the activity. The activity was different from DIF-I since DIF-I activity was eluted with 250 mM NaCl from a DEAE column under the same condition.

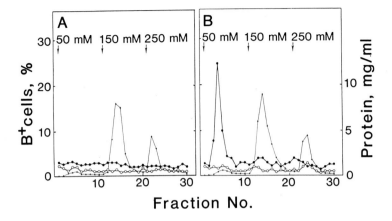

Fig. 4. Erythroid-inducing activity in the cytosol after DEAE column chromatography. MEL (11A2) cells were incubated for 6 hr in the absence (A) and presence (B) of 1.8% (v/v) DMSO. The cytosol fraction (approximately 600 mg total protein) was applied to a DEAE column (20 x 80 mm) and eluted in a step-wise manner with 80 ml each of 50 mM, 150 mM and 250 mM NaCl in basal buffer (20 mM Tris, pH 7.5/ 10% (v/v) glycerol/ 0.25 mM dithiothreitol). Twenty (20 μl) of each fraction (8 ml) were assayed for the erythroid-inducing activity employing UV irradiated permeabilized MEL cells as recipients (7, 8). (●) Erythroid-inducing activity shown as percentage benzidine-positive (B$^+$) cells. The protein concentration of each fraction (▲) is shown (right scale). Data from reference (18).

In order to investigate this activity further, we assayed erythroid inducing activity of the extracts prepared from MEL cells which had been exposed to various inducing agents and inhibitors. The activity was also examined in the extracts from non-erythroid cells (FM3A). The cytosol from each sample was applied to a DEAE column and the activity in the 50 mM NaCl eluate was assayed (Fig. 5). We found that the activity was also induced by HMBA, another potent inducer for erythroid differentiation (Fig. 5C). On the other hand, no activity was detected in the eluate prepared from MEL cells which had been treated with DMSO in the presence of TPA (Fig. 5D) or in the eluate from the cells treated with DMSO in the presence of cycloheximide (Fig.

5E).   No activity was induced in mouse non-erythroid cells (FM3A)
by DMSO (Fig. 5F).

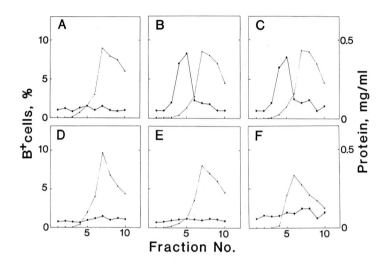

Fig. 5.   Induction of erythroid-inducing activity (DIF-II) under
various conditions. MEL 11A2 cells and non-erythroid FM3A cells
were incubated under various conditions (see below) for 6 hr. The
cytosol fraction ($\sim$ 120 mg of protein) from each preparation was
applied to a DEAE column (12 x 86 mm) and eluted with 50 mM NaCl
in basal buffer. From each fraction (1.25 ml), samples (20 μl)
were taken and assayed for erythroid-inducing activity. (A)
Untreated MEL 11A2 cells (control).   (B) MEL 11A2 cells treated
with 1.8% DMSO plus TPA at 100 ng/ml. (E) MEL 11A2 cells treated
with 1.8% DMSO plus cycloheximide at 10 μg/ml.   (F) FM3A cells
treated with 1.8% DMSO for 6 hr. Protein concentration of each
fraction was measured; protein peaks occur aroud fraction 7. Data
from reference (18).

⎯⎯⎯⎯⎯⎯⎯⎯⎯⎯⎯⎯⎯⎯⎯⎯⎯

        The time course for the induction of DIF-II was studied by
assaying the activity in the 50 mM eluate prepared from MEL cells
which had been exposed to DMSO (1.8%) for various lengths of time.
The activity started to appear soon after exposure to DMSO,
reached a maximum at 6 hr incubation and decreased after 10 hr.
The kinetics, especially its transient nature, was similar to that
observed in the cytoplast fusion experiments.

        These characteristics in the induction of the activity

(effect of inhibitors, species specificity and induction keneties)
were identical with those of the putative second intracellular
factor (DIF-II) implicated by the cell fusion and cytoplast fusion
experiments (4, 17).

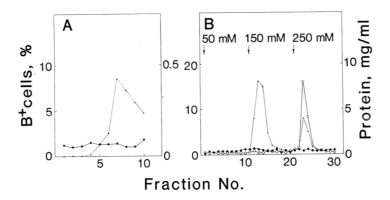

Fig. 6. DIF-II and DIF-I activities in cytosol from a
differentiation defective MEL cell (DR-1). (A) MEL cell line
(DR-1) was incubated in the presence of 1.8% (v/v) DMSO for 6 hr.
The cytosol fraction (approximately 110 mg protein) was applied to
a DEAE column (12 x 75 mm) and eluted with 50 mM NaCl in basal
buffer. From each fraction (2.0 ml), 20 µl was taken and assayed
for erythroid-inducing activity (●) (shown as the percentage
appearance of B⁺ cells). The protein concentration of each
fraction (▲) is shown (right scale).
   (B) MEL cell line (DR-1) was incubated in the presence of
mitomycin C (1.0 µg/ml) for 24 hr. The cytosol fraction
(approximately 110 mg protein) was applied to a DEAE column (12 x
75 mm) and eluted in a step-wise manner with 20 ml each of 50 mM,
150 mM and 250 mM NaCl in basal buffer, respectively. From each
fraction, 20 µl were assayed for DIF-I activity (○) and DIF-II
activity (●). The protein concentration of each fraction is shown
(▲) (right scale). Data from reference (18).

    We examined whether DIF-II activity was present in mutant
MEL cells defective in erythroid differentiation. A mutant
(DR-1) was isolated whose level of erythroid induction was less
than 0.1% after 120 hr incubation with any of the typical inducing
agents such as DMSO, HMBA or sodium butyrate. The results of cell
fusion experiments between DR-1 and parental MEL cells demonstrated that DR-1 was normal for DIF-I induction but defective in
DIF-II. The cytosol from DR-1, which had been exposed to DMSO for
6 hr, was prepared and DIF-II activity in the 50 mM (NaCl) eluate
from a DEAE column was assayed. No activity was detected (Fig.
5A). On the other hand, when cytosol was prepared from MMC
treated DR-1 and assayed for DIF-I activity, a normal level of
DIF-I activity was detected in 250 mM (NaCl) eluate where DIF-I
was expected to be eluted (Fig. 5B). Thus, the mutant is
apparently impaired in the process leading to the induction of
DIF-II. This provides further evidence that DIF-II is directly
involved in in vitro differentiation by DMSO or HMBA.

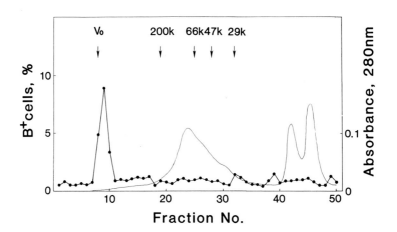

Fig. 7. Gel filtration of DIF-II. The DIF-II fraction eluted
with 50 mM NaCl from a DEAE column was concentrated in a Minicon
(Amicon), and 200 μ l (680 μ g of protein) of the sample was
fractionated through Superose 12 (Pharmacia) at a flow rate of 0.5
ml/min, uaing basal buffer containing 50 mM NaCl. From each
fraction (0.25 ml), 20 μl was assayed for erythroid-inducing
activity (●). Protein concentration of each fraction was
monitored automatically at 280 nm and is shown as a solid line
without symbols. The molecular weight markers used to calibrate

the column were α- amylase (M_r 200,000), bovine serum albumin (M_r 66,000), ovalbumin (M_r 47,000), and carbonic anhydrase (M 29,000). The void volume (V_o) was determined by blue dextran. Data from reference (18).

_____

Intracellularly DIF-II activity was located in cytoplasmic fraction. More than 93% of the activity was present in the cytosol fraction, consistent with the observation from the cytoplast fusion experiments in which DMSO induced activity was located in cytoplasts (17). DIF-II was partially purified from the cytosol by successive column chromatography, including step-wise DEAE-cellulose chromatography, ion-exchange FPLC (Mono Q), hydroxylapatite chromatography, and gel filtration with Superose 12. The partially purified DIF-II exhibited a protein-aceous nature, the erythroid-inducing activity being completely lost when the sample was treated with trypsin (2.0 μg/ml, 5 min at 37°C) or heat (15 min at 56°C). Its activity was nondialyzable and, in contrast to DIF-I, the molecular size of DIF-II was found to be quite large. Its activity was eluted near the void volume of a Superose 12 gel-filtration column (Fig. 6). The large molecular size of DIF-II was also confirmed by glycerol gradient centrifugation in which its activity was detected at the position where proteins with a higher molecular weight than catalase (M_r 246,000) sedimented.

ACKNOWLEDGEMENTS

The authors wish to thank Ms. Y. Okamoto for her excellent editorial assistance. This work was supported in part by a Grant in-Aid from Japanese Ministry of Education and Welfare.

REFERENCES

1. Friend, C., Patuleia, M. C. & de Harven, E. (1966): Natl. Cancer Inst. Monogr., 228:505-520.

2. Friend, C., Scher, W., Holland, J. G. & Sato, T. (1971): Proc. Natl. Acad. Sci. USA, 68:378-382.

3. Gusella, J., Geller, R., Clarke, B., Weeks, V. & Housman, D. (1976): Cell, 9:221-229.

4. Kaneko, T., Nomura, S. & Oishi, M. (1984): Cancer Res., 44: 1756-1760.

5. Leder, A. & Leder, P. (1975): Cell, 5:319-322.

6. Nomura, S. & Oishi, M. (1983): Proc. Natl. Acad. Sci. USA, 80:210-214.

7. Nomura, S., Kamiya, T. & Oishi, M. (1986): Exp. Cell Res., 163:434-444.

8. Nomura, S., Yamagoe, S., Kamiya, T. & Oishi, M. (1986): Cell, 44:663-669.

9. Orkin, S. H., Harosi, F. I. & Leder, P. (1975): Proc. Natl. Acad. Sci. USA, 72:98-102.

10. Reuben, R. C., Wife, R. L., Breslow, R., Rifkind, R. A. & Marks, P. A. (1976): Proc. Natl. Acad. Sci. USA, 73:862-866.

11. Sachs, L. (1978): Nature, 274:535-539.

12. Sasa, S., Granick, S., Chang, C. & Kappas, A. (1975): In: Erythropoiesis: Induction of enzymes of the heme biosynthetic pathway in Friend leukemia cells in culture, edited by K. Nakano, J. W. Fisher & F. Tanaka, pp. 383-396. Univ. of Tokyo Press, Tokyo.

13. Scher, W. & Friend, C. (1978): Cancer Res., 38:841-849.

14. Sugano, H., Frusawa, M., Kawaguchi, T. & Ikawa, Y. (1973): Bibl. Haematol. (Basel), 39:955-967.

15. Takahashi, E., Yamada, M., Saito, M., Kuboyama, M. & Ogasa, K. (1975): Gann, 66:577-580.

16. Terada, M., Nudel, U., Fibach, E., Rifkind, R. A. & Marks, P. A. (1978): Cancer Res., 38:835-840.

17. Watanabe, T., Nomura, S. & Oishi, M. (1985): Exp. Cell Res., 159:224-234.

18. Watanabe, T. & Oishi, M. (1987): Proc. Natl. Acad. Sci. USA, 84:6481-6485.

MECHANISMS OF ACTION AND PHARMACOLOGY OF DIFFERENTIATION INDUCERS

Pharmacology and Mechanisms of Action of Differentiation Agents

J.A. Hickman and R.M. Friedman*

CRC Experimental Chemotherapy Group, Pharmaceutical Sciences Institute,
Aston University, Birmingham, B4 7ET, UK and
*Department of Pathology, F. Edward Hebert School of Medicine,
Uniformed Services University of the Health Sciences,
4301 Jones Bridge Road, Bethesda, MD 20814, USA

The pharmacology of differentiating agents has been reviewed in the past year (41, 69, 87, 98, 122). This chapter presents an analysis of the pharmacology and mechanism of action of agents, which bring about tumor cell differentiation, and attempts to identify whether there are principal questions --and maybe some answers--of common interest to the many investigators now working with different drugs which affect a variety of different models. Articulating these questions--in the end a highly subjective exercise--has proven to be no easy task, and it has to be admitted that there are few definitive answers either. What follows is a personal overview, which of necessity is highly selective in its analysis of the two thousand or so papers which a Medline computer search revealed were published in 1986 and 1987 on the effects of chemical substances on differentiation.

We considered it important to ask whether there is a common mechanism of action associated with the disparate chemical structures which induce the differentiation of some cell lines. For example, we have found 73 different agents described in the literature which induce the terminal differentiation of the HL-60 human promyelocytic leukemia cell line. Although, clearly, these agents must have different primary loci of action in the cell, it seems reasonable to assume that at some point in the HL-60 cell, the consequences of these interactions might converge to initiate a limited number of events which determine commitment to terminal differentiation. The same argument might be put with respect to the murine Friend erythroleukemia (MEL) cell line, where again a bewildering number of compounds are capable of the induction of terminal erythroid differentiation. Some attempt at classification of the inducers of MEL cell differentiation was made by Rovera and Surrey (97) based on cross resistance patterns; only butyrate and hemin (which induces globin synthesis, but does not induce terminal differentiation) were in classes of their own, with the rest of the inducers appearing to work by a common mechanism. Are there

conserved cellular responses leading to leukemic cell
differentiation, which are triggered by a variety of agents,
acting by independent pathways to induce metabolic imbalance?
We shall attempt to tackle this question. In other cell types,
particularly those derived from epithelial cells, it is evident
that few agents are effective in the induction of phenotypic
changes; fewer still successfully induce irreversible
maturation. Here a common mechanism may not exist; therefore,
these systems present a challenge to some of the current dogmas
arising from work on leukemic cell differentiation.

      This brings us to other questions: how do we chose a model
for the identification of potential inducers of terminal
differentiation, or maturation; and, which model may best
illustrate general rules of the mechanism of drug-induced
differentiation? Is it best in screening for new agents to aim
for a broad trawl--as is provided by the HL-60 cell line--or, is
this cell line the "differentiators" equivalent of the
temporarily disgraced murine L1210, recently culled from the
arena of cytotoxic drug screening because it was considered to
be too indiscriminate in the selection of potential chemotherapeutic drugs? Dogma in the choice of a pharmacological
model for screening generally spells missed drugs, and it is
probably best to encourage a multitude of models. This at least
serves the additional purpose of preventing the formulation of
too many dogmas regarding the mechanisms involved, as it is
quite clear that profound differences exist amongst various cell
types. Perhaps the most striking of these has been the recent
description of drastically increased expression of the myc
protooncogene as chronic lymphocytic leukemia cells were induced
to differentiate to plasma cells by a phorbol ester (78), the
antithesis of what has almost become the dogma of myc repression
for cells to become committed to differentiation (see below).
Haematopoetic tumor models of differentiation continue to
dominate the investigations of the pharmacology of tumor cell
differentiation, and much of what follows will of necessity have
to reflect that dominance.

      Although the molecular pharmacology of many of the agents
which induce tumor cell differentiation is relatively well
defined, doubts concerning their precise loci of action
complicate attempts to determine what are the causative
mechanisms of the induction of differentiation. Such doubts
extend to even those agents with a well-defined locus of action,
such as the phorbol esters, which despite having a
characterized--and even cloned--receptor, the enzyme protein
kinase C, appear to induce the monocytic differentiation of
myeloid cells by a mechanism which involves undefined elements
in addition to the activation of protein kinase C and its
sequellae (72, 91, 128). This is discussed further below. The
polar solvents such as dimethylsulfoxide which induce maturation
or terminal differentiation (reviewed in 111) are almost
universally considered to be membrane-active, implying an

interaction with the lipid bilayer. But is this so? In a
studies of the archetypal membrane-active agents, the
anaesthetics, controversy abounds, so that there is now
excellent evidence to suggest that protein targets provide a
more feasible locus for their action (42, 43). It is probably
misleading to consider that we are dealing with drugs with
monovalent and well defined mechanisms, so that studies which
attempt to analyze the molecular events responsible for the
induction of differentiation by pharmacological means, with the
assumption that each agent has a well defined locus of action,
must always be interpreted with caution.

The majority of the agents which induce differentiation are
cytotoxic drugs, and the investigations of the relationship
between the imposition of cellular cytotoxicity and the
induction of differentiation may provide clues as to the events
which lead to the terminal differentiation of some cell types.
One of us (76, 77) recently demonstrated that, for a series of
structurally disparate polar solvents, optimum differentiation
of the HL-60 cell line occurred at a mathematically fixed, and
therefore predictable, fraction of the acutely cytotoxic
concentration. Two recent papers on the mechanism of
cytotoxicity of two types of antiproliferative agent, the
epipodophylotoxins and 5-fluorouracil, tackle the central
question of why cytotoxic drugs which prevent replication should
also bring about cell death. The inhibition by epipodophylo-
toxin of topoisomerase II activity, accompanied by the formation
of double stranded-protein associated breaks, was insufficient
to kill cells when they were subsequently incubated with an
inhibitor of protein synthesis, cycloheximide. This suggested
that the cellular response to damage is important in determining
cell death, and it may be that a cellular response to the
biochemical changes imposed differentiating agents is critical
to the initiation of events which commit a cell to differentiate
(22a). If this is correct, then the task of understanding the
mechanism of action of the disparate agents which induce
differentiation may be somewhat simplified in that there may be
a limited repetoire of cellular responses to a multitude of
drug-induced changes or lesions. Clearly, if we are to
understand the mechanism of action of the cytotoxic drugs which
induce differentiation, a better understanding is required of
the mechanisms by which they cause cell death. For too long,
vague concepts of the induction of "unbalanced growth" have been
promulgated; it is time to define cell mortality in molecular
terms (see also ref. 7).

The molecular events which bring about the commitment of
cells to terminal differentiation are central to an understanding of how pharmacological agents promote tumor cell
differentiation. These events occur relatively early in the
exposure period but may be complicated by the superimposition of
biochemical changes which determine the lineage of cell development (38, 129). A two-step model which consists of the

imposition of a limit to proliferative potential, accompanied by events which induce a commitment to differentiate (126), serves as a useful paradigm in the study of the tumor cell different- iation, at least of haematopoetic tumors.

If it is assumed that the expression of certain oncogenes may be responsible for the malignant phenotype (4, 5), and the impediment to the normal, and balanced maturation of the cells, then clearly early changes in the expression of these genes, or the activity of their products may be important. It should be established whether oncogene regulation is relevant to commit- ment, to the fall in proliferative potential, or is a reflection of the change of differentiated phenotype rather than a causative force in that change (28).

Gene expression is controlled by cellular messages which emanate from the cell surface, so that it is becoming increasingly important that we begin to unravel the mechanism by which intracellular signals (such as changes in ionic composition, or protein phosphorylation) are coupled to the modulation of gene expression. The regulation of proliferation by growth factor receptor cascades at the locus of the cell membrane is reasonably well defined; however, we must ask whether those changes occurring at the cell surface in response to a differentiating agent, are relevant to commitment or to the reduction of proliferative potential. These questions are dealt with more fully elsewhere in this volume.

DRUG-INDUCED COMMITMENT

Analysis of the degree of differentiation induced by the incubation of leukemic cells with differentiating agents for various times suggests that there is a minimum time of exposure which must be maintained before the cells can express markers of a more mature phenotype--that is, before they become committed, generally irreversibly and in a stochastic manner, to terminal differentiation (50,116). It is in this time window of "precommitment" that events occur that are causative in the promotion of differentiation; however, some markers of the mature phenotype may be expressed during the commitment period, so that it is difficult to disentangle causative changes from others. Commitment may precede, and be independent of the fall in proliferative potential: for example, cells treated with concentrations of polar solvents, which do not limit proliferative potential, may be manipulated to undergo many divisions until such time as their proliferation becomes inhibited by nutrient limitation or cell density. At this time, they express markers of the mature phenotype (38, 77, 125). Experiments aiming to isolate the events of commitment from those of a fall in proliferative potential may be helpful in dissecting these two components from each other.

Leukemic cell lines retain a "memory" of their exposure to agents; commitment of HL-60 promyelocytic leukemia cells may be

accumulated through the additive effects of different inducers
(129). Yen et al (13) suggest these events are independent of
lineage determination, so that the type of differentiated cell
which results depends on later lineage development events,
implying that the early stages of commitment do take place by a
common cellular response to different inducers. The process of
commitment of leukemic cell lines has been reviewed recently by
Tsiftsoglou et al (119).

Recent work in two areas may provide valuable clues about the
biochemical nature of the precommitment state and that of
commitment: one concerns the use of agents which inhibit
differentiation; the other, the use of agents which enhance the
level of commitment. The enhancement of commitment,
particularly by biological response modifiers (53) has important
clinical implications, which are discussed elsewhere in this
volume.

INDUCTION OF "ADAPTIVE RESPONSES"

It was noted above that the majority of agents inducing
differentiation of leukemic cell lines are cytotoxic drugs.
Generally, the optimal degree of differentiation is promoted by
prolonged exposure to these agents at concentrations marginally
below those which induce acute toxicity. These are conditions
defined for a variety of toxins to induce an adaptive response
or responses of some type: the amplification of certain genes
in response to antimetabolites (103); the expression of DNA
repair enzymes when drugs interact with chromatin (82); the
synthesis of metallothionines in response to heavy metals (52);
changes in cellular thiol metabolism, particularly the induction
of glutathione transferases in response to electrophiles (18);
the interferon-type response after viral challenge (95); the
synthesis of heat shock proteins subsequent to modifications of
cellular proteins (83); and, the induction of other stress
proteins, for example by glucose deprivation (114). In
addition, Zuckier and Tritton (136) noted that the cytotoxic
drug Adriamycin at sublethal concentrations caused the
up-regulation of epidermal growth factor receptors in actively
growing HeLa and 3T3 cells, presumably as the cells attempted to
overcome a fall in their proliferative potential. Several of
these adaptive responses to toxins, perhaps not surprisingly,
have been identified as early responses of cells to their
exposure to a variety of differentiating agents. Are any of
them necessary or sufficient to bring about the commitment of
the cells to terminal differentiation, as some workers suggest?
It is possible that there is common ground here, and that a
variety of the early changes seen after different inducing
agents are adaptive responses, which may be a part of a
coordinated program coupled to terminal differentiation. As
suggested above, this would shift the pharmacological emphasis
of many studies from what the drugs do (which are likely to be

non-overlapping events), to how the cell responds to the
consequences of drug action. Developmental roles have been
suggested for both the adaptive responses of gene amplification
(113) and the activation of genes which encode heat shock
proteins (6,73,108).

There are some striking similarities in the kinetics of
induction and decay of some of these adaptive responses, and the
kinetics of the induction and decay of precommitment memory.
For example, incubation of Chinese hamster ovary cells with DMSO
or dimethylformamide induces the maximal expression of thermotolerance (reduced susceptibility to elevated temperatures) only
after 24 hours of exposure to the solvent (51). Thermotolerance
then decays over two to three subsequent cell cycles (75).
Additionally, the induction of this type of response is blocked
by incubation with inhibitors of protein synthesis (83), as are
the events leading to commitment (119). Comparable kinetics of
the induction and decay of gene amplification after short-term
exposure to hydroxyurea were reported (57).

GENE AMPLIFICATION

The similarity in protocols used for the induction of precommitment events in leukemic cells and those for the induction
of gene amplification associated with the production of double
minute chromosomes, have been noted by Yen et al (130). They
showed that the precommitment period of two cell cycles for
retinoic acid-induction of HL-60 cell differentiation is reduced
by a pulse exposure of 20 hours to hydroxyurea. It was
suggested that gene amplification may be involved in the S-phase
specific events which lead to commitment. Preliminary analysis
of the DNA content of the cell treated with hydroxyurea
suggested that overreplication of chromosomes had occurred. The
idea that a temporary inhibition of DNA synthesis, induced by
those compounds with S-phase specificity, induces the amplification of genes (and their products?) necessary for commitment, is interesting. These results (130) could also be
interpreted in terms of the effects of a combination of two
inducers of differentiation, since Yen seems to ignore the fact
that hydroxyurea itself induces differentiation (23), and at
marginally effective concentrations, it may be contributing to
precommitment memory events in a manner so well defined by his
group (129). One of us (J.A.H. with F. Richards, unpublished)
analyzed the chromatin of HL-60 cells which had been incubated
with effective concentrations of N-methylformamide, but found no
indication of the formation of double minutes or homologously
staining regions typical of gene amplification. Although Yen et
al (129) point to the effectiveness of a number of antimetabolites as inducers of HL-60 cell differentiation, clearly
many of the other inducers have quite different primary targets,
and may not directly inhibit DNA synthesis. Nevertheless, the
involvement of gene amplification in differentiation is an

attractive hypothesis. Vershavsky (124) had suggested that the phorbol ester tumor promoter and differentiating agent TPA could act as a non-specific "firone," bringing about gene amplifications, but this has been disputed(10).

CHANGES IN CHROMATIN STRUCTURE - DNA STRAND BREAKS

Changes in the structure of chromatin would be required, of necessity, by cells regulating the expression of their genes. Chou et al (22) showed that the chromatin structure of c-myc and c-fos was altered as HL-60 cells were induced to differentiate by phorbol esters, with relaxation of the nucleosomal subunits during their state of active transcription. What types of mechanisms are involved in these changes and might they represent some type of adaptive response?

In an interesting paper by Yoshioka et al (132) the treatment of mouse FM3A cells with toxic concentrations of 5-fluorouracil brought about the formation of distinctive (and possibly non-random) double-stranded DNA breaks, which were not formed by the accumulation of single strand breaks. These accompanied cell death. The breaks and cell death were prevented by incubation with cycloheximide. The authors present a model whereby metabolic imbalance (considered in this case to be triggered by dNTP pool imbalances) activates transcription of an endonuclease responsible for the DNA breaks. In these cells, the breaks are not re-ligated, and they are presumably lethal. Is it possible that in cells undergoing differentiation at marginally subtoxic levels of cytotoxins, the complex patterns of DNA breakage observed promote new gene expression, to ensure continued viability under conditions where strand religation occurs (36, 63)?

It has been suggested that the activity of topoisomerase II may be responsible for the breaks in DNA and, therefore, the relaxation of chromatin in differentiating granulomonocytic precursor cells. Modulation of topoisomerase II activity during TPA-induced differentiation has been investigated by Morin and colleagues (90). The attractiveness of topoisomerases as critical elements, which bridge the membrane-bound signal transduction systems to changes in gene expression, activated at least in part by chromatin relaxation, arises from the observations that topoisomerase II was a substrate for protein kinase C. Specific phosphorylation of topoisomerase II by protein kinase C was observed as HL-60 cells were induced to differentiate to monocytes by TPA (102). In addition, Girard et al (47) recently showed the physical translocation of protein kinase C to the nucleus of TPA-treated cells; however, Morin and coworkers (72, 91) and others (132) have shown that activation of protein kinase C in HL-60 cells by diacylglycerols failed to induce monocytic differentiation, and an analysis of both type I and II topoisomerase activity after diacylglycerol treatment showed that there was an activation equivalent to that produced

by TPA (90). This suggests that the activation of
topoisomerases may be dissociated from differentiation in the
HL-60 cell. One criticism of this work might be that the
treatment of HL-60 cells with non-toxic concentrations of the
diacylglycerols is not likely to be accompanied by conditions
which limit the proliferative capacity of the cells--one of the
ingredients necessary for commitment--so that the cells might
well have had precommitment memory induced but have too high a
proliferative potential for their successful commitment to
terminal differentiation.

Inhibitors of topoisomerase II have been suggested as down
regulators of myeloid cell differentiation (40, 41, 132). These
experiments may assume an unwarranted specificity for the
topoisomerase poisons; for example, Morin et al (90) point to
the inhibition of RNA polymerase by novobiocin (48).

HEAT SHOCK PROTEINS

All eukaryotic cells investigated to date, when exposed to
elevated temperatures synthesise an evolutionarily conserved
family of proteins, the heat shock proteins (83), the role of
which appears to be the association with and stabilization of
cellular proteins (94). The expression of heat shock proteins
may be responsible for subsequent thermotolerance of cells.
Heat shock protein synthesis additionally occurs in certain
cells during their differentiation (6, 73, 108). Transcription
may be cell cycle regulated and, therefore, coupled to proliferation control (62). Gene regulation by steroid hormones in
chick oviducts is associated with tissue-specific transcription
of a 108 kD heat shock protein (2). Generally, these "natural"
inductions of the transcription of heat shock genes seem to be
regulated in a manner which is different from that resulting
from the imposition of a cellular stress.

In K562 cells treated with haemin, a 70 kD heat shock protein
was synthesized (108) which in the developing erythrocyte
appears to act as a clathrin-uncoating ATPase involved in the
removal of transferrin receptors from the mature cells (26).
Since haemin does not terminally differentiate MEL cells, this
may raise doubts about the possible role of heat shock proteins
in the events leading to commitment. Comparison between the MEL
cell and the HL-60 cell, here with respect to heat shock,
highlights a paradox, in so far as hyperthermia was reported to
inhibit DMSO-induced differentiation (as does TPA, vitamin D3,
and butyrate - see below), whereas a more severe heat shock
induced HL-60 cell differentiation: a heat shock of 43.5 C for
1 hour and a variety of agents which induce the expression of
heat shock proteins (sodium arsenite, ethanol, cadmium and
procaine) all induced the granulocytic differentiation of HL-60
cells. Interestingly, although the 1 hour heat shock inhibited
new protein synthesis, up to 36% of cells ceased division and
expressed markers of granulocytic differentiation when assayed

96 h later. This showed that the time required for the treatment to commit the cells to terminal differentiation was very much shorter than that required for agents like the polar solvents (generally 12 hours) (55).

The recent work in the laboratory of one of us (JAH with F. Richards) has shown that treatment of HL-60 cells with N-methylformamide (NMF) at an acutely toxic concentration induced the synthesis of the major heat shock proteins (hsps) at 70, 90 and 110 kD, whereas treatment under conditions of the induction of granulocytic differentiation clearly decreased, within 2 hours, the constitutive synthesis of a 70 kD protein. There is some evidence that transformed cells overexpress heat shock proteins (60). Immunoblotting with an antiserum to a 70 kD hsp showed that cellular levels of this hsp 70 rise after 24 hours of incubation with NMF, with a peak protein level at 36 hours (Richards and Hickman, unpublished). The timescale of these changes was very similar to those of the induction and decline of 2'-5'-oligoadenylate synthetase observed by Schwartz et al (104), which might also be considered to be a stress response.

The actual role of the heat shock proteins in cell different-iation remains to be established. It is interesting that transfection of Chinese hamster ovary cells with myc enhanced transcription of a Drosophila heat shock promoter (66); it is possible that the changes we observe in heat shock proteins are related to the dynamics of myc expression. However, these experiments with myc should be interpreted with some caution, as Anathan et al (1) have recently shown the activation of a heat shock promoter under conditions where cells contain abnormal quantities of proteins.

The hypothesis that the induction of a cellular stress, and some type of response to that stress (an adaptive response) may lead to differentiation, is attractive for some of the leukemic cell lines, but fails, as yet, to explain why in some systems, such as MEL cell treated with retinoic acid (118, 56), or colonic carcinoma cell lines (29), cells may undergo phenotypic and other changes (for example in their cell cycle), under the conditions of marginal cytotoxicity, but fail to terminally differentiate, or may suffer the consequences of cytotoxicity. These are models which should at the molecular level help in the dissection of those crucial events which lead to terminal differentiation, and which are preseumably already pheno-typically programmed to take the pathways of cell death or resistance to the toxins, rather than that of differentiation. Like drug resistant lines, they serve as vital negative controls. However, it is important that they are not viewed too negatively: for example, if a change in an oncogene, or even a stress response, is observed in these lines in the absence of differentiation, this does not necessarily mean that these changes are unimportant for differentiation, but rather that it is possible that the factors which couple them to terminal differentiation may be awry.

BLOCKADE OF COMMITMENT AND ERASURE OF COMMITMENT "MEMORY"

The murine Friend erythroleukemia cell line provides a
classical pharmacological system for the analysis of commitment,
in that the agonists which promote differentiation are themselves antagonized by certain drugs (21, 92, 121). Incubation
of cells with 1 fM dexamethasone prevents the commitment induced
by dimethylsulfoxide (DMSO) and release from this glucocorticoid
block is rapidly followed by terminal differentiation (92). It
was suggested that the events responsible for commitment of the
cells were not steroid-sensitive (i.e. precommitment events),
but instead, that the expression of genes representative of the
mature cell was inhibited (92). Dexamethasone inhibits transcription and post-transcriptional modification of RNA (9),
including that of globin and other RNAs in MEL cells; however,
Levenson and Housman (80) presented evidence that commitment
memory was erased by dexamethasone, implying that the steroid
also inhibited transcription of genes involved in the crucial
precommitment period, the early events which bring about
commitment. Release from a dexamethasone-induced blockade, and
analysis of newly synthesized RNAs should show the specific
transcription of species which play a role in commitment.

One might speculate about whether the accrual and decay of
commitment memory represents the temporal accumulation of
biochemical lesions imposed by prolonged periods of incubation
with differentiating agents, and their subsequent repair, or
whether it represents the accumulation of a cellular response to
these lesions, or both. Inhibition of the accumulation of
memory by cycloheximide and 3-deoxyadenosine (an inhibitor of
RNA transport from nucleus to cytoplasm) suggests that a commitment memory is a protein factor synthesized in response to
drug-induced changes, whose stability is sufficient to allow its
maintenance for several cell cycles, before decay (80). The
induction of protein factors responsible for FEL cell differentiation has been described in cell fusion experiments; it would
be interesting, if one of these was found to resemble the factor
responsible for commitment memory. One factor appears to be
specific for the MEL cell; the second appears to be non-cell
type-specific in that irradiation of other cell types induces
its synthesis (85, 86).

Promotion of differentiation of Friend cells by DMSO is also
inhibited by lithium (46, 133). A kinetic analysis of commitment in these cells suggests that lithium was exerting its
effects early in a precommitment stage, and it was most
effective during the first 10 hours of DMSO treatment before the
cells became committed (133). Lithium inhibits the synthesis of
phosphatidylinositol, a precursor for the release of the intracellular second messengers 1,4,5-inositol trisphosphate and
diacylglycerol (8). One can speculate on the possibility that

commitment may involve modulation of membrane signal cascades. Faletto and Macara (35) had previously shown an early decrease in phosphatidylinositol (PI) metabolism in DMSO treated MEL cells; this suggests that a stimulation (indirectly inhibited by Lithium), followed by a down regulation of PI metabolism may be key events in precommitment. Lithium administered to patients has been reported to increase the circulating levels of GM-CSF, and to decrease the number of committed erythroid stem cells, observations compatible with the effects seen on MEL cells (12).

Analysis of the arrest of biochemical changes in the progress of differentiation of MEL cells imposed by these inhibitors and others such as the phorbol ester TPA (37), procaine (121), hyperthermia (not heat shock) (96), butyrate (24), vitamin D3 (126), or N-6-methyladenosine (119) has not yet provided critical information regarding the events determining the initiation of the commitment to phenotypic change.

POTENTIATION OF COMMITMENT

An alternative way to analyze the biochemical nature of precommitment events is to study conditions where commitment is potentiated. In this respect, there have been a number of recent reports that pretreatment of leukemic cell lines with biological response modifiers induces a sensitization to differentiating agents (3, 10, 21, 45, 54, 70, 115). Recombinant interferon gamma, at concentrations up to 1,000 U/ml had essentially no effects on the morphological maturation or upon certain functional measures of maturity of HL-60 cells, but did produce a moderate increase in non-specific esterase activity, typical of the maturation to monocytes (54). In admixture with a normally suboptimal concentration of retinoic acid, the expression of a full range of markers of maturity was observed. Interferon alpha also potentiated the effects of retinoic acid (71), and increased the rate of expression of markers of maturity, although it was claimed that gamma interferon was 40-fold more potent than alpha interferon (54). Similar potentiation was observed when interferon gamma was used in combination with vitamin D3, and a greater commitment of HL-60 cells to monocytoid differentiation was observed than when either compound was used alone (3). Gamma interferon itself had minimal effect on the human ML-1 myeloblastic leukemic cell line, but strongly enhanced the response of the cells to tumor necrosis factor, which induced monocytic differentiation (115).

Gamma interferon also had complex, but reversible, effects in K562 cells, inducing expression of class I histocompatibility antigens and beta 2-microglobulin, but having no effect on c-myc, gamma globulin, or transferrin receptors (20). The failure of this more primitive cell type to undergo terminal differentiation when treated with gamma interferon (and other agents) makes it an attractive cell type to use in comparison to the HL-60 cell, as the latter system potentially allows a dissection of those events which represent reversible phenotypic changes (albeit to maturity) from those which represent commitment to irreversible differentiation. Further examples of this are discussed below.

Most interestingly, DMSO induction of granulocytic differentiation in HL-60 cells was accompanied by a 25-fold induction of 2'-5'-oligoadenylate synthetase activity, an enzyme associated with the antiproliferative activity of interferons. Activity reached a maximum at 48 hours and declined thereafter. Similar increases in interferon-induced genes, including type I histocompatibility antigen RNA and 2'-5'-oligo (A) phosphodiesterase, were seen in the presence of neutralizing antibodies to interferons (104). Could this be considered as another example of the induction of an adaptive response?

Not only are clinical trials of interferon in combination with potent inducers of differentiation going to be important, but it will be of interest to screen these combinations in model systems in vivo. The standard 80 to 90% differentiation achieved in the in vitro models is unlikely to make any substantial effect on the survival time of the host. If the efficacy can be increased and the precommitment exposure time decreased (to a level compatible with the pharmacodynamics of the agent) by combination with interferon, then major advances might ensue. Clinical trials (see elsewhere in this volume) are underway (45).

BIOCHEMICAL CHANGES ASSOCIATED WITH COMMITMENT. MODULATION OF THE EXPRESSION OF ONCOGENES AND THEIR PRODUCTS

The view that the modulation of oncogene expression plays a pivotal role in the coordinated control of proliferation and differentiation was alluded to above. It has been suggested that regulation of the c-myc oncogene plays a key role in the control of proliferation and differentiation (67), but what that role is remains an enigma, with recent work muddying the picture even further. It has been suggested that the myc product increases the activity of transcriptional promoters for various genes (66) (this experiment was discussed above); on the basis of recent evidence, this appears to be an increasingly attractive tenet.

In MEL (74), HL-60 (39, 49, 93, 110), U937 (32), and DLD-1A colon cells (19) there is a decrease in the expression of myc RNA concommitant with the acquisition of the mature phenotype. In both MEL and HL-60 cells, the changes appear to involve a biphasic response in the early stages of differentiation with an early fall followed by variable, later restoration of expression (33, 74, 131). Yen et al (131) have even suggested that an early rise in HL-60 myc RNA may be related to the acquisition of precommitment memory. Tonini et al (117) recently showed that myc RNA from K562 cells fell only transiently in response to cytosine arabinoside and daunomycin; in later stages of differentiation, when presumably the cells were fully committed, myc m RNA levels rose to those observed in the leukemic cells.

When MEL cells were transfected with the myc gene under the control of a viral promoter, DMSO-induced differentiation was inhibited (30); yet, perhaps paradoxically, in DMSO-resistant cells, both myc and myb RNA decreased after DMSO treatment, in the absence of differentiation (107). Similarly, in a recent paper by Ely et al (33), using a TPA-resistant subline of the HL-60 (HL-60-1E3), the early fall in myc RNA, which was observed in sensitive cells, occurred in the absence of full differentiation. As mentioned above, it is possible that the lesion in these resistant lines may be related to the way that these temporal changes in myc are coupled to subsequent events; therefore, it may be premature to assume that an early fall in myc RNA is not a vital event in the cascade leading to terminal differentiation.

In F9 teratocarcinoma cells, the expression of myc seems to be related to proliferation rather than differentiation (27, 31). Perhaps the most puzzling observations have been those of Larsson et al (78) who have shown that treatment of CLL cells with the phorbol ester TPA produced apparently terminal differentiated, immunoglobulin secreting lymphoblasts and plasmablasts, in which myc RNA levels rose 70-fold, and then remained at a value 20-fold higher than the parent cell. Levels of myc protein also rose. The authors suggest that it is possible that myc gene expression actually promotes differentiation in these cells, and as mentioned above, perhaps the role of myc as an element involved in transcriptional control is more compatible with these observations.

Calabretta (16) has provided evidence that the induction of c-fos, which is observed in the differentiation of myeloid cell lines, may be also dissociated from differentiation. He used lines which do not differentiate after TPA treatment (K562 and K-Gla), and showed an induction of c-fos RNA. Treatment of HL-60 and U-937 cells with diacylglycerols activated protein kinase C, but failed to induce their differentiation despite the expression of c-fos RNA. Experiments of this type with the diacylglycerols were discussed above, and are also open to criticism. Nevertheless, it is clear that the expression of the fos gene is not sufficient in itself to account for the commitment of the cells to terminal differentiation.

These recent studies highlight the need to study different cell types, particularly those which have a natural or induced resistance to an agent, in attempt to test hypotheses that changes in oncogene expression are integrally involved in processes which are driving differentiation. Perhaps one criticism of much of this work is that most studies report changes in the transcription of oncogenes without measuring changes in the protein content of oncogene products, and it is possible that changes regulated posttranslationally may be as important as those at transcription. At this moment in time, it cannot be claimed that a clear role for oncogene expression in differentiation has emerged.

INTERACTIONS BETWEEN INTERFERONS, GROWTH FACTORS, AND ONCOGENES

Proteins encoded by oncogenes might be involved in cell proliferation by:
i) acting as intracellular growth stimulatory substances either in the cytoplasm or in the nucleus; ii) mimicking growth factors; or iii) imitating occupied growth factor receptors (59). Interferons (IFNs) have been shown to affect the expression of oncogenes in each of these groups. In RS485, an LTR-activated c-Ha-ras1-transformed mouse cell line, prolonged interferon treatment resulted in reversion of 1 to 10% of the cells of these cultures. These morphological revertants were then cloned to yield several lines that did not form colonies in soft agar or tumors in nude mice. Analysis of revertants indicated the persistence of the transforming ras DNA, but a 4-8 fold reduction in the Ha-ras mRNA and the Ha-ras encoded p21 protein, as long as the cells were cultured in medium containing interferon (99). This appears to be due to an interferon-mediated transcriptional downregulation of the production of human c-Ha-ras1 mRNA (99, 100). There are a few other reports that interferons can reverse the transformed and tumorigenic phenotype in several cell lines in vitro. Mouse IFN treatment resulted in complete reversion of C3H10T1/2 cells transformed by x-irradiation. Only partial, or no reversion at all was found in the same cell line transformed by methylcholanthrene or SV40 (13, 14).

Other laboratories have reported that the expression of c-Ha-ras and c-src was reduced following interferon treatment of RT4 human bladder carcinoma cells (109); however, interferons were reported to either upregulate the expression of c-Ki-ras (34), or have no effect on c-Ki-ras, c-Ha-ras, or N-ras expression (15). Treatment of Rous sarcoma virus-transformed rat cells resulted in both reduced synthesis of the product of src, pp60^{src}, and decreased expression of the transformed phenotype (8). Treatment of mouse fibroblasts transformed by myeloproliferative sarcoma virus (which contains the v-mos oncogene) with mouse IFN induced morphological reversion and a reduction in cloning efficiency in soft agar and in cell proliferative activity. There was also a selective reduction in all retroviral mRNA levels, possibly due to an inhibition of viral LTR enhancer activity. Upon removal of the interferon, retroviral gene expression increased to pre-treatment levels, and the transformed phenotype reappeared (105). Prolonged treatment with mouse interferon of several cell lines (134), including Balb/c cells transformed by Moloney murine sarcoma virus, also resulted in the appearance of revertant cells. The persistence of the transforming mos oncogene in the Balb/c revertants was indicated by hybridization with a v-mos probe,

focus-formation by transfecting DNA extracted from the
revertants, and the presence of two mos-specific mRNA forms
(106).

Five groups have reported that interferon regulates c-myc
expression (34, 61, 63, 65, 84). Two laboratories have found
that myc inhibition in Daudi cells was due to negative
regulation at a post-transcriptional level (68, 84); one, at the
level of transcription (65). Studies in HeLa cells indicated
that while HuIFN or downregulated c-myc expression, treatment
with HuIFN stimulated it (63).

In the case of oncogenes that simulate growth factors, the
chain of human platelet-derived growth factor (PDGF) closely
resembles the oncogene v-sis (59). PDGF mediates an increase in
the intracellular levels of the mRNAs for actin, c-myc, c-fos,
and ornithine decarboxylase (ODC); interferon antagonizes these
effects of PDGF (65). Recent studes on cell replication have
focused on the effects of oncogenes and growth factors that
stimulate cell proliferation. Interferons inhibit the mitogenic
actions not only of PDGF, but also of various other
growth-stimulatory factors including epidermal growth factor
(EGF) (137). Tumor necrosis factor (TNF) exerts a mitotic
effect on human diploid cells, in which TNF also inhibits virus
growth. Studies indicate that IFN $_2$ induced by TNF is
responsible for the latter activity: antibody to HuIFN $_1$
enhanced the mitogenic activity of TNF suggesting that IFN $_2$
induction by TNF is involved in a negative feedback mechanism
regulating cell growth (70).

Several oncogenes have growth factor receptor activity:
v-erbB, for instance, is homologous to the receptor for EGF.
Short-term treatment with interferon increases EGF binding to
MDBK cells, but longer treatment results in a very significant
decrease in EGF binding, due to decreased EGF receptor number
and affinity (135).

Spontaneous interferon production appears to occur in some
systems where it may be associated with growth regulation.
These studies include growth-arrested mouse leukemic cells
during terminal differentiation (44), density-inhibited human
melanoma cells (25), and the growth of synchronized mouse
fibroblasts (127). A 22,000 Da protein, which was similar to
IL-2, stimulated HuIFN production (123). PDGF also induced
the production of IFN in mouse fibroblasts (137). These
results taken together suggest that some growth factors are
interferon inducers that may exert their regulatory activity at
least in part through their ability to induce interferon.
Specifically, the interferon involved seems to be a species of
IFN , which acts as an autocrine negative regulator of growth
and differentiation. A. Kimchi (personal communication) found
that addition of antibody directed against mouse IFN to
untransformed baby rat kidney cells that had been transfected
with the ras oncogene resulted in their transformation. In
previous studies, transfection by a second oncogene was

necessary for such a transformation to occur. This work suggests that interferon is normally secreted in such a system, and that this interferon is required to maintain the cells in a non-transformed state. Inhibition of the response to endogenous interferon may therefore be a step in the direction of oncogenic transformation, so that autocrine interferon production may be one important mechanism in normal cellular growth regulation.

CONCLUDING COMMENTS

We began this review by asking whether there was any common ground upon which those interested in the mechanism of action and pharmacology of differentiating agents could focus. Certainly, those of us who are interested in the promotion of differentiation by cytotoxic drugs would wish to find common ground with regard to how these drugs bring about cell death--by processes which are largely undefined--and if, and how these events might lead to cell differentiation in selected cell types, when the drugs are used at marginally toxic concentrations. If it is generally true that terminal differentiation requires separable commitment events and a limited proliferative potential, how is it going to be possible to design a drug which promotes terminal differentiation without non-selectively inhibiting the proliferation of normal tissues?

It is the pharmacologists' role to chose models of tumor cell differentiation which might lead to novel, clinically efficacious modes of treatment. There have been few attempts to apply the knowledge of in vitro systems in vivo. Recent understanding of the accumulation of commitment memory suggests that agents like HMBA do not need to be maintained at steady concentrations for extended periods: pulse treatment, to accumulate commitment memory might be as efficacious and less host-toxic, as well as being more compatible with the pharmacokinetic profiles of the agents. The use of biological response modifiers to enhance commitment, and to shorten the period required for accumulation of precommitment memory should lead to dramatic increases of efficacy in this respect.

Finally, in considering differentiation therapy as a potential therapeutic modality, we must ask what we can learn from the 40-year struggle of cancer chemotherapy with the realities of a lack of selectivity, drug-induced resistance, poor drug delivery, and inherent tumor heterogeneity. Is not the induction of differentiation just another way of enhancing cell death? We are likely to face many of the same problems, but at least we have that 40 years' experience to build on!

ACKNOWLEDGEMENTS.

The authors wish to thank the many members of the Pharmacology and Mechanisms of Action Group associated with this meeting for sending their thoughts, unpublished work, and many published papers for us to review. We apologize to them if we have been grossly insensitive to their varied insights, but we are sure they are sympathetic to our plight! JAH wishes to thank Frances Richards for criticism and helpful comments.

REFERENCES

1. Ananthan, J., Golberg, A.L. and Voellmy, R. (1986):Science, 232:522-524.
2. Baez, M., Sargan, D.R., Elbrecht, A., Kulomaa, M.S., Zarucki, Schulz, T., Tsai, M-J. and O'Malley, B.W. (1987):J. Biol. Chem., 262:6582-6588.
3. Ball, E.D., Howell, A.L. and Shen, L. (1986):Exp. Hematol., 14:998-1005.
4. Barbacid, M. (1986):Carcinogenesis, 7:1037-1042.
5. Bishop, J.M. (1987):Science, 235:305-311.
6. Bensaude, O., Babinet, C. and Morange, M. (1983):Nature, 305:31-333.
7. Berger, N.A. (1986):J. Clin. Invest., 78:1131-1135.
8. Berridge, M.J. (1984):Biochem. J., 229:345-360.
9. Beutler, B., Krochin, N., Milsark, I.W., Luedke, C. and Cerami, A. (1986):Science, 232:977-980.
10. Bojan, F., Kinsella, A.R. and Fox, M. (1983): Cancer Res., 43:5217-5221.
11. Bourgeade, M.F., Rousse, T.S., Paulin, D., and Chany, C. (1981):J. Interferon Res., 1:323-332.
12. Brosjo, O., Bauer, H.C., Brostrom, L.A., Nilsson, O.S., Reinholt, F.P. and Tribukait, B. (1987):Cancer Res., 47:258-262.
13. Brouty-Boye, D., Cheng, Y-S.E., and Chen, L.B. (1981):Cancer Res., 41:4174-4184.
14. Brouty-Boye, D. and Gresser, I. (1981):Int. J. Cancer, 28:165-173.
15. Brouty-Boye, D., Wybier-Franqui, J., Nardeux, P., Daya-Grosjean, L., Andeol, Y. and Suarez, H.G. (1986):J. Interferon Res., 6:461-471.
16. Calabretta, B. (1987):Mol. Cell Biol., 7:769-774.
17. Chany, C. and Vignal, M. (1970):J. Gen. Microbiol. 7:203-210.
18. Chasseaud, L.F. (1979):Adv. Cancer Res., 29:175-274.
19. Chatterjee, D., Shank, P.R. and Savarese, T.M. (1986):Proc. Amer. Assoc. Cancer Res., 27:9.
20. Chen, E., Karr, R.W., Frost, J.P., Gonwa, T.A. and Ginder, G.D. (1986): Mol. Cell Biol., 6:1698-1705.
21. Chen, Z-X., Banks, J., Rifkind, R.A. and Marks, P.A. (1982):Proc. Natl. Acad. Sci., USA, 79:471-475.
22. Chou, R.H., Chen, T.A., Churchill, J.R., Thompson, S.W. and Chou, K.L. (1986):Biochem. Biophys. Res. Commun., 141:213-221.
22a. Chow, K-C and Ross, W.E. (1987):Mol. Cell Biol., 7:3119-3123.

23. Collins, S.J., Ruscetti, F.W., Gallagher, R.E. and Gallo, R.C. (1978): Proc. Natl. Acad. Sci., USA, 75:1458-2462.
24. Corin, R.E., Haspel, H.C., Peretz, A.M., Sonenberg, M. and Rifkind, R.A. (1986):Cancer Res., 46:1136-1141.
25. Creasey, A.A., Eppstein, D., Marsh, Y.V., Khan, F., and Merigan, T. (1983):Mol. Cell. Biol., 3:780-786.
26. Davis, J.Q., Dansereau, D., Johnstone, R.M. and Bennett, V. (1986):J. Biol. Chem., 261:15368-15371.
27. Dean, M.A., Levine, R.A. and Campisi, J. (1986):Mol. Cell Biol., 6:518-524.
28. Deusberg, P.H. (1985):Science, 228-669-677.
29. Dexter, D.L., Barbosa, J.A. and Calabresi, P. (1979):Cancer Res., 39:1020-1025.
30. Dmitrovsky, E., Kuehl, W.M., Hollis, G.F., Kirsch, I.R., Bender, T.P. and Segal, S. (1986):Nature, 322:748-750.
31. Dony, C., Kessel, M. and Gruss, P. (1985):Nature, 317:636-639.
32. Einat, M., Resnitzky, D. and Kimchi, A. (1985):Nature, 313-597-600.
33. Ely, C.M., Leftwich, J.A., Chevenix-Trent, G., Hall, R.E. and Westin, E.H. (1987):Cancer Res., 47:4595-4600.
34. Emanoil-Ravier, R., Pochart, F., Canavet, M., Garcette, M., Tobaly-Tapierd, J. and Peries, J. (1985):J. Interferon Res., 5:613-619.
35. Falletto, D.L. and Macara, I.G. (1985):J. Biol. Chem., 260:4884-4889.
36. Farzaneh, F., Meldrum, R., and Shall, S. (1987) Nucleic Acids Res., 24:3493-3502.
37. Fibach, E., Gambari, R., Shaw, P.A., Maniatis, G., Reuben, R.C., Sassa, S., Rifkind, R.A. and Marks, P.A. (1979):Proc. Natl. Acad. Sci., USA, 76:1906-1910.
38. Fibach, E., Peled, T., Treves, A., Kornberg, A. and Rachmilewitz, E.A. (1982):Leuk. Res., 6:781-790.
39. Filmus, J. and Buick, R.N. (1985):Cancer Res., 45:822-825.
40. Francis, G.E., Berney, J.J., North, P.S., Khan, Z., Wilson, E.L., Jacobs, P. and Ali, M., Leukemia, in press. 41.
41. Francis, G.E. and Pinsky, C., Growth and differentiation control. In EORTC Cancer chemotherapy and biological response modifiers Annual 9, Eds. Pinedo, H.M., Chabner, B.A. and Longo, D.L., Elsevier, Amsterdam, in press.
42. Franks, N.P. and Lieb, W.R. (1984):Nature, 310:599-601.
43. Franks, N.P. and Lieb, W.R. (1986):Arch. Toxicol., Suppl. 9, 27-37.
44. Friedman-Einat, M., Revel, M., and Kimcai, A. (1982): Mol. Cell. Biol., 2:1472-1480.
45. Gallagher, R.E., Lurie, K.J., Leavitt, R.D. and Wiernik, P.H. Leukemia Res., in press.
46. Gallicchio, V.S. (1985):Exp. Cell. Biol., 53:287-293.
47. Girard, P.R., Stevens, V.L., Blackshear, P.J., Merrill, A.H., Wood, J.G. and Kuo, J.F. (1987):Cancer Res., 47:2892-2898.

48. Gottesfeld, J.M. (1986):Nucl. Acids Res., 14:2075-2088.
49. Grosso, L.E. and Pitot, H.C. (1984):Biochem. Biophys. Res. Commun., 119:473-480.
50. Gusella, J., Geller, R., Clarke, B., Weeks, V. and Housman, D. (1976):Cell, 9:221-229.
51. Hahn, G.M., Shiu, E.C., West, B., Goldstein, L. and Li, G.C. (1985): Cancer Res., 45:4138-4143.
52. Hamer, D.H. (1986):Ann. Rev. Biochem., 55:913-951.
53. Hawkins, M.J., Hoth, D.F. and Wittes, R.E. (1986):Sem. Oncol. 13:132-140.
54. Hemmi, H. and Breitman, T.R. (1987):Blood, 69:501-507.
55. Hickman, J.A. and Richards, F.M. (1987):Proc. Amer. Assoc. Cancer Res., 28:46.
56. Higgins, P.J. (1986):Int. J. Cancer, 38:889-899.
57. Hill, A.B. and Schimke, R.T. (1985):Cancer Res., 45:5050-5057.
58. Huberman, E. and Callaham, M.F. (1979):Proc. Natl. Acad. Sci. USA, 76:1293-1297.
59. Hunter, T. (1985):Trends Biochem., 10:275-280.
60. Imperiale, M.J., Kao, H-T., Feldman, L.T., Nevins, J.R. and Strickland, S. (1984):Molec. Cell. Biol., 4:867-874.
61. Jonak, G.J. and Knight, E., JR. (1984):Proc. Natl. Acad. Sci. USA, 81:1747-1750.
62. Kaczmarek, L., Calabretta, B., Kao, H-T., Heintz, N., Nevins, J. and Baserga, R. (1987):J. Cell. Biol. 104:183-187.
63. Kelly, J.M., Gilbert, C.S., Stark, G.R., and Kerr, I.M. (1985):Cur. J. Biochem., 153:367-371.
64. Khan, Z. and Francis, G.E. (1987):Blood. 69:1114-1119.
65. Kimchi, A., Yarden, A., Gat, G. and Resnitzsky, D. (1985):In:The 2-5A System: Molecular and Clinical Aspects of the Interferon Regulated Pathway, edited by B.R.G. Williams and R.H. Silverman, pp 185-202. Alan R. Less, Inc. New York.
66. Kingston, R.E., Bladwin, A.S. JR. and Sharp, P.A. (1984): 312, 280-282.
67. Klein, G. and Klein, E. (1985):Nature, 315:190-195.
68. Knight, E. JR., Anton, E.D., Fahey, D., Friedland, B.K. and Jonak, G.J. (1985):Proc. Natl. Acad. Sci. USA, 82:1151-1154.
69. Koeffler, H.P. (1986):Semin. Hematol., 23:223-236.
70. Kohase, M., Henrickson-Destefano, D., May, L.T., Vilcek, J. and Sehgal, P.B. (1986):Cell, 45:659-666.
71. Kohlhepp, E.A., Condon, M.E. and Hamburger, A.W., (1987):Exp. Haematol., 15:414-418.
72. Kreutter, D., Caldwell, A.B. and Morin, M.J. (1985):J. Biol. Chem., 260:5979-5984.
73. Kurtz, S., Rossi, J., Petko, L. and Lindquist, S. (1986):Science, 231, 1154-1157.
74. Lachman, H. M. and Skoultchi, A.I. (1984):Nature, 310:592-594.

75. Landry, J. and Chretien, P. (1983):Can. J. Biochem. Cell
    Biol., 61:428–437.
76. Langdon, S.P. and Hickman, J.A. (1987):Cancer Res.,
    47:140–144.
77. Langdon, S.P., Richards, F.M. and Hickman, J.A. Leukemia
    Res., in press.
78. Larsson, L–G., Gary, H.E., Totterman, T., Pettersson, U. and
    Nillson, K. (1987):Proc. Natl. Acad. Sci. USA,
    84:223–227.
79. Levenson, R. and Housman, D. (1979):Cell, 17:485–490.
80. Levenson, R. and Housman, D. (1981):Devel. Biol. 86:81–86.
81. Lin, S.L., Garber, E.A., Wang, E., Calguiri, L.A.,
    Schellekens, H., Goldberg, A.R. and Tamm, I. (1983):Mol.
    Cell. Biol., 13:1656–1664.
82. Lindahl, T. (1987):Br. J. Cancer, 56:91–95.
83. Lindquist, S. (1986):Ann. Rev. Biochem., 55:1151–1191.
84. Mechti, N., Blanchard, J.M., Picchaczyk, M., Dani, C.,
    Jeantelle, P and Lebleu, B. (1985):In: The Interferon
    System, edited by F. Dianzani and B.B. Ripsi, pp.
    423–428, Raven Press, New York.
85. Nomura, S. and Dishi, M. (1983):Proc. Natl. Acad. Sci. USA.,
    80:210–214.
86. Nomura, S., Yamagoe, S., Kamiya, T. and Oishi, M.
    (1986):Cell, 44:663–669.
87. Marks, P.A., Sheffrey, M. and Rifkind, R.A. (1987): Cancer
    Res., 47:659–666.
88. Milarski, K.L. and Morimoto, R.I. (1986):Proc. Natl. Acad.
    Sci. USA, 83:9517–9521.
89. Mitchell, T., Sariban, E. and Kufe, E. (1986):Mol.
    Pharmacol., 30:398–402.
90. Morin, M.J., Cross, S.M. and Squinto, S.P. (1987):Proc.
    Amer. Assoc. Cancer Res., 28:47; and personal
    communication.
91. Morin, M.J., Kreutter, D., Rasmussen, H. and Sartorelli,
    A.C. (1987):J. Biol. Chem., 262:11758–11763.
92. Murate, T., Kaneda, T., Rifkind, R.A. and Marks, P.A.
    (1984):Proc. Natl. Acad. Sci. USA., 81:3394–3398.
93. Okazaki, R., Mochizuku, T., Tashima, M., Sawada, H. and
    Uchino, H. (1987):J. Cell Physiol., 131:50–57.
94. Pelham, H.R.B. (1986):Cell, 46:959–961.
95. Pestka, S., Langer, J.A., Zoon, K.C. and Samuel, C.E.
    (1987):Ann. Rev. Biochem., 56:727–777.
96. Raaphorst, G.P., Azzam, E.I., Borsa, J. Einspenner, M. and
    Vdasz, J.A. (1984):Canad. J. Biochem. Cell. Biol.,
    62:1091–1096.
97. Rovera, G. and Surrey, S. (1978):Cancer Res., 38:3737–3744.
98. Sachs, L. (1986):Cell Biophys., 9:225–242.
99. Samid, D., Chang, E.H. and Friedman, R.M. (1984):Biochem.
    Biophy. Res. Comm., 119:21–28.

100. Samid, D. and Friedman, R.M. (1986):In: <u>Interferons As Cell Growth Inhibitors and Antitumor Factors</u>, edited by R.M. Friedman, T. Sreevalsen, and T. Merigan, pp. 413-422. Alan R. Liss, Inc. New York.

101. Sartorelli, A.C., Ishiguro, K., King, C.L., Morin, M.J. and Reiss, M. (1986):Adv. Enzyme Regul., 25:507-529.

102. Sahyoun, N., Wolf, M., Besterman, J., Hsieh, T-S., Sander, M., Levine, H., Chang, K-J. and Cuatrecasas, P. (1986):Proc. Natl. Acad. Sci. USA., 83:1603-1607.

103. Schimke, R.T. (1984):Cancer Res., 44:1735-1742.

104. Schwartz, E.L. Maher, A. and Nilson, L. (1987):Proc. Amer. Assoc. Cancer Res., 28:43, and personal communication.

105. Selinger, B., Krupa, G., and Peizenmaur, K. (1987):J. Virol., 61:2567-2572.

106. Sergiescu, D., Gerfaux, J., Joret, A.M., and Chang, C. (1986):Proc. Natl. Acad. Sci. USA, 83:5764-5768.

107. Sherman, M.L., Yee, N.S. and Kufe, D.W. (1987):Proc. Amer. Associ. Cancer Res., 28:195.

108. Singh, M.K. and Yu, J. (1984):Nature, 309:631-633.

109. Soslaw, G., Bogucki, A.R., Gillespie, D. and Bubbell, H.R. (1984):Biochem. Biophys. Res. Comm., 119:941-948.

110. Slungaard, A., Confer, D.L. and Schuback, W.H. (1987):J. Clin. Invest., 79:1542-1547.

111. Spremulli, E.N. and Dexter, D.L. (1984):J. Clin. Oncol., 2:227-241.

112. Steinbertz, P.G., Rosen, G., Gharimi, F., Wany, Y. and Miller, D.R. (1980):J. Pediat., 96:923-927.

113. Strom, C.M. and Dorfman, A. (1976):Proc. Natl. Acad. Sci. USA., 73:3428-3432.

114. Subjeck, J.R. and Thung-Tai, S. (1986):Am. J. Physiol., 250:C1-C17.

115. Takuma, T., Takeda, K. and Konno, K. (1987):Biochem. Biophys. Res. Commun., 145:514-521.

116. Tarella, C., Ferrero, D., Gallo, E., Pagliardi, G.L. and Ruscetti, F.W. (1982):Cancer Res., 42:445-449.

117. Tonini, G.P., Radzioch, D., Gronberg, A., Clayton, M., Blasdi, E., Bennetton, G. and Varesio, L. (1987): Cancer Res., 47:4544-4547.

118. Traganos, F., Higgins, P.J., Bueti, C., Darzynkiewicz, Z. and Melamed, M.R. (1984):J. Natl. Cancer Inst., 73:205-218.

119. Tsiftsoglou, A.S., Hensold, J., Robinson, S.H. and Wong, W., in New Avenues in Developmental Cancer Chemotherapy, pp. 205-227, Academic Press, New York, 1987.

120. Tsiftsoglou, A.S., Housman, D. and Wong, W. (1984):Proc. Amer. Assoc. Cancer Res., 25:47.

121. Tsiftsoglou, A.S., Mitrani, A. and Housman, F. (1981): J. Cell Physiol., 108:327-335.

122. Tsiftsoglou, A. S. and Wong, W. (1985):Anticancer Res., 5:81-100.

123. Van Damme, J., Opdenakker, G., Billeau, A., Desomer, P., Dewit, L., Poupart, Pond Content, J. (1985):J. Gen. Virol. 66:693-700.
124. Varshavsky, A. (1981):Proc. Natl. Acad. Sci. USA., 78:3673-3677.
125. Von Melchner, H. and Hoffken, K. (1985):J. Cell Physiol. 125:573-581.
126. Wang, J.K. Johnson, M.D., Morgan, J.I. and Spector, S. (1986): Mol. Pharmacol. 30:639-642.
127. Wells, V. and Mallucci, L. (1985):Exp. Cell Res., 159:27-36.
128. Yamamoto, S., Gotoh, H., Aizu, E. and Katoh, R. (1985):J. Biol. Chem., 260:14230-14234.
129. Yen, A., Forbes, M., DeGala, G. and Fishbaugh, J. (1987):Cancer Res., 47:129-134.
130. Yen, A., Freeman, L. and Fishbaugh, J. (1987):Leukemia Res., 11:63-71.
131. Yen, A., Guernsey, D., Burtraw, G. and Fischbaugh, J. (1987):Proc. Amer. Assoc. Cancer. Res., 28:163.
132. Yoshioka, A., Tanaka, S., Hiraoka, O., Koyama, Y., Hirota, Y., Ayusawa, D., Seno, T., Garret, C. and Wataya, Y. (1987):J. Biol. Chem., 262:8235-8241.
133. Zaricznyj, C. and Macara, I.G. (1986): Exp. Cell Res., 168: 402-410.
134. Zilberstein, A., Ruggieri, R. and Revel, M. (1985):In: The Interferon System, edited by F. Dianzani and G.B. Rossi, pp. 73-83. Raven Press, New York.
135. Zoon, K.C., Karasaki, Y., Zurnedden, D.L., Hu, R. and Arnheiter, H. (1986):Proc. Natl. Acad. Sci. USA, 83:8826-8830.
136. Zuckier, G., and Tritton, T.R. (1983): Exp. Cell Res., 148:155-161.
137. Zullo, J.N., Cochram, B.H., Huang, A.S. and Stiles, C.D. (1985):Cell, 43:793-800.

Induced Differentiation of Human Urinary Bladder Carcinoma

R.A. Rifkind, P. Russo and P.A. Marks

*The DeWitt Wallace Laboratory of Developmental Cell Biology
and the Urology Service, Department of Surgery, Memorial
Sloan-Kettering Cancer Center, New York, NY 10021*

Evidence from studies on murine erythroleukemia cells (MELC) and a broad range of other transformed cell lines of human origin and non-human species indicate that the transformed phenotype can be altered by exposure to one of the polar-planar group of differentiation inducers, including hexamethylene bisacetamide (HMBA) (26,27). Recent studies with MELC have defined early changes in cell function and gene expression, which occur in HMBA-exposed MELC during the period prior to irreversible commitment to terminal cell division and differentiation and prior to the onset of accelerated transcription of those genes, such as the globin genes, which characterize the differentiated state (27). Evidence that HMBA-mediated MELC differentiation involves a protein-kinase C-related mechanism and, in particular, the activity of the proteolytically activated, Ca^{2+} and phospholipid independent, form of that kinase, has been presented (30). In addition, early modulation of expression of several of the nuclear oncogenes, including c-myb, c-myc, c-fos and the p53 protein has been detected in several laboratories (21,22,34,37,41). Although gene transfection studies have shown that perturbing the expression of c-myc can modify the kinetics of induced differentiation (6,11,23), the mechanisms linking these early c-onc responses following HMBA administration to the eventual commitment of MELC to terminal differentiation have not yet been established. Nevertheless, taken together, these investigations and a broad array of data from related systems, have prompted the implementation of further studies designed to test the potential of differentiation inducers, particularly HMBA, as a modality for altering the oncogenicity of human tumor cells in the clinical setting. As a first step, phase I clinical trials designed to establish toxicological constraints and dosage parameters have been undertaken at a number of institutions, and these are reported elsewhere in this volume (Egorin et al; and 4,12,35).

We have initiated a combined laboratory and clinical program, designed to focus on a clinically significant cancer apparently well-suited as a candidate for the application of differentiation therapy employing HMBA or other differentiating agents. The condition selected is carcinoma-in-situ (CIS) of the urinary bladder, chosen because it answers to a number of criteria which appear of importance to a clinical trial designed to elicit potential efficacy.

What are reasonable criteria for design of a useful advanced Phase I/Phase II study of a candidate differentiation agent? These could include:

1. A tumor from which there can be developed an in vitro, cell culture-based system with which to determine phenotypic characteristics that can be measured as evidence of the biological activity of the agent and in which to study the effects of the differentiation agent upon the tumor cells. Although preliminary studies can employ transformed human cell lines from the organ in question, the use of relatively freshly explanted tumor cells, growing under conditions which allow sufficient time for in vitro testing, is important in order to validate the induced phenotypic change in cells most closely approximating those found in the original tumor, and in order to develop a predictive assay for the purpose of screening potentially sensitive tumors.

2. A readily measurable set of markers which can identify malignant and differentiated cells of the tumor lineage. Some of these should be characteristics other than the criterion of growth potential. Although growth potential might appear to be the most significant criterion for an effective strategy, our experience with differentiation agents and clinical tumors is too limited to close our judgment to the implications of other characteristics of phenotypic modulation and their potential impact on the natural history of a cancer. Furthermore, such markers may provide a relatively simple means for evaluating success or failure in terms of successful or unsuccessful phenotypic modulation of the tumor during clinical administration of the agent, and provide criteria for adjusting the rate of administration of the agent. Indeed, it may be anticipated that these markers could provide important early evidence of efficacy, long before assessment of changes in the natural history of the tumor may be possible.

3. A tumor site which can be regularly sampled during the course of therapy in order to observe directly the modulation of phenotype. The least invasive approach possible

is clearly desirable as are procedures employed routinely in the normal management and follow-up of the disease.

    4. A tumor site to which adequate levels of the agent can be delivered without undue toxicity. With respect to HMBA, there is a relatively sharp peak of effective concentration, based on in vitro studies of MELC and other cell lines (26). To date, such levels (4-5mM) have not been achieved in patients due to reversible but unacceptable toxicity at rates of administration of the agent which result in serum levels above 1-2mM (12,35), including acidosis, neurological symptoms and thrombocytopenia.

    5. A tumor for which development of alternative therapy remains an imperative.

In the context of these criteria, carcinoma of the urinary bladder provides an attractive target for study of the potential effects of the differentiation agent, HMBA, for a number of reasons. Bladder .cancer is the third most prevalent malignant disease among men and tenth among women (13), with over 40,000 new cases reported annually in the United States. Of these, 70-80% are superficial (stages Ta, CIS and T1)); the rest are invasive (T2-4), accounting for about 10,000 deaths each year (39). Therapy for CIS, a high grade malignancy confined to the urothelial lining of the bladder is far from satisfactory (29); following transurethral resection alone the recurrence rate is 90% and in 50% there is progression to invasion and metastasis. Resection plus intravesical BCG, the current standard, still leaves recurrence in 40% (17). Failure at this stage leaves only radical cystectomy and urinary diversion or experimental chemotherapies.

Cancer of the urinary bladder can be, and is routinely, diagnosed and followed on a regular basis by cystocoscopy, during which shed malignant cells are recovered in significant quantities, by saline barbotage or by biopsy. These shed cells are routinely made available for diagnostic cytometry (flow cytometry for DNA content) and cytology; they can, in addition, be a source of cells for the establishment of short term cultures in vitro (36). Furthermore, bladder urothelial cells have been extensively studied with respect to their expression of a variety of antigens detectable by monoclonal antibodies, and patterns of expression characteristic of normal differentiation and malignant transformation have been described (5,7,8,9,14,15,24). These antigens include the blood group antigens, some relatively specific urothelial antigens, as well as less specific epithelial antigens such as the intermediary filaments.

Finally, although optimally effective serum concentrations

of HMBA (4-5mM) have not yet been achieved, as already noted, the urine is the principle route of excretion of unaltered HMBA and its major, active metabolites (3,28,35) and Egorin and co-workers (personal communication) have determined that effective levels are readily achieved in bladder urine following parenteral administration of relatively low, non-toxic doses of the agent.

Malignant (10,31,32) and normal (18,19) urothelial cells have been successfully grown in tissue culture on glass and plastic substrates, but more efficient growth requires an extracellular matrix (ECM) substrate, secreted by endothelial cells such as from the bovine cornea (1,16,33). Under these conditions bladder urothelium derived from barbotage (saline irrigation) during cystoscopy will attach and initiate a culture which can be sustained for 6 weeks or more in a standard medium (αMEM, penicillin, streptomycin and 20% fetal calf serum) with passages upon confluency (36). Unlike cultures derived from biopsy material, these cultures are free of fibroblast contamination and do not become over-grown as is the common experience with bladder biopsy cultures. Five of the 7 cases, which constitute our preliminary experience with this system, displayed a fraction of distinctly aneuploid (hyperdiploid) cells on DNA cytofluorometry of the cells recovered at cystoscopy. Following culture, a marked increase in the aneuploid cell population was observed in the cultures, even when the original fraction of aneuploid cells was very small or undetectable.

Two different differentiation-inducing agents were selected for the preliminary study of CIS urothelium in vitro, cis-retinoic acid (RA), which can initiate phenotypic changes in embryonal carcinoma lines (40), HL-60 human leukemia (2,20), melanoma (25) and neuroblastoma (38), and HMBA, whose actions have been described above. Following successful culture of cells recovered from cystoscopy, $1.5-2.5 \times 10^4$ tumor cells were plated on ECM coated 35 mm petrie dishes in the presence and absence of HMBA (5mM) or RA (5×10^{-8}M). Individual plates were harvested on every 2nd day and cell counts and trypan blue exclusion determined to establish the effect of the differentiation inducers on proliferation and viability. After 6 days in culture cells growing in slide-quality growth chambers were subject to immunoperoxidase staining with a panel of monoclonal antibodies to detect effects of the inducers on the expression of a selected group of antigens (36), which include:

1. Prekeratin intermediate filaments, characteristic of epithelial cells, not fibroblasts or lymphoid cells.
2. MoAb T16-reactive ubiquitous bladder urothelial antigen.

3. MoAb T43-reactive antigen found on invasive and metastatic bladder urothelium.

4. The blood group precursor Type I, expressed in many malignant bladder urothelia, but not expressed in normal urothelium.

5. The blood group substance, Lewis^X, expressed predominantly in malignant bladder urothelium.

Within 2-4 days of culture with HMBA, cell growth essentially ceased, in all 7 cases, without evidence of cytotoxicity, as measured by dye exclusion. With RA, on the other hand, the growth response was inconstant; growth was increased (compared to control cells) in one, unaltered in 4, and decreased in two. With respect to the antigenic markers, a fairly constant pattern of response to HMBA was detected, which included suppressed expression of the T16 urothelial antigen, the blood group precursor and Lewis^X. Several of the cultures displayed a change in the intracellular staining pattern for the intermediate filaments, namely a marked perinuclear reorganization of the filaments. The marker for high grade invasive malignancy, T43, was expressed in 3 of the 7 cases, and expression was markedly diminished by HMBA, in two of these three. On the other hand, RA had only inconstant effects on the antigenic phenotype; there was increased expression of the blood group precursor and another malignancy-related antigen, in several instances, and no significant effect on the other antigens.

Taken together, these preliminary studies suggest that bladder urothelial cells, obtained by a relatively non-invasive and routine clinical procedure, can be propagated in vitro under conditions in which aneuploid, presumptive malignant cells are the predominant population. These cells can be tested for their responsiveness to differentiation inducers with respect both to growth potential and to phenotype, expressed as reactivity to a panel of monoclonal antibodies for a number of specific and less specific urothelial antigens. Retinoic acid caused little or no change in growth pattern (indeed, there was accelerated growth in one instance), nor in antigen expression (in fact, augmented expression of two antigens associated with high grade malignancy was detected). HMBA, on the other hand, regularly suppressed growth (without overt cytotoxicity) and altered expression of the antigen pattern in a fashion consistent with progression toward a less malignant, more normal urothelial phenotype.

Based upon these observations, an advanced Phase I study is currently in progress at Memorial Sloan-Kettering Cancer Center, designed to define the tolerability of chronic, low dosage HMBA, given in three 30-day courses, by continuous infusion, to patients with CIS of the urinary bladder. This study examines the ability of HMBA to alter the proliferative capacity and antigenic profile of each patient's bladder urothelium, in vivo, and will address the duration of persistence of phenotypic change, if there is such, after cessation of HMBA administration, as well as the reproducibility of the effect during repeated courses of therapy. This study will also provide evidence as to the predictive value of in vitro screening of shed urothelium with regard to the effectiveness of HMBA as a clinically effective phenotype modifier. The experimental design also provides a potentially effective approach to the study of more complex combinations of differentiation agents and other chemotherapeutic agents. Longer range studies, directed at detecting modification of the natural history of CIS of the urinary bladder, await the results of these preliminary investigations.

This work was supported, in part, by grants from the National Cancer Institute (CA-31768 and CA-08748) and the Samuel and May Rudin Foundation.

1. Bulbul, M., Pavelic, K., Slocrum, H., Frankfurt, O., Rustam, Y., Huben, R., and Bernacki, R. (1980): J. Urol., 136:512-516.
2. Breitman, T.R., Selonick, S.E., and Collins, S.J. (1980): Proc. Nat. Acad. Sci. USA, 77:2936-2940.
3. Callery, P.S., Egorin, M.J., Geelhaar, L.A., and Nayar, M.S. (1986): Cancer Res., 46:4900-4903.
4. Chun, H., Leyland-Jones, B., Hoth, D., Schoemaker, D., Wolpert-DeFiliposes, M., Grieshaber, C., Cradock, J., Davignon, P., Moon, R., Rifkind, R., and Wittes, R.E. (1986): Cancer Treatment Reports, 70:991-996.
5. Coon, J.S., Pauili, B.U., and Weinstein, R.S. (1983): Cancer Surveys, 2:479-494.
6. Coppola, J.J., and Cole, M.D. (1986): Nature (Lond.), 760-763.
7. Cordon-Cardo, C., Lloyd, K., Finstad, C.L., McGroaty, M.E., Reuter, V.E., Bander, N.H., Old, L.J., and Melamed, M.R. (1986): Lab. Invest., 55:444-453.
8. Cordon-Cardo, C., Reuter, V.E., Lloyd, K., Fair, W.R., Old, L.J., and Melamed, M.R. (1987): Cancer Res. (in press).
9. Davidson, I. (1972): Am. J. Clin. Path., 57:715-719.
10. Dittrich, C., Schmidhauer, C., Havelec, L., Lenzhofer, R., Brecyer, S., Porpaczy, P., and Moser, K. (1986): Oncology, 43:40-45.
11. Dmitrovsky, E., Kuehl, M., Hollis, G.F., Kirsch, I.R., Bender, T.P. and Segal, S. (1986): Nature (Lond.), 322:748-750.

12. Egorin, M., Sigman, L.M., Van Echo, D.A., Forrest, A., Whitacre, M.Y., and Aisner, J. (1987): Cancer Res. 47:617-623.
13. Feldman, A.P., Kessler, L., Myers, M.H., and Naughton, M.D. (1986): New Eng. J. Med., 1394-1397.
14. Fradet, Y., Cordon-Cardo, C., Whitmore, W.F., Melamed, M.R., and Old, L.J. (1984): Proc. Nat. Acad. Sci. USA, 81:224-228.
15. Fradet, Y., Cordon-Cardo, C., Whitmore, W.F., Melamed, M.R. and Old, L.J. (1986): Cancer Res. 46:5183-5188.
16. Gospodarowicz, D., Delgado, D., and Yodavsky, I. (1980): Proc. Nat. Acad. Sci. USA, 77:4094-4098.
17. Herr, H.W., Pinsky, C.M., Whitmore, W.F., Oettgen, H.F., and Melamed, M.R. (1983): Cancer, 51:1323-1326.
18. Herz, F., Suhermer, A., and Koss, L.G. (1979): Proc. Soc. Exp. Biol. Med., 161:153-157.
19. Herz, F., Gazivods, P., Paperhausen, P., Katsuyama, J., and Koss, L. (1985): Lab. Invest., 53:571-574.
20. Imaizumi, M., Uozumi, J., and Breitman, T.R. (1987): Cancer Res. 47:1434-1440.
21. Kirsch, I.R., Bertness, V., Silver, J., and Hollis, G. (1985): In: Leukemia: Recent Advances in Biology and Treatment, pp 91-98. Alan R. Liss, Inc., New York.
22. Lachman, H.M., and Skoultchi, A.I. (1984): Nature (Lond.), 310:592-594.
23. Lachman, H.M., Cheng, G.H., and Skoultchi, A.I. (1986): Proc. Nat. Acad. Sci. USA, 83:6480-6484.
24. Lloyd, K. (1987): Am. J. Clin. Path., 87:129-139.
25. Lotan, R. (1980): Biochem. Biophys. Acta, 605:33-91.
26. Marks, P.A., and Rifkind, R.A. (1978): Annu. Rev. Biochem., 47:419-448.
27. Marks, P.A., Sheffery, M., and Rifkind, R.A. (1987): Cancer Res., 47:659-666.
28. Meilhoc, E., Moutin, M.J., and Osborne, H.B. (1986): Biochem. J., 238:701-707.
29. Melamed, M.R., Vontsa, N.G., and Grabstald, H. (1964): Cancer, 17:1533-1545.
30. Melloni, E., Pontremoli, S., Michetti, M., Sacco, O., Cakiroglu, A.G., Jackson, J.F., Rifkind, R.A., and Marks, P.A. (1987): Proc. Nat. Acad. Sci. USA, 84:5282-5286.
31. Messing, E.M., Fahrey, J.L., Dekernion, J.B., Bhuta, S.M. and Bubbers, J.E. (1982): Cancer Res., 42:2392-2397.
32. Niell, H., Soloway, M.S. and Nissenkorn, I. (1982): J. Urol., 127:668-670.
33. Pode, D., Alon, Y., Horowitz, A., Vlodausky, I.J., and Baionan, S. (1986): J. Urol. 136:482-486.
34. Ramsay, R.G., Ikeda, K., Rifkind, R.A., and Marks, P.A. (1986): Proc. Nat. Acad. Sci. USA, 83:6849-6853.
35. Rowinsky, E.K., Ettinger, D.S., Grochow, L.B., Brundett, R.B., Cates, A.E., and Donehower, R.C. (1986): J.

Clin. Oncol. 4:1835-1844.
36. Russo, P., Sheinfeld, J., Cordon-Cardo, C., Fair, W.R., Marks, P.A. and Rifkind, R.A. (1987): Surgical Forum (in press).
37. Shen, D-W., Real, F.X., DeLeo, A.B., Old, L.J., Marks, .P.A., and Rifkind, R.A. (1983): Proc. Nat. Acad. Sci. USA, 80:5919-5922.
38. Sidell, N. (1982): J. Nat. Cancer Inst., 68:589-593.
39. Silverberg, E. (1984): CA-A Cancer Journal, 34:7-23.
40. Stickland, S., and Mahdavi, V. (1978): Cell, 15:393-403.
41. Todokoro, K., and Ikawa, Y. (1986): Biochem. Biophys. Res. Commun., 135:1112-1118.

DESIGN OF IN VIVO MODELS FOR DIFFERENTIATION THERAPY

In Vivo Model Systems for Differentiation Therapy of Leukemia and Solid Tumors

T.R. Breitman[1] and M.I. Sherman[2]

[1]*Laboratory of Biological Chemistry, Developmental Therapeutics Program, Division of Cancer Treatment, National Cancer Institute, National Institutes of Health, Bethesda, Maryland 20892 and*
[2]*Department of Oncology and Virology, Roche Research Center, Nutley, New Jersey 07110*

INTRODUCTION

It is clear from other contributions at this conference that there has been considerable effort to clarify mechanisms of action of differentiation inducers on both normal and malignant cell types and to discover new agents, both natural and synthetic, that induce this phenomenon. While progress is encouraging, application for treatment of human malignancies is still at an early stage.

One hurdle for the application of differentiation therapy is the development of in vivo models to study if agents active under the relatively controlled conditions in vitro are also active in the more complex and less predictable animal environment. For example, many studies in vitro are performed with defined culture conditions that are manipulated easily. In addition, in vitro systems are amenable to a battery of tests for differentiation. Thus, even "a little differentiation" is usually observed in vitro. Studies in vivo do not have a comparable experimental luxury.

There are many animal models for cytotoxic cancer chemotherapy. While animals bearing some tumors are cured with cytotoxic drugs, the direct application of these results to treatment of patients has had limited success. Furthermore, attempts to establish and to test cytotoxic therapies with human tumors in in vivo models has been even more difficult. Although these results are discouraging, the benefit expected from studies in vivo justifies the continuation of efforts in this area.

Our subgroup formed in 1986 at the First Conference on Differentiation Therapy to evaluate in vivo models for differentiation therapy. Implicit in our discussions then, and during the year, was the need to define appropriate in vivo systems for growing and monitoring the cells, as well as for establishing appropriate markers for the assessment of differentiation. During our subgroup meeting we decided to consider solid and hematopoietic tumors separately since problems and procedures were often quite different for these two tumor classes. Certain critical issues were emphasized by the end of our discussions. Among them were the following:

(1) What are the most desirable models for in vivo evaluation of differentiation of neoplastic cells and particularly cells of human origin?

(2) How should evaluation and end points of in vivo differentiation therapy differ from cytotoxic therapy; in which ways should they be the same?

(3) Is it possible to narrow the number of protocols or model systems for in vivo evaluation of differentiation therapy with neoplastic hematopoietic cells or solid tumors?

(4) What approaches can identify and test endogenous differentiation inducers or modulators whose functions might be to promote differentiation during development and whose actions might be relatively cell-type specific, thus reducing the likelihood of adverse side-effects?

(5) Because of possible side-effects, how might in vivo models include approaches to monitor differentiation-inducing effects upon normal somatic or stem cells of the tumor-bearing host?

MODELS FOR IN VIVO DIFFERENTIATION OF
HEMATOPOIETIC CELLS

There are two general categories of models suggested for studying differentiation of leukemia cells: a) animal leukemia cells carried in syngeneic animals and b) human leukemia cells, either from cell lines or from patients, carried in athymic nude mice or in immunosuppressed mice. The mouse is so universally used that reference to an animal system is essentially synonymous with a murine system. The catalog of in vivo models does not have an animal system in which acute myeloid leukemia develops spontaneously at a high incidence. Thus, for the acute myeloid leukemias we do not have an animal model for studying prevention or treatment that is comparable to the lymphoid AKR mouse model.

Growth of Leukemia Cells in vivo

The absence of a "natural model" requires compromises in comparison to the human disease. One major compromise is the "unnatural site" chosen for leukemic cell growth. Sites used for studying differentiation of leukemia cells in animals are: i.p., s.c., i.v., and implantation i.p. of diffusion chambers inoculated with tumor cells. Each of these conditions has advantages and disadvantages based on considerations including: how well the tumor cells grow; assessibility for measurements of growth and differentiation; localization of the differentiating agent or its metabolite(s) at the site; the half-life of the agent at the site; whether the tumor cells interact with host cells or with factors produced by the host that may play a role in modulating differentiation; ability to measure metastatic potential; the length of time that effects can be monitored; both the technical ease and the cost of performing the experiments; the response of the host to the tumor; and if the desired effects are achieved.

Differentiation in vivo of murine leukemia cells.

The initial experiments on in vivo induction of differentiation used diffusion chambers inoculated with clones of the myeloid leukemia cell line Ml implanted i.p. (20,25). These studies show that diffusible endogenous factors in mice promote differentiation of Ml cells to granulocytes and macrophages with loss of growth potential. An involvement of the immune system in the production of these factors is suggested strongly by the findings that differentiation is depressed in athymic or immuno-suppressed hosts and is restored in immunodepressed hosts and promoted in normal animals by injection of purified colony stimulating factor, differentiation factor(s), antigens or even normal cells producing these factors (22,24,25,27,28). The question of an involvement in differentiation of cell-to-cell contact of leukemia cells with host cells is not easily addressed using the diffusion chamber technique. Thus, while cell-to-cell interaction is not obligatory for differentiation in vivo, an assessment of the possible role of this interaction needs further study.

Ml cells injected i.p., s.c., or i.v. also differentiate in response to factors produced by the immune system (18,27). The advantages of these routes of administration are that effects on life-span and metastasis can be measured. However, it is more difficult to evaluate whether the effects observed are indeed due to differentiation.

Agents inducing differentiation of murine leukemia cells in vitro are also active in vivo. Thus, dexamethasone, $1\alpha,25$-dihydroxyvitamin D_3, alkyl ethylene-glycophospholipids, butyric acid, propionic acid, 5-fluorodeoxyuridine, and actinomycin D induce differentiation of Ml or WEHI-3B cells measured in diffusion chambers or as an increase in life-span of the host (19-23,27,35). In addition, there is some evidence that combinations of differentiation inducers or differentiation inducers with cytotoxic agents are more effective than these agents alone (19,23,27).

Differentiation in vivo of human leukemia cells.

Fresh human normal and leukemia cells differentiate in diffusion chambers implanted i.p. in mice (3,9,17,42). Fresh

leukemia cell preparations contain various concentrations of
normal immature cells. Therefore, in studies with leukemia cells
it is difficult to control for the contribution of normal cell
maturation to the differentiated pool. In some cases the
leukemia cells have specific markers and leukemia cell differentiation is substantiated (3). Because easily measured markers of
leukemia cells are not generally available, the routine use of
fresh leukemia cells for studying differentiation in an in vivo
model is severely restricted.

Some of the complications of working with fresh human leukemia
cells are reduced by using established cell lines. Cells from the
human promyelocytic leukemia line HL60 differentiate in diffusion
chambers implanted i.p. into normal mice (26,28). Differentiation is markedly enhanced by pre-immunizing the mice or by
transferring spleen cells enriched for T lymphocytes from immu-
nized mice to the non-immunized hosts (28). Thus, the immune
system appears to be involved in the differentiation of HL60
cells in vivo in a manner similar to that shown with murine
leukemia cells.

HL60 cells form nonmetastatic tumors when injected s.c. into
athymic nude mice (5,16,36,37). The efficiency of induction of
tumors s.c. is increased approximately two-fold by cyclophos-
phamide-priming of the host (36). In one study the tumors were
not serially transplantable for more than three generations (16).
In another study HL60 was established as serially transplantable
ascites and solid human tumor xenograft lines in non-immuno-
suppressed athymic nude mice (5). Nonmetastatic tumors are also
established in immunosuppressed mice injected s.c. with cells
from the human leukemia lines U937, K562, or KGl (36).

There have been a limited number of studies on the effects in
vivo of agents that are active inducers of differentiation in
vitro. The active vitamin D_3 metabolite $1\alpha,25$-dihydroxyvitamin
D_3 decreases markedly the number of tumors arising from s.c.
injection of K562 or HL60 cells but has no effect on tumors
derived from U937 cells (36). Retinoic acid, hexamethylenebisacetamide (HMBA), and combinations of HMBA and cytoxan significantly increase survival times of mice implanted i.p. with
HL60 cells (5). In neither of these studies was differentiation
determined to be the mechanism for the anti-tumor effects. In one
study with athymic nude mice carrying HL60 tumors i.p., retinoic
acid therapy neither increased the lifespan nor induced differentiation of HL60 cells (45).

It is clear that more models and more effort are needed for
studying differentiation therapy of human leukemia cells. A
mouse model recently described by Fingert and co-workers (11,12
and this volume) has yielded encouraging preliminary results. It
is our hope that efforts will continue to develop in vivo assay
systems that are predictive for differentiation therapy of
various human malignancies. A less obvious but important point
is that it may also be fruitful to understand the reasons for

negative results in a system in vivo in which tumor cells continue to proliferate in the presence of differentiation inducers.

MODELS FOR IN VIVO DIFFERENTIATION
OF SOLID TUMORS

In vivo evaluation of differentiation inducers on solid tumors presents a different spectrum of technical considerations and concerns when compared with hematopoietic tumors, and often necessitates different strategies. An important issue is that there is a much broader spectrum of solid tumor types than hematopoietic tumors. It must, therefore, be decided which tumor types are most appropriate for testing various differentiation inducers and what criteria should be used in making such choices. An obvious approach to the selection of in vivo tumor models would be to draw from results of in vitro studies. Alternatively, as we learn more about the nature of endogenous differentiation inducers, and about the response of normal cells to exogenous effectors of differentiation (see, e.g., 13,14) we can be guided by this information. Although we would now be loath to draw conclusions about the antineoplastic potential of a cytotoxic agent until it has been evaluated in several tumor models, differentiation-inducing agents might be considerably more specific in their spectrum of action than are many cytotoxics. After the tumor types have been chosen for study, different variables remain to be decided upon, including site and method of tumor introduction, markers of differentiation to be followed, methods for scoring differentiation and the endpoints to be used. No single experimental approach appears to be suitable for all solid tumors or for all objectives. It should be stressed that there has been a paucity of experimental data or experience with differentiation of most solid tumor types in vivo. Thus, much work remains to be done to establish and evaluate potentially useful model systems.

Inoculation of Tumor Cells

The means of inoculating malignant hematopoietic cells is critical from the point of view of retrieving the cells after treatment. This is not usually a concern with solid tumors since they tend to give rise to primary growths at the site of administration. Of greater concern with solid tumors is the influence of the environment at the site of injection and the shape and size of the tumor masses. With regard to the former variable, tumors are often inoculated subcutaneously. The advantage of this approach is that a single mass is often formed at the injection site and its growth is easy to monitor by palpation. One disadvantage is that clinically relevant tumors, unlike subcutaneous ones, are subject to interactions with extracellular matrices and cells of the organs in which they reside and such interactions are known to facilitate differentiation in many instances (see, e.g., 15). Location could, therefore, markedly influence how the cells would respond to administered differentiation-inducing agents. Achievable concentrations of these agents might be different in subcutaneous vs other sites.

In vitro studies with embryonal carcinoma cells (the stem cells of teratocarcinomas) suggest that the organization of the cells (monolayer culture vs free-floating aggregates) strongly influences the extent and direction of differentiation (e.g., 30). Although organization of tumor cells is unlikely to be so divergent in various in vivo sites, more subtle differences could have an important effect upon the capacity for differentiation. For example, cells from several embryonal carcinoma lines grow as small ascitic aggregates rather than large tumors when inoculated intraperitoneally. Whereas the patterns of differentiation in solid subcutaneous growths are disorganized and vary in type and extent depending upon the cell line (e.g., 31), intraperitoneal aggregates from some lines tend to contain much more organized, predictable and limited patterns of differentiation (e.g., 29); such aggregates from other cell lines show no signs of differentiation even though they can differentiate to some degree subcutaneously (29,31).

Somewhat more sophisticated models have been utilized by some groups to evaluate antineoplastic compounds. For example, Bogden has developed a subrenal capsule assay (see 4). Tumors become well vascularized under the kidney capsule and appear not to have a significant lag time before growth occurs following implantation. Intimate tumor-organ interaction can be quickly established. Recent studies indicate that cytotoxic drug potency can often be evaluated in as little as six days (4). Depending upon the endpoint of the test, such short-term assays could be ideal for evaluating differentiation-inducing agents. An obvious disadvantage of this model system is that implanting the tumors is labor intensive and requires some degree of surgical skill.

Since primary tumors are often resected in patients, there might be substantial clinical relevance in evaluating effects of differentiation-inducing agents upon the incidence and growth of metastases or small residual foci. In fact, it would not be unreasonable to expect that differentiation therapy might be more effective in a post-surgical, adjuvant setting than against untreated primary tumors. Metastasis models share with the subrenal capsule system the advantage of close tissue interaction and good access to vascularization. Several rodent metastasis models, both experimental and spontaneous, have been described and they are often reasonably simple to generate and to evaluate.

It is often supposed that human tumors are more relevant than rodent ones for drug evaluation. The requirement for athymic or chemically immunosuppressed mice for in vivo human tumor models makes evaluation in these systems expensive and necessitates appropriate animal facilities. The use of immunocompromised mice might in some instances fail to reveal the full therapeutic potential of a differentiation-inducing agent, since such an agent might alter surface macromolecular properties of the tumor cells so as to render them more susceptible to immune surveillance. It is conceivable that potent combinations of biological response modifiers such as interferon-α and interleukin-2 (8,44) act synergistically for this reason. Recent studies with the subrenal capsule model have suggested the feasibility of transplanting human tumors to normal immunocompetent mice for short-term assays of antineoplastic agents (4). Such a model might be particularly appropriate for evaluating the full potential of differentiation inducers on certain human tumors. Finally, although it has been notoriously difficult to obtain metastases with human tumors in athymic mice, Fidler and his colleagues (10) have demonstrated that this can be achieved with some tumor types by implanting the cells in the spleen or kidney.

None of the approaches so far described might be considered ideal for evaluation of effects of differentiation inducers on skin tumors, which are for several reasons attractive targets for this type of therapy. Fusenig and his coworkers (see 15) have established methods for evaluating differentiation and invasiveness of squamous carcinoma cells on subdermal graft beds of granulation tissue. This procedure has recently been modified for use in less hardy athymic mice (7). The subdermal system is particularly appropriate for studies to evaluate effects of other cell types and extracellular matrices on differentiation of skin tumor cells. A skin graft model developed by Yuspa and his coworkers (38, and this volume) is attractive for evaluating the effects of differentiation inducers upon skin tumors because agents can be applied topically, biopsies are easily obtained and tumor growth can be followed by visual inspection.

Markers of Differentiation

The differentiation of many cell types has been monitored with a large variety of markers. Morphology is a classical and convenient approach to evaluating differentiation. In tumors such as teratocarcinomas, in which heterogeneity of differentiated cell types is characteristic, morphology is a particularly appropriate criterion since individual markers of differentiation would be unlikely to detect all cell types. In tumors where particular differentiation events are expected, enzymes or antigens can be used with more confidence to measure differentiation. Appearance or disappearance of these markers can be monitored. Recently, cDNA probes have become available for measuring expression of genes which discriminate between undifferentiated cells and their differentiated progeny (e.g., 1,2).

Enzymes, antigens and mRNAs can be measured in tumor sections (by histochemistry, immunohistology or in situ hybridization, respectively) or biochemically in tumor homogenates or extracts. The differentiation marker and method of choice depends in large part upon assay availability and the degree of quantitation required in the scoring process (see below).

It should be pointed out that differentiation patterns and phenotypes need neither faithfully nor fully reflect those observed in normal tissues. For example, Müller and Wagner (34) have obtained, by transfection of cultured embryonal carcinoma cells with the c-<u>fos</u> oncogene, cells which have clearly lost their undifferentiated characteristics but which appear to have acquired a mixed phenotype. Since the cells have lost the transformed phenotype of their undifferentiated progenitors, this differentiation process, albeit aberrant, could be adequate to suppress malignant growth of the cells in vivo.

Scoring of Differentiation

Realistic endpoints for the evaluation of the efficacy of antineoplastic drugs in the clinic are tumor regression, extended survival and quality of life. It can, therefore, be argued that similar criteria should be placed insofar as possible upon the preclinical assessment of candidate drugs. Thus, the most desirable experimental endpoints for a conventional antineo-plastic agent would be regression of the tumor (as opposed to simple inhibition of growth), increased survival time and a favorable therapeutic index (difference between effective and toxic doses). At the final stages of evaluation, a differ-entiation-inducing agent should ideally satisfy these same cri-teria with the exception that simple inhibition of tumor growth rather than regression might be acceptable if all the tumor cells were terminally differentiated.

There are, however, justifications for using endpoints other than tumor size to evaluate the effects of differentiation inducers. For example, in vitro studies suggest that there is often a relatively small difference between the concentration of an inducer which is optimal for differentiation and that which is cytotoxic. Thus, in initiation of in vivo studies with an inducer it is desirable to attempt to test whether the inducer interferes with tumor growth primarily by promoting differentiation; such conclusions are not always readily drawn (e.g., see 39). In a study by McLean and Freshney (33), it was observed that dexa-methasone induced diffferentiation of WIL lung adenocarcinoma cells in vitro. In vivo, dexamethasone caused a pattern of tumor necrosis which suggested to the authors that the agent was interfering with tumor growth by inhibiting angiogenesis rather than by promoting differentiation (although differentiation of tumor cells could have reduced their production of angiogenic and/or chemotactic agents). On the other hand, as mentioned above, interactions of tumor cells with extracellular matrices or normal host cells could easily increase their propensity for differentiation upon exposure to exogenous inducers.

There is no single prescribed method for scoring tumor cell differentiation. Several approaches can be used and each has its advantages and disadvantages. The benefits of using sectioned material for evaluation are the relative ease and convenience of the procedures involved and the ability to take into account in the scoring process quantitative or qualitative heterogeneity of differentiation (types of cells formed and "maturity" of the differentiation phenotype) in different parts of the tumor. However, many sections of a tumor might have to be studied to provide an accurate estimation of heterogeneity.

Biochemical analyses more easily address needs for quantitative assessments of differentiation but provide only an average value. Distorted data could result from the presence of normal host cells (hematopoietic cells, vascular cells, fibrous and adjacent normal tissue) and necrotic cells which are often found in the central region of tumors due to interruption of vascularization. Removal of dead and non-malignant host cells prior to scoring requires disaggregation of the tumor cells, a tedious process which can itself introduce inaccuracies into the evaluation. Biochemical analyses could be of limited value if the differentiated cell types formed were heterogeneous as, e.g., with teratocarcinomas or skin carcinomas. Unless one can reliably measure the disappearance of one or more enzymatic or antigenic markers which are invariably and uniquely associated with the undifferentiated phenotype, a variety of differentiation markers might have to be used to measure extent of differentiation. It is probably desirable to assess tumors by histology in initial studies to determine the degree to which biochemical analyses would be compromised by the problems discussed. In later studies involving dose responses or combination therapy, biochemical analyses might provide a more accurate quantitative assessment of efficacy. As mentioned above, however, in later stages of evaluation it would be most expedient, practical and meaningful to monitor tumor growth and survival times as endpoints.

Chemoprevention

The emphasis in this volume has been on the role of differentiation inducers in tumor therapy. Extensive in vitro and in vivo studies have been carried out on the effects of retinoids on differentiation of embryonal carcinoma cells (32,40). Some successes in controlling teratocarcinoma growth with retinoic acid have been reported (41,43). In other studies, it has been found that although this agent is a potent inducer of differentiation in vitro, and can often increase levels of differentiation in vivo, it generally fails to interfere markedly with growth of tumors generated by these cells (32). In vitro studies suggest that cells can become refractory at relatively high frequencies to the differentiation-inducing effects of retinoids at both genetic and epigenetic levels (40). One could predict from these results that differentiation agents might meet with only limited success in tumor therapy because persistence and expansion of refractory tumor cell populations could commonly occur. In view of this, and the fact that some differentiation inducers are potent at non-toxic concentrations, it might be reasonable to expect that such agents would be considerably more successful and effective in preventing, rather than curing, cancer. Indeed, numerous studies with retinoids have led to the compelling conclusion that these agents are generally more effective in suppressing the growth of preneoplastic lesions and in preventing their progression than in countering frank neoplasias (see 6). A great deal might be gained by expanding our efforts on the in vivo effects of differentiation agents to include meaningful chemoprevention models as well as those designed to evaluate therapeutic effects.

ACKNOWLEDGEMENTS

We thank Drs. D. Dexter, M. Hozumi, J. Lotem, I. Freshney, F. Takaku, N. Fusenig, and C. Chomienne for many of the helpful suggestions incorporated into this report.

REFERENCES

1. Augenlicht, L.H., Bogen, M., Halsey, H., Anderson, L., and Taylor, J. (1987): Proc. Am. Assoc. Cancer Res., 28:44.

2. Augenlicht, L.H., Wahrman, M.Z., Halsey, H., Anderson, L., Taylor, J., and Lipkin, M. (1987): Cancer Res., in press.

3. Boecker, W.R., Ohl, S., Hossfeld, D.K., and Schmidt, C.G. (1978) Lancet 1:267-268.

4. Bogden, A.E. (1987): In: Fundamentals of Cancer Chemotherapy, edited by K. Hellmann and S.K. Carter, pp. 173-179. McGraw-Hill, New York.

5. Bogden, A.E., Cobb, W.R., Breitman, T.R., Wolpert-DeFilippes, M.K., DeLarco, B., Venditti, J.M., Plowman, J., and Shoemaker, R.H. (1985): Proc. Am. Assoc. Cancer Res., 26:34.

6. Bollag, W. and Hartmann, H.R. (1983): Cancer Surv., 2:293-314.

7. Boukamp, P., Rupniak, H.T.R.R., and Fusenig, N.E.F. (1987): Cancer Res., 45:5582-5592.

8. Brunda, M.J., Bellantoni, D., and Sulich, V. (1987): Int. J. Cancer, 40:365-371.

9. Fauerholdt, L. and Jacobsen, N. (1975): Blood, 45:495-501.

10. Fidler, I.J. (1986): Cancer Metastasis Rev., 5:29-49.

11. Fingert, H.J., Treiman, A., and Pardee, A.B. (1984): Proc. Natl. Acad. Sci. USA, 81:7927-7933.

12. Fingert, H.J., Chen, Z., Mizrahi, N., Gajewski, W.H., Bamberg, M.P., and Kradin, R.L. (1987): Cancer Res., 47:3824-3829.

13. Francis, G.E., and Berney, J.J. (1986): First Conf. Diff. Ther., Abstr. 34.

14. Fuchs, E., and Green, H. (1981): Cell, 25:617-625.

15. Fusenig, N.E. (1986): In: Biology of the Integument, vol. 2, edited by J. Bereiter-Hahn, A.G. Matoltsy, and K.S. Richards, pp. 409-442. Springer-Verlag, Berlin.

16. Gallagher, R., Collins, S., Trujillo, J. McCredie, K., Ahearn, M., Tsai, S., Metzgar, R., Aulakh, G., Ting, R., Ruscetti, F., and Gallo, R. (1979): Blood, 54:713-733.

17. Hoelzer, D., Kurrle, E., Schmucker, H., and Harriss, E.B. (1977): Blood, 49:729-744.

18. Honma, Y., Hayashi, M., Kasukabe, T., and Hozumi, M. (1982): Leukemia Res., 6:117-122.

19. Honma, Y., Hozumi, M., Abe, E., Konno, K., Fukushima, M., Hata, S., Nishii, Y., DeLuca, H.F., and Suda, T. (1983): Proc. Natl. Acad. Sci. USA, 80:201-204.

20. Honma, Y., Kasukabe, T., and Hozumi, M. (1978): J. Natl. Cancer Inst., 61:837-840.

21. Honma, Y., Kasukabe, T., Okabe-Kado, J., Hozumi, M., Tsushima, S., and Nomura, H. (1983): Cancer Chemother. Pharmacol., 11:77-79.

22. Honma, Y., Kasukabe, T., Okabe, J., and Hozumi, M. (1979): Cancer Res., 39:3167-3171.

23. Kasukabe, T., Honma, Y., Hozumi, M., Suda, T., and Nishii, Y. (1987): Cancer Res., 47:567-572.

24. Lotem, J., Ben-Nun, A., and Sachs, L. (1986): Leukemia Res., 10:1165-1168.

25. Lotem, J. and Sachs, L. (1978): Proc. Natl. Acad. Sci. USA, 75:3781-3785.

26. Lotem, J. and Sachs, L. (1979): Proc. Natl. Acad. Sci USA, 76:5158-5162.

27. Lotem, J. and Sachs, L. (1981): Int. J. Cancer, 28:375-386.

28. Lotem, J. and Sachs, L. (1985): Leukemia Res., 9:1479-1486.

29. Martin, G.R. (1978): In: Development in Mammals, vol. 3, edited by M.H. Johnson, pp. 225-265. Elsevier/North Holland, Amsterdam.

30. McBurney, M.W., Jones-Villeneuve, E.M.V., Edwards, M.K.S., and Anderson, P.J. (1982): Nature, 299:165-167.

31. McCue, P.A., Matthaei, K.I., Taketo, M., and Sherman, M.I. (1983): Devel. Biol., 96:416-426.

32. McCue, P.A., Thomas, R.A., Schroeder, D., Gubler, M.L., and Sherman, M.I.: submitted for publication.

33. McLean, J.S., Frame, M.C., Freshney, R.I., Vaughan, P.F.T., Mackie, A.E., and Singer, I. (1986): Anticancer Res., 6:1101-1106.

34. Müller, R., and Wagner, E.F. (1984): Nature, 311,438-442.

35. Okabe, J., Honma, Y., Hayashi, M., and Hozumi, M. (1979): Int. J. Cancer, 24:87-91.

36. Potter, G.K., Mohamed, A.N., Dracopoli, N.C., Groshen, S.-L.B., Shen, R.N., and Moore, M.A.S. (1985): Exp. Hematol., 13:722-732.

37. Potter, G.K., Shen, R.N., and Chiao, J.W. (1984): Am. J. Pathol., 114:360-366.

38. Roop, D.R., Lowy, D.R., Tambourin, P.E., Strickland, J., Harper, J.R., Balaschak, M., Spangler, E.F., Yuspa, S.H. (1986): Nature, 323:822-824.

39. Sherman, M.I., Thomas, R.A., Schroeder, D., and McCue P.A. (1987): First Conf. Diff. Ther., Abstr. 115.

40. Sherman, M.I. (1988): In: Advanced Research on Animal Cell Technology, edited by A.O.A. Miller. Martinus Nijhoff, Hingham, Mass., in press.

41. Speers, W.C. (1982): Cancer Res., 42:1843-1849.

42. Steele, A.A., Sensenbreener, L.L., and Young, M.G. (1977): Exp. Hematol., 5:199-210.

43. Strickland, S., and Sawey, M.T. (1980): Devel. Biol., 78:76-85.

44. Truitt, G.A., Stern, L.L., and Bontempo, J. (1987): Proc. Am. Assoc. Cancer Res., 28:369.

45. Uozumi, J., Imaizumi, M., and Breitman, T.R. (1986): Proc. Am. Assoc. Cancer Res., 27:44.

In Vivo Model for Differentiation Therapy of Leukemia and Solid Tumors

H.J. Fingert, M.L. Sherman* and Z. Chen

Department of Surgery, Massachusetts General Hospital Cancer Center,
Boston Massachusetts 02114 and
*Laboratory of Clinical Pharmacology, Dana-Farber Cancer Institute, Boston,
Massachusetts 02115

INTRODUCTION

The preclinical study of differentiation therapies has been a challenging endeavor, especially those studies aimed to evaluate treatment response and mechanism in a living host.

Prior in vivo models for differentiation therapy include the suspension of leukemia cells in a bone marrow clot or diffusion chambers, and the subcutaneous, intravenous, or intraperitoneal injection of tumor cells into athymic nude or syngeneic mice (7,9,18,21). However, these models have been limited due to high expense and fastidious care requirements of nude mice, thus limiting their use for many broad-scale experiments, such as those required for combination treatment protocols. Furthermore, these methods are often technically cumbersome, and they are not easily reproduced with a variety of histologic cell types or clinical tumor material.

IN VIVO GROWTH OF HUMAN TUMORS IN THE SUBRENAL CAPSULE ASSAY (SRCA)

A short-term method for the growth of a wide variety of human tumors in mice was developed by Castro and Cass (6) and later refined by Bogden et al. (3). The SRCA is used by numerous research institutions to screen the activity of new anticancer agents against human tumor xenografts (20). In addition, this assay is used for individual selection of chemotherapy based on specific drug sensitivities of clinical tumor samples (2,3,27). In contrast to the diffusion chamber technique (11), several laboratories have found the SRCA practical and feasible for more broad-scale studies with new anticancer drugs, using both transplantable and primary human tumors

(3,4,16,26,28). Using athymic nude mice, this method has been used extensively for screening *in vivo* antitumor activity of new drugs by the Division of Cancer Treatment of the National Cancer Institute and other research institutions (16,20,29). However, the validity of this assay largely depends on positive tumor growth in control (untreated) animals, necessitating the use of nude mice to avoid immunologic regression of human tumor grafts.

The SRCA is an *in vivo* method which permits precise *in situ* measurements of human tumor grafts implanted under the renal capsule of mice (3,4) (Fig. 1). Preselected 1 mm fragments of viable tumor tissue are implanted under the renal capsule, a site presumed superior for delivery of nutrients and drugs. Precise measurement (accurate to 0.1 mm) of graft size *in situ* is readily accomplished by a stereomicroscope with an ocular micrometer, and each engrafted animal provides its own baseline for evaluating drug activity. In contrast to the subcutaneous site, which often requires several weeks or months for appreciable tumor growth, the SRCA can quantify statistical changes in tumor size after 6-12 days. In nude mice, 7-fold greater blood flow has been demonstrated for SRCA-implanted as compared to subcutaneous tumors, suggesting that the SRCA is advantageous for delivery of nutrients and systemic antitumor agents (25). In normal immunocompetent mice, human tumors can be studied 4-6 days after implantation before major immune rejection, providing economic advantages over use of nude mice (3,4,27).

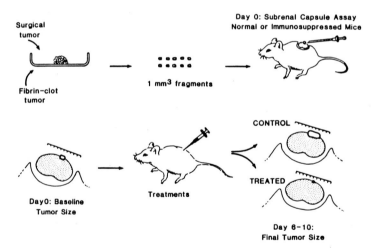

FIG. 1. Protocol for subrenal implantation and growth of human tumors. By using immunosuppressed mice, greater growth of control (untreated) tumors is achieved, improving discrimination of treatment response in the assay period.

The SRCA has not been well described as an *in vivo* model to study differentiation therapies. A major drawback has been the inability to implant and monitor tumor cells that are common targets for experimental differentiation therapy, i.e., cultured cell lines or leukemic blasts which display a differentiated phenotype when exposed to differentiating agents *in vitro* (7,9,15). In the past, this SRCA technique required a solid tumor matrix for accurate implantation and serial measurement. We recently described (14) a simple, rapid technique for direct implantation and quantitative analysis of cultured epithelial cancer or leukemia cells in the SRCA (Fig. 2). These studies demonstrated that a) stepwise additions of fibrinogen and thrombin provide a solid fibrin clot as a tumor cell matrix; b) the fibrin clot matrix maintains homogeneity and viability of implanted tumor cells; c) rapid growth *in vivo* is observed by diverse types of human or rodent epithelial and leukemia cell lines; and d) these tumors display histological features that characterize malignant growth *in vivo*, including frequent tumor mitoses, neovascularization, and invasion into normal tissues (14).

PROTOCOL FOR FIBRIN-THROMBIN CLOT OF TUMOR CELLS

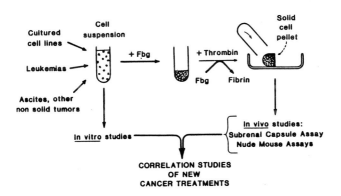

FIG. 2. Protocol for fibrin-thrombin clot of tumor cells. The tumor or leukemic cells are obtained from passaged cell lines and resuspended in the presence of fibrinogen. Thrombin is added to initiate enzymatic formation of a fibrin clot, which is cut with a scalpel blade into homogeneous 1 mm fragments for implantation into the SRCA.

TUMOR GROWTH VS. IMMUNOLOGIC REJECTION IN THE SRCA MODEL

We (13,14) and others (1,2,26) found that immunosuppression of normal host mice a) further extends the duration of tumor growth beyond the six day period; b) improves discrimination of active treatments, and c) greatly improves histologic validity of tumor grafts. Immunosuppression of host CD-1 mice can be achieved by whole-body irradiation (WBI) given before tumor implantation, cyclosporine given daily after tumor implantation, or cyclophosphamide given preimplantation combined with cyclosporine (13,14,26).

In order to investigate the kinetics of tumor growth vs. graft rejection in the SRCA, we utilized HL-60 human promyelocytic leukemic cells transplanted from suspension culture to normal or irradiated mice. Figure 3 reveals two phases of tumor growth which we observed in these and other experiments (13,14): a) days 0 to 6 post-implantation into control mice shows a "slow-growth" phase, wherein tumors increased only by about 30% (average diameters) compared to the initial size, and b) rapid growth beyond day 6 was observed in mice immunosuppressed with non-lethal whole-body irradiation (600 rads given 4-16 hrs before tumor implantation). In contrast, tumors regressed after day 6 in control mice without irradiation, corresponding to histologic graft rejection (13).

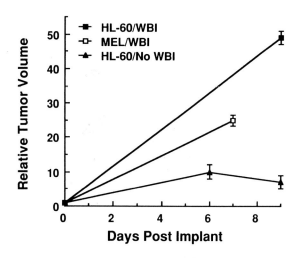

FIG. 3. Effect of immunosuppression on growth of leukemic cells in the SRCA. HL-60 cells in normal mice, HL-60 cells in mice pretreated with whole body irradiation (WBI) or MEL cells in mice pretreated with WBI were implanted in the SRCA and assayed at various times following implantation. Mean ± SEM.

Other laboratories have confirmed growth of several human tumors in irradiated or cyclosporine-treated mice (2,26). These studies and others from our own laboratory (13,14) have led to the following conclusions: a) although the 6-day SRC model allows analysis of some tumor growth with rodent or human tumor implants, greater discrimination of viable vs. nonviable tumors could be achieved by extending the model to 9 to 12 days; b) immunosuppression can preserve the rapid-growth phase of implanted tumors, and thereby vastly improve the discrimination of active treatment. Immunosuppression of host mice by irradiation or cyclosporine had no antitumor effect per se, allowing extended treatment after tumor implantation.

In addition to leukemic cells, this assay can be used to monitor both *in vivo* growth and treatment response for a wide variety of tumor types. Table 1 lists the relative increase in tumor volumes observed with numerous human or rodent tumor cells implanted in the SRCA. As previously reported (13,14), histologic analysis of growing tumors revealed frequent mitoses and neovascularization. Furthermore, certain cell types displayed rapid invasion into the kidney.

TABLE 1. Growth of human or rodent tumor cells in the SRCA[a]

Cell Type	Relative tumor volume (V_f/V_i)	Day of Assay
Human		
HL60 promyelocytic leukemia	50	9
CX1 colon carcinoma	10	9
LOX melanoma	20	10
A431 vulvar carcinoma	24	9
T24 bladder carcinoma	24	6
RT112 bladder carcinoma	5	9
Rodent		
PC4 mouse erythroleukemia	25	7
MCB sarcoma	36	6
B16 melanoma	50	10

[a]Cells were implanted directly from monolayer or suspension cell culture by the fibrin clot protocol, and tumor volumes were computed by the formula (Volume = Length x Width x Width/2). Relative tumor volumes were calculated as the ratio of the average final volume (V_f) to the average initial volume (V_i), using 5-6 mice per group.

GROWTH FACTORS AND CELL-CELL INTERACTIONS IN THE SRCA

In several *in vitro* models, the initial growth of human tumor or leukemic cells is often greatly enhanced by addition of specific growth factors. Welte et al. (30) found that granulocyte-macrophage colony stimulating factor (GM-CSF) promotes growth of passaged and primary human leukemic cells. GM-CSF is produced in the culture media of several epithelial cancer cell lines, one of the highest producers being the 5637 bladder carcinoma cell line. We studied the capacity of the 5637 cells to provide a "feeder" effect and, thus, promote the *in vivo* growth of human leukemia cells in the SRCA. These studies used the KG-1 human myelocytic cell line, which is known to contain GM-CSF receptors and maintains better growth *in vitro* in the presence of this growth factor (19). As shown in Fig. 4, KG-1 cells alone demonstrated less than a 2-fold increase in tumor size on day 6 after implantation into the SRC of irradiated mice. In contrast, addition of irradiated 5637 cells to the KG-1 cells (ratio of 19 KG-1 to 1 5637 cells in the fibrin clot) showed a 5-fold increase in tumor volume (p < 0.01). Irradiation of the 5637 cells (600-900 rads) was shown to be cytostatic in culture, but allowed continued production of GM-CSF into the culture media as measured by a bioassay (17).

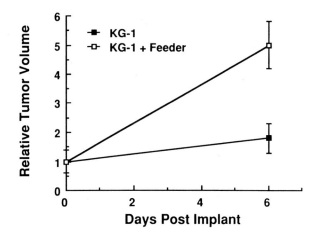

FIG. 4. Effect of irradiated 5637 cells on KG-1 cell growth. KG-1 cells alone or KG-1 cells mixed with GM-CSF producing 5637 cells were implanted in the SRCA and assayed on day 6 for relative tumor volume. Mean ± SEM.

HEXAMETHYLENE BISACETAMIDE

Hexamethylene bisacetamide (HMBA, NSC 95580) is a polar-planar compound structurally similar to dimethyl sulfoxide (DMSO). DMSO was observed to induce erythroid differentiation of Friend-virus infected murine erythroleukemia (MEL) cells (15). Later studies demonstrated that HMBA was a more potent inducer of MEL cells as well as HL-60 human promyelocytic leukemia cells at a concentration two orders of magnitude lower than DMSO (δ, 2,22,23). HMBA is currently in clinical Phase I - II trials (10,24).

In recent studies, Egorin et al. (5) demonstrated rapid formation of numerous HMBA metabolites after systemic administration *in vivo.* Furthermore, high concentrations of HMBA produced a metabolic acidosis, attributed to formation of acidic metabolites as well as renal tubular changes. Although extensive work has been done *in vitro* with HMBA as the parent compound, few experiments have been designed to study these numerous byproducts and other *in vivo* metabolic effects.

We investigated HMBA in our modified SRCA model, using either HL-60 or MEL cells implanted by the fibrin clot technique described above. Fig. 5 demonstrates a significant antiproliferative effect (p < 0.01) with HMBA (2000 mg/kg/d on days 1-5 after tumor implantation) given either subcutaneous (s.c.) or intraperitoneal (i.p.). Similar results were obtained with MEL cells, as shown in Fig. 6. The MEL experiments were terminated on day 7, since overgrowth of control tumors occurred after this period leading to inaccuracy of tumor volume measurements. Further studies in progress include histochemical and genetic analyses of HMBA-treated and control tumor grafts.

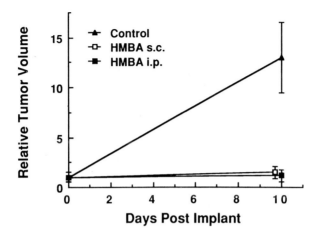

FIG. 5. Effect of HMBA on HL-60 cells in the SRCA. Mice were treated with HMBA (2000 mg/kg/d for 5 days after tumor implantation) administered either subcutaneous (s.c.) or intraperitoneal (i.p.). Mean ± SEM.

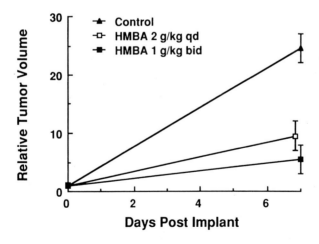

FIG. 6. Effect of HMBA on MEL cells in the SRCA. Mice were treated with HMBA at 2000 mg/kg daily (q.d.) or 1000 mg/kg twice a day (b.i.d.). Mean ± SEM

The plasma pharmacokinetics of HMBA were examined in non-tumored mice after subcutaneous injection (2000 mg/kg). Plasma levels were measured by gas chromatography as described (5,10). These experiments demonstrated that the mice rapidly attained plasma levels exceeding 1 mM after a single injection of 2000 mg/kg s.c. (Fig. 7). These concentrations are similar to those reported in recent clinical studies with HMBA administered by infusion technique (10,24). The plasma half-life in mice was calculated to be approximately 50 minutes. While a HMBA dose of 2000 mg/kg daily was well tolerated with no animal deaths, more frequent dosing produced weight loss and occasional mortality. Doses of 1000 mg/kg twice a day were well tolerated.

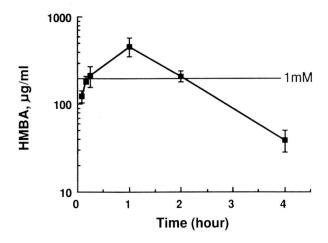

FIG. 7. Pharmacokinetics of HMBA in mice. A single dose of 2000 mg/kg HMBA was administered subcutaneously in non-tumored mice. Three mice were injected per time point. Mean ± SEM. The limit of detection was 10 µg/ml.

SUMMARY

The preclinical development of differentiation therapies requires the demonstration of drug activity in both *in vitro* and *in vivo* model systems. *In vivo* models provide valuable experimental tools to investigate drug metabolism and distribution, organ toxicity, *in vivo* growth and biologic characteristics of targeted tumor grafts, and other variables relevant to clinical application of new cancer therapies (7). A major advantage of the SRCA is the ability to investigate drug activity against a wide variety of tumor histologies, and thus compare *in vivo* treatment response to the same differentiation therapies. By use of immunosuppressed mice, the SRCA allows broad-scale experimentation with far greater economy than similar studies with athymic mice. Our fibrin-clot protocol (14) also provides a technique to examine cell-cell interactions, and the effects of tumor microenvironment on *in vivo* growth or treatment response. Furthermore, the direct use of passaged cell lines provides a simple, rapid methodology for mechanistic studies and *in vitro-in vivo* drug activity correlations. Our present studies suggest that GM-CSF-producing feeder cells promote growth of some human leukemia cells in the model. Our studies also demonstrate antiproliferative effects by HMBA at doses that provide plasma levels in mice relevant to ongoing clinical trials.

ACKNOWLEDGMENTS

This research was supported in part by PHS grant numbers CA42802 and CA01092 awarded by the National Cancer institute, DHHS. The authors thank Dr. M. Moore for 5637 cells, Dr. H.P. Koeffler for KG-1 cells, and Dr. M. Egorin for assistance with HMBA assays. We also thank Dr. J. Griffin for performing GM-CSF assays and Dr. D. Kufe for helpful discussions and review of the manuscript.

REFERENCES

1. Basler, G.A., Schurig, J.E., Henderson, A.J., Schlein, A., Farwell, A.R., Rose, W.C., and Bradner, W.T. (1986): *Proc. Am. Assoc. Cancer Res.*, 27:410.
2. Bennett, J.A., Pilon, V.A., Briggs, D.R., and McKneally, M.F. (1985): *J. Natl. Cancer Inst.*, 75:925-936.
3. Bogden, A.E., Haskell, P.M., LePage, D.J., Relton, D.E., Cobb, W.R., and Esber, H.J. (1979): *Exp. Cell Biol.*, 47:281-293.
4. Bogden, A.E., Cobb, W.R., LePage, D.J , Haskell, P.M., Gulkin, T.A., Ward, A., Kelton, D.E., and Esber, H.J. (1981): *Cancer*, 48:10-20.
5. Callery, P.S., Egorin, M.J., Geelhaar, L.A., Balachandran Nayar, M.S. (1986): *Cancer Res.*, 46:4900-4903.
6. Castro, J.E., and Cass, W. (1974): *Br. J. Surg.*, 61:421-426.
7. Cheson, B.D., Jasperse, D.M., Chun, H.G., and Friedman, M.A. (1986): *Cancer Treat. Rev.*, 13:129-145.
8. Collins, S.J., Bodner, A., and Ting, R. (1980): *Int. J. Cancer*, 25:213-218.
9. Dexter, D.L., and Hager, J.C. (1980): *Cancer*, 45:1178-1184.
10. Egorin, M.J., Sigman, L.M., Van Echo, D.A., Forrest, A., Whitacre, M.Y., and Aisner, J. (1987): *Cancer Res.*, 47:617-623.
11. Fauerholdt, L. and Jacobsen, N. (1975): *Blood*, 45:495-501.
12. Fibach, E., Reuben, R., Rifkind, R.A., and Marks, P.A. (1977): *Cancer Res.*, 37:4440-444.
13. Fingert, H.J., Treiman, A., and Pardee, A.B. (1984): *Proc. Natl. Acad. Sci. USA*, 81:7927-7931.
14. Fingert, H.J., Chen, Z., Mizrahi, N., Gajewski, W.H., Bamberg, M.P., and Kradin, R.L. (1987): *Cancer Res.*, 47:3824-3829.
15. Friend, C., Scher, W., Holland, J., and Sato, T. (1971): *Proc. Natl. Acad. Sci. USA*, 68:378-382.
16. Giovanella, B.C., Stehlin, J.S., Jr., Shepard, R.C., and Williams, L.J., Jr. (1983): *Cancer*, 52:1146-1152.
17. Griffin, J.D., Sullivan, R., Beveridge, R.D., Larcom, P., and Schlossman, S.F. (1984): *Blood*, 63:904-911.

18. Hoelzer, D., Kurrle, E., Schmucker, H., and Harriss, E.B. (1977): *Blood,* 49:729-744.
19. Koeffler, H.P. (1983): *Blood,* 62:709-719.
20. National Cancer Institute, (1984): *In Vivo Cancer Models.* National Institutes of Health Publication 84-2635, Bethesda, Maryland.
21. Preisler, H.D., Bjornsson, S., Mori, M., and Lyman, G.H. (1976): *Br. J. Cancer,* 33:634-645
22. Reuben, R.C., Khanna, P.L., Gazitt, Y., Breslow, R., Rifkind, R.A., and Marks, P.A. (1978): *J. Biol. Chem.,* 253:4214-4218.
23. Reuben, R.C., Wife, R.L., Breslow, R., Rifkind, R.A., and Marks, P.A. (1976): *Proc. Natl. Acad. Sci. USA,* 73:862-866.
24. Rowinsky, E.K., Ettinger, D.S., Grochow, L.B., Brundrett, R.B., Cates, A.E., and Donehower, R.C. (1987): *J. Clin. Oncol.,* 4:1835-1844.
25. Sands, H., Jones, P.J., Neacy, W., Shah, S.A., and Gallagher, B.M. (1984): *Cancer Lett.,* 24-:65-72.
26. Schurig, J.E., Basler, G.A., Henderson, A.J., Hirth, R.S., Mahrt, C.R., and Bradner, W.T. (1985): *Proc. Amer. Assoc. Cancer Res.,* 26:361.
27. Stratton, J.A., Kucera, P.R., Micha, J.P., Rettenmaier, M.A., Braly, P.S., Berman, M.L., and DiSaia, P.J. (1984): *Gynecol. Oncol.,* 19:336-347.
28. Stratton, J.A., Rettenmaier, M.A., Braley, P.S., and DiSaia, P.J. (1983): *J. Biol. Response Mod.,* 2:272-279.
29. Venditti, J.M. (1981): In: *Design of Models for Testing Cancer Therapeutic Agents,* edited by I. Fidler and R.J. White, pp. 80-94. Van Nostrand Reinhold, New York.
30. Welte, K., Platzer, E., Lu, L., Gabrilove, J.L., Levi, E., Mertelsmann, R., and Moore, M.A.S. (1985); *Proc. Natl. Acad. Sci USA,* 82:1526-1530.

Detection of *In Vivo* Differentiation in Myeloid Leukemias

A. Raza, N. Mandava, S. Gezer, A. Hassan, N. Soni,
C. Grande, and H.D. Preisler

Department of Hematologic Oncology, Roswell Park Memorial Institute
666 Elm Street, Buffalo NY, 14263

INTRODUCTION

Aberrations of proliferation and differentiation appear to be two fundamental defects that underlie the process of neoplastic conversion in a cell. Careful evaluation of these processes in the most frequently occurring neoplasms have been seriously compromised because of the difficulties encountered in studying solid tumors. Hematopoietic malignancies, though less commonly seen, offer an advantage over solid tumors in that the malignant cells are present in suspension form and are readily accessible for repeated samplings. Thus, the myeloid leukemias have provided an excellent model system for the investigation of both proliferation and differentiation. Unfortunately, even here, progress has been restricted due to a lack of adequate methodologies. For example, studies of cell cycle kinetics in acute myeloid leukemia (AML) have mostly assessed the simplest measurement of proliferation, i.e. the percentage of cells actively synthesizing DNA (labeling index or LI) in bone marrow aspirates (BM) in vitro (11,18). Little information exists on more complex measurements such as the duration of S-phase (Ts) or total cell cycle time (Tc) of myeloblasts in AML. So much so that most conclusions regarding the proliferative properties of myeloblasts in AML that include measurements of LI as well as Ts and Tc have been based on data obtained from 20 newly diagnosed patients who received tritiated thymidine (^{3}HTdr) infusions in nine separate studies (1,2,7,8,9,10,13,15,26). Therefore, correlations of these data with either the course of the disease or response to therapy have yielded inconsistent results.

The study of differentiation is even more complex. The possibility that malignant cells can be induced to differentiate is therapeutically appealing. It has been extensively investigated, but most of the studies have involved either tissue culture lines (6,25) or manipulations of freshly obtained human cells in vitro (3,14). Both these latter systems may not accurately reflect in vivo events. Ideally, we should develop the ability to test the efficacy of a differentiating agent in vivo. Unfortunately, this has not materialized thus far because no specific tumor marker has been identified which would identify malignant cells and thereby allow one to follow their course in vivo.

In an attempt to improve the methodologies available for investigation of both cellular proliferation and differentiation in the myeloid leukemias, we took advantage of the unique properties of the thymidine analogue bromodeoxyuridine (BrdU). This halogenated pyrimidine can be incorporated into newly synthesized DNA in the place of thymidine. A monoclonal anti-BrdU antibody is then used to identify the S-phase cells, cells which have incorporated BrdU (22,23). Once BrdU is incorporated into a cell, it becomes an integral part of the genome and can be used as a label to identify cells and a marker to follow their course in vivo. We have administered 1 or 2 hour infusions of BrdU to patients with florid AML who subsequently received induction chemotherapy. Given that very few, if any, normal progenitor cells would be labeled by BrdU in a floridly leukemic marrow, and given that chemotherapy would almost certainly destroy any maturing normal cells, it is likely that the subsequent appearance of BrdU in terminally differentiated cells such as granulocytes indicates in vivo differentiation of leukemic cells (20).

In this paper, we would like to describe our observations in serial weekly bone marrow samples obtained from AML patients who were given BrdU immediately prior to remission induction chemotherapy. The detection of BrdU labeled blast cells, the appearance of BrdU-labeled granulocytes, their clinical and biological significance and their utility as a determinant of prognosis for the patient will be discussed.

MATERIALS AND METHODS

The BrdU protocol was reviewed and approved by the Roswell Park Memorial Institute's Clinical Investigation Committee as well as the National Cancer Institute (NCI) and the Federal Drug Administration (FDA). The BrdU used in this study was supplied by the NCI. Informed consent as per guidelines required by the NCI and FDA was obtained from every patient prior to the administration of BrdU. The dose of BrdU employed in the first 20 patients at Roswell Park was 200 mg/M^2 intravenously over 2 hours. This was subsequently lowered to 100 mg/M^2 intravenously over 1 hour without jeopardizing results. Finally, the dose has been further reduced to 50 mg/M^2 intravenously over 30 minutes for patients with CML, and once again no compromise in the clarity of labeling has been noted. The reason for successive reductions in the BrdU was to identify the minimal possible dose of a potentially mutagenic agent which was necessary for labeling S-phase cells. It must be noted that no toxicity was observed at 200 mg/M^2 of BrdU or at either of the lower doses.

A total of 20 patients are being presented in this paper. These 20 patients are retrospectively selected from a total of

26 patients studied since 6 did not survive therapy. All patients had a diagnosis of AML and were studied either at the time of diagnosis, or relapsed leukemia. BM aspirate and biopsy samples were obtained immediately at the end of the BrdU infusion. BM biopsies were embedded in plastic using glycol methacrylate (GMA) and all samples were processed by the monoclonal anti-BrdU antibody as described before (19,21). Additionally, serial biopsy specimens were obtained and processed in GMA from all 20 AML patients on a weekly basis after start of chemotherapy. Remission induction chemotherapy was administered to all twenty patients. Twelve received a combination of cytosine arabinoside (araC) and an anthracycline, seven received araC in "high doses" with or without daunomycin and one patient received mitoxantrone and 5-azacytidine. Responses were defined by the criteria described earlier (16) and treatment failures were classified according to our previously reported system (17).

RESULTS

Figure 1 shows an immediate post-BrdU infusion BM aspirate that has been processed by the anti-BrdU antibody. Since the secondary antibody here was conjugated to peroxidase, the S-phase cells show bright reddish-brown staining over the nuclei. By morphology, all the S-phase cells labeled by BrdU appear to be blasts. Following intensive induction chemotherapy, a second BM aspirate was obtained, which was also processed by the anti-BrdU antibody.

Figure 2 shows this sample in which granulocytes labeled with BrdU are clearly visible. Of note in Fig. 2 is the fact that the peroxidase labeling in the granulocyte is not as bright as in cells of Fig. 1 which indicates that dilution of the BrdU label must surely have occurred as the cell underwent several divisions prior to differentiation.

Figure 3 shows an immediate post-BrdU infusion biopsy section in which the S-phase cells show marked peroxidase labeling around the nuclear membrane. This is not a surprising finding, since it has been previously reported that the initiation sites for replicons may be in this region. Serial BM biopsies in these individuals demonstrated several interesting features. These will be summarized as follows:
1. BrdU labeled cells were detected one week following chemotherapy in more than one-half of the patients with AML. The pattern of labeling in these BrdU positive cells was quite different than that observed in day 0 or immediate post-BrdU infusion biopsies. The majority of cells had more homogenous staining of the nucleus indicating that DNA synthesis was completed in these cells. However, occasional cells continued to demonstrate the persistent BrdU-labeling around the nuclear membrane indicating that these cells were arrested in S-phase. Hence it is

FIGURE 1.

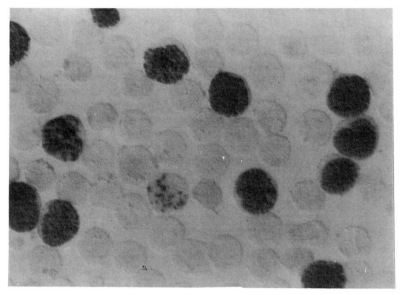

S-phase myeloblasts labeled by peroxidase-conjugated secondary antibody and the primary monoclonal anti-BrdU antibody in an immediate post-BrdU infusion BM aspirate.

FIGURE 2.

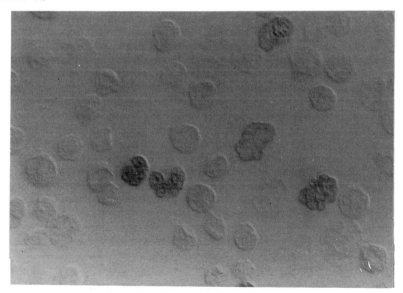

Granulocytes labeled by the anti-BrdU antibody are clearly visible in this BM aspirate from the same patient as in Fig. 1. This sample was obtained after induction chemotherapy was administered.

possible to recognize cells arrested in S-phase but not killed by chemotherapy. If present in a large enough number, this may be an important finding since such cells may resume DNA synthesis at a later date and prevent the patient from entering CR, or perhaps be responsible for early relapse of the disease.

2. Appearance of BrdU labeled granulocytes was noted in seven AML patients in serial biopsies. Interestingly, labeling by anti-BrdU antibody was frequently restricted to one or two lobes of polymorphonuclear leukocytes (PMN). Figure 4 shows a granulocyte labeled by BrdU in two lobes.

3. The clinical significance of detecting BrdU labeled cells in post therapy biopsies is shown in Table 1. Here, it is interesting to note that if no BrdU labeled cells were detected in the day 17 biopsy, then the incidence of CR or RD was almost equal (3 CR's, 2 RD's). When BrdU labeled blasts were persistently detected in day 17 biopsies, 8 of 8 patients demonstrated resistance to therapy. On the other hand, the appearance of BrdU labeled PMN's in these patients seemed to indicate a favorable outcome since 7 of 7 patients entered CR. In some individuals, both labeled blasts and PMN's were noted in earlier biopsies, but by day 17, at least in the patients being reported here, either only persistent blasts remained or labeled granulocytes appeared. The number of labeled PMN's was however much less compared to the number of persistent blasts in the RD patients.

TABLE 1. Relationship of residual BrdU labeled cells following chemotherapy to clinical outcome in AML patients who survived an induction course.

	Complete Remission (No of Pts.)	Resistant Disease (No of Pts)
No labeled cells	3	2
BrdU labeled Blasts	0	8
BrdU labeled Granulocytes	7	0

DISCUSSION

Despite immense interest in the question, until quite recently direct evidence to substantiate the capability of malignant cells to undergo differentiation has been lacking. With the rapid proliferation of novel technologies, at least two separate lines of proof have been forwarded by Fialkow et al (5) and Fearon et al (4) to provide incontrovertible evidence that granulocytes from many patients with AML originate from the malignant clone. Our approach is quite different

FIGURE 3.

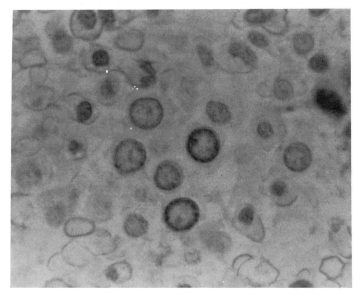

Immediate post-BrdU infusion BM biopsy showing labeling of S-phase cells most prominent around the nuclear membrane.

FIGURE 4.

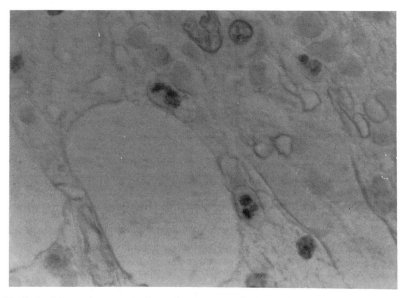

BrdU labeling is restricted to two lobes in this granulocyte seen on a day 17 biopsy section.

from the techniques employed by others. BrdU infusions were administered prior to therapy. Following chemotherapy, serial biopsy specimens were obtained and processed by the monoclonal anti-BrdU antibody to permit identification of labeled cells.

Interestingly, we saw many patterns in these follow-up biopsies. Firstly, there were a number of patients in whom no BrdU-labeled cells were detectable by day 17. Others had persistence of BrdU labeled myeloblasts or the appearance of granulocytes containing BrdU. Since granulocytes are terminally differentiated cells and do not enter DNA synthesis phase, the BrdU must have been incorporated in these cells at an earlier stage such as at the blast, promyelocyte or myelocyte level. Hence the appearance of granulocytes labeled by BrdU indicates the presence of in vivo differentiation. Several questions can be asked at this point:

1) Do these BrdU labeled granulocytes represent terminal differentiation of the leukemic cells or co-existence of residual normal hematopoiesis? BrdU was administered at the time when patients had florid leukemia, therefore it is difficult to imagine that many normal progenitor cells would be actively synthesizing DNA in such a leukemic marrow.

2) Did leukemic cells undergo differentiation because of or despite chemotherapy? All the patients reported here received remission induction chemotherapy and survived the course so that an outcome of CR or RD was available in each case. Most of the patients received cytosine arabinoside (araC) either as a single agent in "high doses" or as part of conventional dose combination therapy with an anthracycline. Therefore, it is possible that araC which has been thought to induce differentiation in some leukemic patients may be similarly active here. (12). However, because it is an S-phase specific agent, it is surprising that all the BrdU labeled cells were not killed by araC. There are several possible explanations. Firstly, chemotherapy was not always administered immediately at the end of the BrdU infusion. In some cases, more than 24 hours elapsed before therapy was actually started, therefore it is likely that the S-phase cells labeled during the BrdU infusion were not in S-phase at the time araC was given. Secondly, it is possible that BrdU-labeled cells which continued to proliferate and re-entered a second S-phase during araC administration were killed. However, cells that were destined to follow the maturation pathway to become promyelocytes, myelocytes and so on did not enter DNA synthesis again. These would not be killed by araC. In other words, araC therapy may have killed all proliferating cells, but all differentiating cells would survive. Therefore, in addition to the possibility of inducing cells to differentiate, surviving mature cells may be selected because of araC therapy.

This latter observation identifies patients in whom the differentiation pathway is intact. It appears to be a very important finding since all the patients who demonstrated this intact pathway (Table 1) (recognized by demonstrating BrdU-labeled granulocytes) entered remission. Such individuals would benefit by araC therapy at more than one level since not only will all the rapidly proliferating cells be killed, but cells capable of following a normal differentiation pathway would survive. On the other hand, patients who do not have an intact differentiation pathway may respond to chemotherapy in the classical sense, i.e. leukemic cells are killed, but may be less able to achieve remission because the surviving leukemic cells cannot undergo maturation. This seems to be the case in patients with blastic crisis of CML where aplasia is often achieved in response to intensive chemotherapy, but normal hematopoietic cells fail to repopulate the marrow.

3) The clinical significance of BrdU labeled cells in post-therapy biopsies is apparent from Table 1. For all the reasons mentioned above, it is clear that whether the BrdU labeled granulocytes are derived from the leukemic clone, or represent normal residual hematopoiesis, their presence following chemotherapy is associated with a positive response. We are now conducting a large scale study of these parameters as determinants of response at the Leukemia Intergroup level (LIG). We expect to utilize these data prospectively in the near future to alter therapeutic plans of individual patients.

The appearance of all the BrdU label in one or two lobes of granulocytes sheds new light on the organization of DNA during S-phase. Since most patients only received a 1 hour infusion of BrdU, whereas S-phase duration on an average is approximately 20 hours in myeloblasts, only 1/20 of the newly synthesized DNA would be labeled by BrdU (24). Following differentiation, the appearance of all this label in 1 or 2 lobes of granulocytes suggests a novel nature of DNA synthesis and organization. The biological significance of this finding is unclear at the present time, but it is possible that DNA synthesized early in S-phase belongs to one lobe whereas late S-phase DNA belongs to another. These possibilities are being tested in vitro in HL-60 cells that are being induced to differentiate with retinoic acid.

In summary, therefore, we have used the presence of BrdU in cells as a label to follow their course in vivo. AML patients were given BrdU infusions followed by remission induction chemotherapy. Serial bone marrow samples were obtained which revealed interesting findings that appear to be of clinical significance. The persistence of BrdU labeled blast cells indicates the presence of residual leukemia and is associated with resistant disease. The appearance of BrdU labeled granulocytes, indicating in vivo differentiation, usually precedes achievement of complete remission. Similar data are being gathered on large numbers of patients with the expectation that the information thus obtained can be used to tailor therapy in individual cases.

REFERENCES

1. Clarkson, B., Ohkita, T., Ota, K., Fried, J. (1967): J. Clin. Invest., 46: 506-529.
2. Clarkson, B., Strife, A., Fried, J., Sakai, Y. (1970): Cancer, 26: 1237-1260.
3. Collins, S., Gallo, R., Gallagher, R. (1977): Nature, 270:347-349.
4. Fearon, E.R., Burke, P.J., Schiffer, C.A., Zehnbauer, B.A., Vogelstein, B. (1986): New Engl. J. Med., 315:15-24.
5. Fialkow, P.J., Singer, J.W., Raskind, W.H., Adamson, J.W., Jacobson, R.J., Bernstein, I.D., Dow, L.W., Majfeld, V., Veith, R. (1978): New Engl. J. Med., 317:468-473.
6. Friend, C., Patuleia, H., Haroen, E. (1966): Natl. Cancer Inst. Monogr., 22:505.
7. Gavosto, F., Pileri, A., Bachi, C., Pegoraro, L. (1964): Nature, 203:92-94.
8. Gavosto, F., Pileri, A., Gabutti, V., Masera, P. (1967): Nature, 216:188-189.
9. Gavosto, F., Pileri, A., Gabutti, V., Masera, P. (1967): Eur. J. Cancer, 3:301-307.
10. Greenberg, M.L., Chanana, A.D., Cronkite, E.P. (1972): Lab. Invest., 26:245-252.
11. Hart, J.S., George, S.E., Frei, E. III, Bodey, G.P., Nickerson, R.C., Freireich, E.J. (1977): Cancer, 39:1603-1617.
12. Housset, M., Daniel, M.T., Degos, L. (1982): Br. J. Haemat., 51:125-129.
13. Killman, S.A., Cronkite, E.P., Robertson, J.S., Fliedner, T.M., Bond, V.P. (1963): Lab. Invest., 12:671-684.
14. Koeffler, H., Golde, D. (1978): Science, 200:1153-1154.
15. Mauer, A., Fisher, V. (1966): Blood, 28(3):428-445.
16. Ohnuma, T., Rosner, F., Levy, R.N., Cuttner, J., Moon, J.H., Silver, R.T., Bloom, J., Falkson, G., Burningham, R., Glidewell, O., Holland, J.F. (1971): Cancer Chemother. Rep., 55: 269-275.
17. Preisler, H.D. (1978): Med. Pediatr. Oncol., 4:275-278.
18. Preisler, H.D., Azarnia, N., Raza, A., Grunwald, H., Vogler, W.R. (1984): Br. J. Haematol., 56:399-407.
19. Raza, A., Spiridonidis, C., Ucar, K., Bankert, R., Mayers, G., Preisler, H.D. (1985): Cancer Res. 45:2283-2287.
20. Raza, A., Preisler, H.D. (1986) Cancer J., 1:15-18.
21. Raza, A., Maheshwari, Y., Ucar, K., Mayers, G., Preisler, H.D. (1987): Acta Haemat., 77:140-145.
22. Raza, A., Maheshwari, Y., Preisler, H.D. (1987) Blood, 69:(6)1647-1653.
23. Raza, A., Maheshwari, Y., Brereton, W., Preisler, H.D. (1987): Am. J. Hematol., 24: 65-75.
24. Raza, A., Mandava, N., Maheshwari, Y., Yasin, Z. (1987): Proc. Am. Assoc. Cancer Res., 28:38, 152a.

25. Rovera, G., Santoli, D., Damsky, C. (1979): Proc. Natl. Acad. Sci. USA, 76:2779-2783.
26. Saunders, E.F., Lampkin, B.C., Maurer, A.M. (1967): J. Clin. Invest. 46:1356-1362.

DESIGN OF COMBINATION
DIFFERENTIATION THERAPY

Combination Differentiation Therapy

M. Wiemann, P. Alexander* and P. Calabresi

Department of Medicine
Roger Williams General Hospital and Brown University
Providence, Rhode Island 02908, USA;
*Faculty of Medicine, University of Southampton, Southampton, S09 4XY U.K.

With only a few exceptions, the successful use of cytotoxic drugs in the treatment of patients with cancer requires that combinations of two or more drugs be used. It, therefore, is not surprising that early clinical trials with drugs that induce tumor cells to differentiate suggest that these agents may also need to be administered in combination if their activity in the laboratory is to be translated into the clinic. For example, Phase I studies with the polar-planar compound N-methylformamide (NMF) demonstrated that the concentrations required for the induction of differentiation in vitro could not be achieved in patients (40). The administration of hexamethylene bisacetamide (HMBA), another low molecular weight polar-planar compound, as a five-day continuous infusion at the maximal tolerated dose achieved steady-state concentrations only minimally effective at inducing in vitro differentiation (13). The administration of HMBA by a ten-day infusion at the maximally tolerated dose produced even lower steady-state concentrations than the five-day schedule (32). Similarly, low-dose cytosine arabinoside, a putative inducer of granulocytic differentiation in myelodysplatic syndromes and acute myeloid leukemia, produces significant toxicity (6).

Advantages of using cytotoxic drugs in combination include the ability to achieve maximal killing of tumor cells with doses of each drug that are tolerated by the patient and the potential to eliminate drug-resistant populations present within heterogeneous tumors. Combining differentiation-inducing drugs may also enhance their anticancer effect with doses of the drugs that are not excessively toxic. The use of these drugs in combination may also reduce existing drug-resistant populations and limit the development of acquired resistance.

The principles that have evolved for the design of effective combinations of cytotoxic drugs may be used, with some modifications, to select differentiation-inducing drugs for combination therapy programs (Table 1). For example, in combining differentiation-inducing drugs, it may not be necessary to include only compounds with activity as single agents, as is usually done in designing multi-drug anticancer therapies. Differentiation-inducers that are only marginally effective or ineffective as single agents may be active in combination with other drugs. Recombinant human leukocyte interferon (IFN-αA) does not induce terminal differentiation of the human promyelocytic leukemic cell line HL-60. When IFN-αA, however, is combined with agents that do induce differentiation of HL-60 cells, such as 12,13-<u>cis</u>-retinoic acid (RA), NMF, or HMBA, induction of differentiation is markedly increased (18, 43).

TABLE 1. <u>Principles for designing differentiation therapy combinations.</u>

---

1. Drugs that are ineffective or only marginally effective as single agents may be active when included in combinations.
2. Drugs selected from different classes of inducers are more likely to be effective in combination than drugs from the same group.
3. Differentiation inducers may be combined effectively with other treatment modalities, e.g., cyotoxic drugs, irradiation, biological agents.
4. Select drugs with toxicities that do not overlap.
5. Optimal doses and schedules of administration must be used.

Drugs from several classes of compounds, as well as certain cytokines, are able to induce a more differentiated phenotype in susceptible human tumor cell lines. These include polar-planar compounds, inhibitors of DNA synthesis, inhibitors of DNA methyltransferase, agents that interfere with microtubule assembly, retinoids, analogs of vitamin D_3, interferons, and hematopoietic growth factors. Agents that act by different mechanisms of action are most likely to be synergistic when used together. The most effective cytotoxic drug regimens, such as the combination of mechlorethamine, vincristine, procarbazine, and prednisone (MOPP) used to treat patients with advanced stages of Hodgkin's disease, include drugs with different mechanisms of action. Similarly, combinations that include differentiation agents from more than one class or differentiation-inducing drugs combined with other chemotherapeutic agents (e.g. cis-platinum) are most likely to be effective.

As with cytotoxic drugs, combinations of differentiation-inducing agents should include drugs with toxicities that do not overlap. The dose-limiting toxicities of several of the clinically available differentiation-inducers are sufficiently varied that combinations can be designed without including drugs with overlapping toxicities.

The efficacy of combinations of cytotoxic drugs is dose and schedule dependent. The effects of several of the differentiation inducers, used either as single agents or in combinations, are strictly dependent upon the schedule of administration. The favorable phenotypic changes induced by N,N-dimethylformamide (DMF), a polar-planar compound with properties similar to NMF, in human colon cancer cell lines, for example, are reversed once DMF is removed from the culture medium (11). The effects of interferons on cell differentiation are also reversible once it is no longer present (31). In vitro and in vivo studies have demonstrated the importance of schedule of administration for the combination of NMF and irradiation. Optimal radiosensitization by NMF is achieved when the drug is administered both before and after irradiation (24). The determination of optimal doses and schedules for differentiation-inducing drugs used in combinations will depend upon carefully designed clinical trials. Laboratory investigations that utilize either human tumor cell lines that can be induced to differentiate or tumor cells freshly isolated from patients are providing information necessary for the design of clinical studies.

Only a small number of Phase I and II clinical trials of differentiation-inducing drugs administered as single agents are complete. NMF, HMBA, and 13-cis-retinoic acid have received the most extensive clinical study. The clinical evaluation of differentiation agents in combinations is, therefore, only now beginning. Although the results from just a few of these trials are available, a number of laboratory studies have demonstrated the effectiveness of combination differentiation therapy. In the sections below, we will discuss several approaches to the development of combination therapies that include differentiation-inducing agents and their potential for the treatment of patients with cancer.

DIFFERENTIATION AGENTS AND CYTOTOXIC DRUGS

A number of biochemical effects produced by drugs that induce the differentiation of tumor cells suggest that these agents might potentiate the activities of conventional anticancer drugs. The polar-planar compound NMF causes several alterations in cancer cells that indicate it may be a particularly attractive candidate for testing in combination with cytotoxic drugs.

Polar compounds alter the fluidity of the membranes of tumor cells and may facilitate the uptake of cytotoxic drugs. Dimethylsulfoxide (DMSO), a polar compound with properties similar to NMF, produces single-strand breaks in DNA (33). NMF induces sister chromatid exchanges in tumor cells and probably damages DNA in a manner similar to DMSO (34). The production of single-strand breaks may alter the tertiary structure of DNA by inducing the unwinding of complimentary strands and changing the structure of chromatin (33). By inducing alterations in the structural integrity of DNA, NMF could render it more susceptible to attack by the active species of a cytotoxic drug.

The polar compound DMF, of which NMF is a metabolite, modulates the activities of enzymes of purine and pyrimidine metabolism in cultured human tumor cells (10,29). Such alterations could result in the potentiation of purine and pyrimidine analogs by either increasing their activation or decreasing their catabolism. For example, the antitumor activities of a number of adenosine analogs, such as arabinosyladenine, are limited because they are rapidly deaminated to inactive metabolites by the enzyme adenosine deaminase. Exposure of the human colon carcinoma cell line clone A to DMF reduced the activity of adenosine deaminase eleven-fold, as compared to untreated controls (10). This suggests that colon cancer cells from some patients could be rendered sensitive to adenosine analogs by pretreatment with this differentiation-inducing drug.

In addition to potentiating damage to DNA by cytotoxic drugs, NMF may also inhibit its subsequent repair. Studies of the combination of NMF and radiation demonstrated a drug-induced enhancement of tumor cell kill in the low-dose shoulder region of the X-ray cell survival curve (25,27). This suggest that NMF may inhibit the repair of radiation-induced sublethal damage. Pretreatment of murine hepatocarcinoma cells with NMF enhanced the cell kill produced by 1,3-bis(2-chloroethyl)-1-nitrosourea, cis-platinum, and melphalan (34). As with radiation, NMF modified the low-dose region of the cell survival curves. Decreases in the shoulder regions of these curves suggest that NMF may also interfere with the repair of drug-induced damage to DNA.

Solid Tumors

At the Roger Williams Cancer Center, we are studying the effect of NMF on the chemosensitivity of human solid tumor cell lines, particularly colon carcinomas and melanomas. Solid tumors are an especially appropriate target for studies of chemosensitization because of their resistance to conventional treatment modalitites. The intratumor heterogeneity that is characteristic of solid tumors is a major obstacle to their successful treatment. Differentiation therapy may provide a means to limit heterogeneity.

Human cancers are composed of heterogeneous subpopulations of cells, each possessing particular phenotypic traits. Heterogeneity exist within a single tumor for a number of cellular characteristics that influence response to different therapeutic modalities. These important manifestations of tumor heterogeneity include growth rate; cell surface receptors for hormones and growth factors; antigenic and immunogenic properties; metastatic ability; and sensitivities to chemotherapeutic drugs, x-irradiation, and hyperthermia.

The emergence of populations of neoplastic cells

resistant to drugs that previously induced a regression of the tumor mass is a common occurrence in the treatment of patients with solid tumors. The development of drug resistance may be associated with a variety of karyotypic and biochemical changes within the cell. Decreased drug transport, changes in the activities of target or catabolic enzymes, and the appearance of amplified genes as homogeneously staining regions or double minute chromosomes are among the alterations observed in drug-resistant populations. Drug resistance is a manifestation of tumor heterogeneity that arises, as do other phenotypic changes, as a consequence of spontaneous genetic mutations. These mutational changes are heritable and, through clonal expansion, lead to the development of resistant subpopulations.

We have previously suggested that differentiation inducing agents might favorably modulate characteristics of tumor heterogeneity that are responsible for drug resistance (7). For example, in a breast carcinoma that contains subpopulations of cells heterogeneous for the expression of hormone receptors, treatment with an inducer of differentiation might convert receptor-negative cells to a receptor-positive phenotype and render them susceptible to subsequent hormonal therapies. The treatment of cultured human colon cancer cells with DMF increases the expression of several cell-surface antigens including carcinoembryonic antigen (CEA) (19). The ability to predictably modulate the expression of tumor-associated antigens could improve the efficacy of monoclonal antibodies as diagnostic and therapeutic agents.

Differentiation-inducing drugs, therefore, could improve the efficacy of other therapeutic modalities by reducing the existing heterogeneity of a solid tumor to a more homogeneous population. The administration of a differentiation-inducing drug between cycles of cytotoxic therapy might also limit the dynamic evolution of new drug-resistant clones (30).

The treatment of cultured human solid tumor cells with NMF does not induce terminal differentiation, as occurs in certain leukemic cell lines. NMF does, however, induce changes suggestive of a more differentiated phenotype. These phenotypic alterations include changes in morphology, decreased growth rate _in vitro_ and _in vivo_, decreased clonogenicity, decreased tumorigenicity in athymic mice, alterations in cell surface antigens, and the production of specialized cell products (12,23). The ability of NMF to induce chemosensitization in these human tumor cell lines is being tested.

In these experiments, human colon cancer or melanoma cells are cultured for three to five passages in a concentration of NMF that is optimal for the induction of differentiation. These concentrations of NMF produce an increase in cell-doubling times but are not cytotoxic. Subsequent sensitivity to cytotoxic drugs is assessed by cell survival and clonogenic assays. For the human colon cancer cell lines clone A, clone D, and HCT-15, pretreatment with NMF caused a ten-fold increase in the activities of cis-platinum and etoposide (39).

The combination of NMF and doxorubicin, however, does not always enhance cytotoxicity. Pretreatment with NMF increased the sensitivity in vitro of the human melanoma cell line Tang to doxorubicin by greater than two-fold (23). NMF, however, induced significant resistance to doxorubicin in the colon carcinoma cell lines clone A and clone D (14).

Although, for each of the colon cancer and melanoma cell lines tested, NMF induced similar changes in growth kinetics and other cellular characteristics indicative of a more differentiated phenotype, its effect on chemosensitivity varied with the tumor cell line being studied and the cytotoxic drug included in the combination.

Other investigators have also demonstrated that NMF can potentiate the response of tumor cells in vitro and in vivo to cytotoxic drugs (20, 34). NMF-induced enhancement occurs for drugs that are both effective and ineffective as single agents. The combination of NMF with cis-platinum appears to be particularly active and has produced either additive or synergistic effects in each tumor cell system tested.

Several possible mechanisms for potentiation of cytotoxic drugs by NMF are discussed above. It is also reported that NMF reduces the intracellular glutathione levels of clone A colon carcinoma cells (9). Depletion of glutathione might be expected to increase sensitivity to doxorubicin. The significance of changes in the levels of glutathione as a mechanism of NMF-mediated chemosensitization, however, remains unclear. Arundel and Tofilon (3) reported that, after correction for the increased cell volume produced by exposure to NMF, the glutathione content of clone A cells was not altered by the drug. Clone A and clone D cells, in addition, were rendered more resistant to doxorubicin by pretreatment with NMF (14).

NMF may, as mentioned above, alter the fluidity of cell membranes and increase the uptake of cytotoxic drugs. We are determining the effect of pretreatment with polar-planar differentiation-inducing drugs on the uptake of cis-platinum (DDP) by human colon cancer cells (38). Intracellular platinum (Pt) levels are measured by plasma emission spectroscopy. After correction for drug-induced increases in cell volume, neither NMF nor HMBA, at concentrations tested, increased the uptake of cis-platinum in these two colon cancer cell lines (Table 2).

TABLE 2.   Platinum uptake by colon cancer cells

Treatment	[Pt] (ppm)	p[a]	Cell Size	p[b]
Clone A:				
DDP (15 μg/ml)	1.5 ± 0.2		5.3 ± 0.6	
DDP + NMF (1%)	3.3 ± 0.2	<0.01	17.2 ± 0.2	<0.01
DDP + HMBA (5 mM)	1.5 ± 0.2	0.80	10.8 ± 1.1	0.01
Clone D:				
DDP (15 μg/ml)	1.7 ± 0.1		3.3 ± 0.1	
DDP + NMF (1%)	1.6 ± 0.2	0.75	5.1 ± 0.3	<0.01
DDP + HMBA (5 mM)	1.6 ± 0.2	0.68	5.2 ± 1.3	0.12

[a]Results of t-test between DDP and DDP + 2nd drug group
[b]mg/10^6 cells.

In vitro and in vivo studies with additional tumor cell lines, other cytotoxic drugs, and schedules of administration are being conducted to further evaluate the effects of polar-planar compounds on the uptake of conventional chemotherapeutic agents.

The results of these studies suggest that NMF may potentiate the activities of cytotoxic drugs against human tumors. The potential for inducing drug resistance indicates the need for additional in vitro and in vivo studies to identify characteristics of tumors and drugs that will predict for sensitization. The dose-limiting toxicity of NMF is hepatotoxicity and it does not produce myelosuppression or nephrotoxicity (42). It should be possible, therefore, to include NMF in combinations that contain the most frequently used drugs, without producing additive toxicities. By altering the blood-brain barrier, polar compounds such as NMF may also facilitate the entry of anticancer drugs into the central nervous system and prove useful in combination therapies of patients with gliomas or tumors metastatic to the brain (5).

Myelodysplasia and Acute Leukemia

A large number of agents induce differentiation of murine and human leukemic cell lines (8, 36). Neoplastic and dysplastic cells from patients with either acute myeloid leukemia or myelodysplastic syndromes can also be induced to granulocytic differentiation in vitro (16). The myelodysplastic syndromes are a group of clonal hematopoietic diseases characterized by defective maturation and ineffective hematopoiesis (6). There is no effective treatment and patients often die of the complications of cytopenias or the disease may evolve into acute myeloid leukemia that is usually refractory to therapy.

There have been several clinical trials of differentiation-inducing drugs administered as single agents in patients with myelodysplastic syndromes. Cytosine arabinoside administered in low-dose and 13-cis-retinoic acid are active in these diseases (4, 17). The responses are of brief duration, however, and the toxicities of both drugs are substantial. Whether low-dose cytosine arabinoside induces differentiation or acts primarily as a cytotoxic drug is uncertain.

Using short-term suspension cultures of bone marrow from patients with myelodysplastic syndromes and myeloid leukemias, Francis et al. (15, 16) systematically analyzed the interactions of differentiation-inducing agents used in combination with conventional chemotherapeutic drugs.

Detailed statistical analyses of the interactions of these agents demonstrated that combinations of differentiation-inducing drugs (retinoic acid and NMF) with inhibitors of DNA synthesis (6-mercaptopurine, cytosine arabinoside, and aphidicolin) produced a differentiation-inducing effect equivalent to that of 10 to 100, or even 1000-fold higher concentrations of single agents (16). The combination of retinoic acid and vincristine was also identified as synergistic (15). These combinations also did not produce synergistic myelotoxicity in vitro.

The identification of synergistic combinations of differentiation-inducing agents and conventional chemotherapeutic drugs is a potentially important advance in the therapy of patients with myelodysplastic syndromes or myeloid leukemias. Clinical trials of combinations of 13-cis-retinoic acid with 6-thioguanine, cytosine arabinoside, or vincristine are now in progress.

DIFFERENTIATION AGENTS AND X-IRRADIATION

In addition to augmenting the sensitivity of tumor cells to cytotoxic drugs, some differentiation-inducing agents also enhance the toxicity of ionizing radiation. For the past several years, investigators at the Roger Williams Cancer Center, as well as other laboratories, have studied the radiation sensitization properties of differentiation-inducing drugs, particularly DMF and NMF.

Initially, studies of two subpopulations of cells isolated from a heterogeneous mouse mammary adenocarcinoma demonstrated that growth of the cells in medium containing noncytotoxic concentrations of DMF prior to irradiation favorably enhanced the x-ray survival response of the more inherently radioresistant clone (25). The modifying effect of DMF occurred in the low-dose shoulder region of the survival curve. Pretreatment with DMF had little effect on the more radiosensitive of the two subpopulations.

DMF also sensitized two subpopulations, clones A and D, of a heterogeneous human colon carcinoma cell line to irradiation (26). Pretreatment with DMF enhanced the radiation response of both cell lines by a factor of 1.3, as compared to untreated controls. If the tumor cells were also maintained in DMF-containing medium after irradiation, there was a further augmentation of the enhancement factor to 2.3 and 1.5 for clones A and D, respectively. As in the experiments with the murine tumor cell lines, the greatest effects occurred in the clinically relevant low-dose region of the x-ray survival curve. The more radioresistant line, clone A, showed the greater radiosensitization response. The observation that maximal radiosensitization occurred when the cells were exposed to DMF both before and after irradiation has important implications for the design of clinical trials.

Arundel et al. (1) demonstrated a similar degree of radiosensitization by NMF in primary human tumor cell cultures. NMF-mediated radiosensitization was not dependent on the histologic cell type of the tumor. Similar to the results obtained with human tumor cell lines, the dose-enhancement factors in the sensitized primary cultures ranged from 1.3 to 2.5 and the radiosensitization resulted from a modification of the shoulder region of the survival curve. These results support the data from experiments with established cell lines and suggest that the combination of NMF and radiation may be active against a variety of tumor types.

If a radiation sensitizer is to be useful in the treatment of patients, it must selectively enhance the radiation response of tumor cells without significantly potentiating radiation damage to normal tissues. Iwakawa et al. (24) demonstrated that the systemic administration of NMF to mice at a dose sufficient to sensitize the FSA fibrosarcoma and its pulmonary metastases to radiation did not affect the radiosensitivity of the gut or testes. These results indicate that, at least in this model, the combination of NMF with radiation produces a therapeutic gain.

Although it is now well-established that DMF and NMF can sensitize human tumor cells in vitro and in vivo to irradiation, the mechanisms responsible are not yet defined. Exposure to NMF may result in differentiation but not radiosensitization (3). NMF causes the formation of DNA-protein crosslinks at doses of radiation that do not induce this form of damage to DNA in control cells. This modification of radiation-induced DNA-protein crosslinks suggest that NMF alters the relationship between DNA and chromatin (3). In human colon cancer cells, DMF increases the rate and extent of potentially lethal damage recovery (2). The role of fluctuations of intracellular glutathione levels in the radiosensitization produced by the polar compounds remains controversial (3, 9).

The potential for NMF to increase the radioresponsiveness of human tumors has been demonstrated. Preclinical studies indicate that the effectiveness of the combination is maximal when the differentiating agent is administered both before and after radiation. A Phase I study of the combination of NMF and radiotherapy in patients with advanced cancer is now in progress at Brown University.

Combinations that include NMF, irradiation, and cytotoxic drugs also appear to have synergistic activity against human tumor cells (27). Other differentiation inducing agents are also being evaluated in the laboratory for radiosensitizing activity.

COMBINATIONS OF DIFFERENTIATION AGENTS

The availability of leukemic cell lines, such as the promyelocytic HL-60, that can be induced to terminal differentiation by a large number of drugs has stimulated the evaluation of combinations that include two or more differentiation-inducing agents. The goal of these studies is to identify combinations that synergistically inhibit growth and induce differentiation, using concentrations of each drug that are tolerated by normal tissues (21, 35, 37).

At the Roger Williams Cancer Center, we are also evaluating the effects of combinations of differentiation-inducing drugs on human leukemic cell lines. Our particular emphasis is to combine drugs that are already in clinical trials as single agents. We have chosen this approach because: [1] When synergistic combinations are identified, clinical trials may be initiated more rapidly; and [2] Because the toxicities of these drugs are known, we are able to design combinations that do not have prohibitive overlapping toxicities.

In addition to the HL-60 cell line, we are using the unique, inducible chronic myeloid leukemic cell line RWLeu-4 (22, 41). In a pattern similar to HL-60, a number of drugs induce RWLeu-4 cells to either myeloid or macrophage differentiation.

As single agents, both NMF and HMBA induce myeloid differentiation of RWLeu-4 cells. Although these two drugs belong to the same class of compounds, their mechanisms of action may be different. Phase I trials of different schedules of NMF and HMBA are completed and their dose-limiting toxicities are different.

When increasing concentrations of NMF, 25, 75, 100 or 150 mM, were combined with HMBA, 1mM, myeloid differentiation was enhanced at each concentration of NMF. The enhancement factors ranged from 1.7 to

2.0.   Similar results occurred when the NMF concentration was kept constant, either 25 or 75 mM, and the HMBA concentration was escalated, 0.5, 1.0 1.5, or 2.0 mM. The enhancement factors ranged from 1.3 to 3.2.

For the RWLeu-4 cell line, therefore, combinations of NMF and HMBA are more effective than either drug used alone. At concentrations of NMF and HMBA that were ineffective as single agents, the addition of the other drug resulted in the induction of differentiation.   We are now evaluating this combination against RWLeu-4 cells growing as chloromas in athymic mice.

The growing number of drugs and biological agents capable of inducing maturation in leukemic cell lines presents multiple possibilities for the design of combination differentiation therapy regimens. Laboratory studies with inducible cell lines and leukemic cells obtained from patients will provide the foundation for the design of clinical trials.

CONCLUSIONS

It is likely that drugs that induce the differentiation of tumor cells will achieve their full potential when used in combination therapy regimens. Because of their diverse mechanisms of action and biological effects, it is expected. that numerous synergistic combinations will be identified. If combination differentiation therapies are able to limit the evolution of tumor heterogeneity, as is suggested by preclinical studies, the efficacy of existing drugs may be significantly enhanced. The role of these regimens as components of adjuvant therapy programs is yet to be explored but offers exciting possibilities. Combination differentiation therapy has the potential to become a significant addition to our anticancer armamentarium.

REFERENCES

1. Arundel, C.M., Bock, S., Brook, W.A., and Tofilon, P.J. (1987): Int. J. Radiat. Oncol. Biol. Phys., 13:753-757.
2. Arundel, C.M., Glicksman, A.S. and Leith, J.T. (1985): Cancer Res., 45:5557-5562.

3. Arundel, C.M. and Tofilon, P.J. (1987): <u>Radiat.</u> <u>Res.</u>, (In Press).

4. Bacarrani, M., Zaccaria, A., Bandini, G., Cavazzini, G., Fanin, R., and Tura, S. (1983): <u>Leuk. Res.</u>, 7:539-545.

5. Broadwell, R.D., Salcman, M., and Kaplan, R.S. (1982): <u>Science</u>, 217:1164-1166.

6. Buzaid, A.C., Garewal, H.S., and Greenberg, B.R. (1986): <u>Am. J. Med.</u>, 80:1149-1157.

7. Calabresi, P.and Wiemann, M.C. (1986): In: <u>Principles of Internal Medicine. Update VII Oncology</u>, edited by J. Mendelsohn, R.G. Petersdorf, R.D. Adams, E. Braunwald, K.J. Isselbacher, J.B. Martin, and J.D. Wilson, pp. 61-79. McGraw-Hill Book Company, New York.

8. Collins, S.J. (1987): <u>Blood</u>, 70:1233-1244.

9. Cordeiro, R.F. and Savarese, T.M. (1986): <u>Cancer Res.</u>, 46:1297-1305.

10. Crabtree, G.W., Dexter, D.L., Stoeckler, J.D., Savarese, T.M., Ghoda, L.Y., Rogler-Brown, T.L., Calabresi, P., and Parks, R.E., Jr. (1981): <u>Biochem, Pharmacol.</u>, 30:793-788.

11. Dexter, D.L., Barbosa, J.A., and Calabresi, P. (1979): <u>Cancer Res.</u>, 39:1020-1025.

12. Dexter, D.L. and Calabresi, P. (1982): In: <u>Pancreatic Tumors in Children</u>, edited by G.B. Humphrey, pp. 45-56. Martinus Nijhoff, The Hague.

13. Egorin, M.J., Sigman, L. M., Van Echo, D.A., Forrest, A., Whitacre, M.Y., and Aisner, J. (1987): <u>Cancer Res.</u>, 47:617-623.

14. Ferrari, L.A., Bliven, S.F., Wiemann, M.C., Calabresi, P., Glicksman, A.S. and Leith, J.T. (1986): <u>Cancer Treat. Rep.</u>, 70:1177-1180.

15. Francis, G.E. and Berney, J.J. (1986): In: <u>Experimental Haematology Today - 1985</u>, edited by S.J. Baum, D.H. Pluznik, and L.A. Rozenszajn, pp. 82-89. Springer-Verlag, Berlin, Heidelberg.

16. Francis, G.E., Guimaraes, J.E.T.E., Berney, J.J., Wing, M.A. (1985): In: <u>Haematology and Blood Transfusion Vol. 29 Modern Trends in Human Leukemia VI</u>, edited by R. Neth, R. Gallo, J. Greaves, and S. Janka, pp.402-408. Springer-Verlag, Berlin, Heidelberg.

17. Gold, E.J., Mertelsmann, R.H., Itri, L.M., Gee, T., Arlin, Z., Kempin, S., Clarkson, B., and Moore, M.A.S. (1983): Cancer Treat Rep., 67:981-986.
18. Grant, S., Bhalla, K., Weinstein, I.B., Pestka, S., Mileno, M.D., and Fisher, P.B. (1985): Biochem. Biophys. Res. Comm., 130:379-388.
19. Hager, J.C., Gold, D.V., Barbosa, J.A., Fligiel, Z., Miller, F., and Dexter, D.L. (1980): J. Natl. Cancer Inst., 64:439-446.
20. Harpur, E.S., Langdon, S. P., Fathalla, S.A.K., and Ishmael, J. (1986): Cancer Chemother. Pharmacol., 16:139-147.
21. Hemmi, H. and Breitman, T.R. (1987): Blood, 69:501-507.
22. Huhn, R.D., Posner, M.R., Foulkes, G., Rayter, S., and Frackelton, A.R., Jr. (1987): Proc. Natl. Acad. Sci. (USA), 84:4408-4412.
23. Ingber, S., Wiemann, M.C., Campagnone, N., and Calabresi, P. (1985): Clin. Res., 33:453A.
24. Iwakawa, M., Milas, L., Hunter, N., and Tofilon, P. J. (1987): Int. J. Radiat. Oncol. Biol. Phys., 13:55-60.
25. Leith, J. T., Brenner, H.J., DeWyngaert, J.K., Dexter, D.L., Calabresi, P., and Glicksman, A.S. (1981): Int. J. Radiat. Oncol. Biol. Phys., 7:934-947.
26. Leith, J. T., Gaskins, L.A., Dexter, D.L., Calabresi, P., and Glicksman, A.S. (1982): Cancer Res., 42:30-34.
27. Leith, J.T., Lee, E.S., Leite, B.S., and Glicksman, A.S. (1986): Int. J. Radiat. Oncol. Biol. Phys., 12:1423-1427.
28. Leith, J.T., Lee, E.S., Vayer. A.J., Dexter, D.L., and Glicksman, A.S. (1985): Int. J. Radiat. Oncol. Biol. Phys., 11:1971-1976.
29. Naguib, F.N.M., Niedzwicki, J.G., Iltzsch, M.H., Wiemann, M.C., el Kouni, M.H., and Cha, S. (1987): Leuk. Res., 10:855-861.
30. Nicolson, G.L. and Lotan, R. (1986): Clin. Expl. Metastasis, 4:231-235.
31. Rossi, G.B. (1985): Interferon, 6:31-68.
32. Rowinsky, E.K., Ettinger, D.S., McGuire, W. P., Noe, D.A., Grochow, L.B., and Donehower, R.C. (1987): Cancer Res., 47:5788:5795.
33. Scher, W. and Friend C. (1978): Cancer Res., 38:841-849.

34. Tofilon, P.J., Vines, C.M., and Milas, L. (1986): Cancer Chemother. Pharmacol., 17:269-273.
35. Trinchieri, G., Rosen, R., and Perussia, B. (1987): Blood, 69:1218-1224.
36. Waxman, S., Scher, W., and Scher, B.M. (1986): Cancer Detection and Prevention, 9:395-407.
37. Weinberg, J.B. and Larrick, J.W. (1987): Blood, 70:994-1002.
38. Wiemann, M.C., Belliveau, J.F., Posner, M.R., Weitberg, A.B., O'Leary, G.P., and Calabresi, P. (1987): Proc. Fifth Internat. Symp. on Platinum, 5:231-232.
39. Wiemann, M.C. and Calabresi, P. (1986): Proc. First. Conf. Diff. Ther., 1:89.
40. Wiemann, M.C., Cummings, F.J., Posner, M.R., Weens, J.H., Crabtree, G.W., Birmingham, B.K., Moore, A., and Calabresi, P. (1985): Proc. Am. Soc. Clin. Oncol., 4:38.
41. Wiemann, M.C., Hollmann, A., Posner, M., Arlin, Z., Friedland, M., and Calabresi, P. (1985): Clin. Res., 33:461A.
42. Wiemann, M.C., Michael, P., Cummings, F.J., Spremulli, E.N., Posner, M.R., Griffin, W.C., Matook, G.M., Birmingham, B.K., and Calabresi, P. (1984): Proc. Am. Soc. Clin. Oncol., 3:41.
43. Wiemann, M.C., Poisson, L., and Calabresi, P. (1987): Clin. Res., 529A.

Control of Proliferation of Myeloid Leukemia Cells by Treatment with Differentiation Inducers in Combination with Anti-Leukemic Drugs *In Vitro* and *In Vivo*

M. Hozumi, T. Kasukabe, Y. Honma, J. Okabe-Kado,
M. Hayashi, Y. Yamamoto-Yamaguchi and M. Tomida

*Department of Chemotherapy, Saitama Cancer Center Research Institute,
Ina, Saitama 362, Japan*

INTRODUCTION

Various types of leukemia cells can be induced to differentiate into cells with similar characteristics to mature myeloid and lymphoid cells(1,6,7,17). On differentiation, the cells cease to proliferate and lose their leukemogenicity. These findings suggest that in vivo induction of terminal cell differentiation by certain compounds, that is differentiation therapy of leukemia, is a possible method for leukemia therapy (1,6,7,17).

In fact, some inducers of differentiation have been reported to be effective in experimental animals inoculated with various myeloid leukemia cell lines and in patients with acute myelogenous leukemia(1,6,7,17). However, the therapeutic effects of the differentiation inducers alone are rather weak and are limited to certain types of myelogenous leukemia. In an attempt to improve the strategy for differentiation therapy of myeloid leukemia, we have been studying the basic problems of this therapy mainly using mouse myeloid leukemia M1 cells as an experimental model(6,7).

Although most M1 cells can be induced to differentiate into nonproliferating mature macrophages and granulocytes, frequently some populations of cells remain unresponsive to the differentiation inducers (3,4,6-9,15,16,18,21,22). Induction of differentiation of all the unresponsive cells is difficult with the highest tolerable concentration of the inducer for the cells. Therefore, we examined the characteristics of the resistant clones of M1 cells that appeared during long-term culture of sensitive M1 cells(4,6-8,15,16,

22). We isolated several variant clones that were resistant to either dexamethasone or a protein inducer
(differentiation inducing factor, D-factor)from ascitic
fluid(4,6,7). All the dexamethasone-resistant clones
showed less response than the sensitive cells to the
protein inducer, but some clones that were resistant to
induction of differentiation by the D-factor were induced to differentiate by dexamethasone, suggesting
that these different inducers have different targets in
the cells(4,6,7).

On the other hand, the resistant M1 cell clones, but
not the sensitive M1 cell clones, were found to produce
an inhibitory protein factor (I-factor) for induction
of differentiation of M1 cells(6,7,15). We recently
purified a factor from the main fraction of the I-
factor in conditioned medium (CM) of a resistant M1
cell clone and estimated its apparent molecular weight
as 68,000(8). Production of the I-factor by the resistant cells was closely associated with resistance of
the cells to differentiation inducers, since inhibition
of synthesis of this I-factor by a low concentration of
actinomycin D concomitantly restored the sensitivity
of the resistant cells to the inducers(6,7). Other
inhibitors of RNA or protein synthesis also sensitized
resistant clones of M1 cells to the D-factor(6,7).
Furthermore, anticancer agents, interferon, and
dimethylsulfoxide also sensitized resistant M1 cells to
the D-factor, although none of these substances alone
induced differentiation of the cells(6,7). These findings suggest that some anticancer drugs in combination
with a differentiation inducer control proliferation of
leukemic cells by inducing differentiation of the cells
as well as by their cytotoxic actions.

We recently examined the effects of differentiation
inducers on proliferation of M1 cells and human myeloid
leukemia cells in long-term cultures to develop a more
effective strategy for therapy with differentiation
inducers. We found in studies using a constant product
of time and concentration (total dose) of drug, that
proliferation of M1 cells was inhibited most effectively by continuous treatment with differentiation in-
ducers such as $1\alpha,25$-dihydroxyvitamin D_3 $(1\alpha,25(OH)_2D_3)$
and dexamethasone(9). Nevertheless, resistant M1 cells
appeared during long-term (25 days) treatment with
$1\alpha,25(OH)_2D_3$ and growth of these cells was not suppres-
sed(9). However, when we treated M1 cells continuously
with $1\alpha,25(OH)_2D_3$ in combination with a noncytotoxic
low dose of cytosine arabinoside (Ara-C) or daunomycin,
the resistant cells did not appear for at least 35
days(9). Moreover, $1\alpha,25(OH)_2D_3$ and cytotoxic drugs
were found to have similar effects on proliferation of

human monoblast-like U937 cells(9).

Based on these in vitro experiments, we examined the effect of 1α-hydroxyvitamin D_3 (1α(OH)D_3) in combination with daunomycin on the survival of syngeneic SL mice inoculated with M1 cells. The survival of the mice was prolonged more by treatment with both 1α(OH)D_3 and daunomycin than by treatment with either drug alone(9). Similar enhancing effects of other differentiation inducers (lipopolysaccharide (LPS), alkylethyleneglycophospholipid and protein inducer) and anticancer drugs (actinomycin D and cyclophosphamide) on prolongation of the survival of the mice were observed previously(6,7). This paper reviews these results and suggests that treatment of myeloid leukemia cells with a differentiation inducer in combination with a low dose of some anticancer drug is more effective therapeutically than treatment with the differentiation inducer alone.

HETEROGENEITY IN RESPONSIVENESS OF MYELOID LEUKEMIA CELLS TO DIFFERENTIATION INDUCERS

The effects of numerous humoral factors and chemicals on the proliferation and differentiation of various human and murine myeloid leukemic cells have been studied by quantitative determinations of phenotypic changes in the differentiating cells(1-4, 6-9,11-19,21). These studies have shown that the proportion of differentiating cells among the total cells depends on the concentration of inducer and that the cell population does not differentiate synchronously (3,6,7,9,21). Similar asynchronous differentiation has been observed in colonies of normal hematopoietic cells in semisolid agar as well as in clonal leukemic cell populations(13). However, details of the kinetics of proliferation and differentiation of myeloid leukemia cells and the mechanisms of induction of this asynchronous differentiation in the cells are unknown. We examined the mechanisms regulating the kinetics of proliferation and differentiation of M1 B24 clone cells, a clone of M1 cells that is highly responsive to D-factor in CM of embryo cells, forming only macrophage-like cells(3). In quantitative studies on change in morphology of the cells, we found that the process of differentiation of M1 B24 cells was promoted by increasing the concentration of the inducer. Moreover, our results showed that the transition of the cells from the undifferentiated state to the differentiated state occurred in a stochastic manner and

that the proportion of well-differentiated cells in
the whole cell population was higher with a higher
concentration of the inducer. The transit time along
the differentiation pathway of the cells also became
shorter with increase in concentration of the inducer
(3).

We also found that heterogeneous populations of M1
B24 cells with different responses to the inducer
appeared during culture of the cells in the presence
of a relatively low concentration of the inducer(3).
When the M1 B24 cells were cultured for 4 days with
2.5% CM of embryo cells, two subpopulations appeared :
cells in an intermediate stage of differentiation with
a higher ratio of nuclear area to cell area NCR (60-
35%) and well-differentiated cells with a lower NCR
(35-12.5%). In tests with various concentrations of
the inducer (CM) we found that through asynchronous
cell differentiation, the proportions of well-differentiated and partially differentiated subpopulations
were regulated dose-dependently by the concentration
of the inducer(3).

The proliferative activity of individual M1B24
cells, measured as the labelling index of the cells
with $[H^3]$thymidine, decreased at a specific stage of
differentiation at which the NCR of the cells was between 50 to 30%, and no proliferative activity was observed in cells in which the NCR had decreased to below
30%(3). These results indicate that each cell loses
the ability to enter the S phase at some specific stage
of differentiation, and that the suppression of proliferation of cells by the differentiation inducer is
due to decrease in the proportion of undifferentiated
and proliferating cells in the whole cell population.

We recently examined the effect on M1 cells of
recombinant human granulocyte colony-stimulating factor
(G-CSF), produced by the gene encoding human G-CSF
from a cDNA library constructed from mRNA in macropha-
ges(21). The recombinant human G-CSF induced differentiation of M1 cells into cells that were functionally, biochemically and morphologically similar to macrophages. Although the half-maximal concentration of
purified D-factor for inducing differentiation of M1
cells was $2X10^{-11}M$, the half-maximally effective concentration of G-CSF was $5.3X10^{-10}M$(21). On the other hand,
on morphological analysis of changes of M1 cells treated with D-factor or G-CSF for 4 days, we found that the
NCRs of the cells treated with D-factor were less than
40%, while those of cells treated with G-CSF were
widely distributed between 20% and 70%(21). These
findings suggest that the response of M1 cells to G-
CSF with weak activity for inducing differentiation

is distinctly heterogeneous.

Heterogeneity in responsiveness to differentiation inducers (GM-CSF in impure or purified form) was also demonstrated by Metcalf(11) in another mouse myelo-monocytic leukemia WEHI-3B cell line, even when the cells were cloned and individual colonies (clones) were analyzed. Metcalf(11) observed that not all the colonies of WEHI-3B cells could be induced to differentiate by purified GM-CSF and that differentiation was associated with marked suppression of the generation of colony-forming cells within the colonies. Later, Metcalf(12) found that the fraction of colony-froming cells in a WEHI-3B cell population gradually decreased and eventually completely disappeared during serial recloning in the continuous presence of postendotoxin serum containing GM-CSF and other differentiation stimulating factors. These results suggest that a number of factors including GM-CSF in the serum are effective for clonal extinction of leukemia cells, even when the leukemia cells are a heterogeneous population with respect to responsiveness to differentiation inducers.

CHARACTERIZATION AND SENSITIZATION OF MYELOID LEUKEMIA CELL CLONES RESISTANT TO DIFFERENTIATION INDUCERS

Binding of Differentiation Inducers

The responsiveness of myeloid leukemia cell lines to differentiation inducers is heterogeneous and unstable and during long-term culture, subpopulations of cells that are resistant to the inducers tend to appear either spontaneously or during treatment with low concentrations of some differentiation inducers. These variant leukemia cells were isolated by cloning and their characteristics were examined.

We isolated several variant clones that were resistant to either dexamethasone (six clones, DR-1 to DR-6) or D-factor (R,R1,R2,R4,R15 and R18) from ascitic fluid of hepatoma bearing rats(4,6,7). The dexamethasone-resistant clones did not show any defect in penetration of glucocorticoid or cytoplasmic receptor binding, but their number of nuclear receptor binding sites for [^{3}H]dexamethasone was markedly less than that of sensitive clones of M1 cells(4,6,7). The binding of dexamethasone to cytoplasmic or nuclear receptor sites in dexamethasone-resistant clones of M1 cells has also been examined by others, who could not detect any defect(18).

Then, we compared the sensitivities of the clones of M1 cells that are resistant to glucocorticoids and D-factor with those of sensitive cells. Although all the dexamethasone-resistant clones showed less response than the sensitive cells to the D-factor, some clones that were resistant to the D-factor were induced to differentiate by dexamethasone(4,6,7). These results suggest that the steroid and the D-factor have different targets in the cells.

We recently purified D-factor to homogeneity for M1 cells from CM of mouse Ehrlich ascites tumor cells and iodinated it without detectable loss of its biological activity(20,22). Then, we examined the specificity of binding of the ^{125}I-D-factor to various cell lines, including several sensitive and resistant clones of M1 cells (Table 1)(22).

TABLE 1. Binding of ^{125}I-D-factor to leukemia cell lines(22)

Cell line	Type of leukemia	^{125}I-D-factor specifically bound/2×10^6 cells (cpm±SE)
Mouse		
M1 cell clone	Myeloid	
Sensitive		
T-22		709 ± 18
B-24		610 ± 85
Resistant		
R-1		394 ± 33
R-4		370 ± 11
DR-3		376 ± 22
Mm-1	Macrophage-like	-41 ± 65
YAC-1	Lymphoma	39 ± 13
Human		
HL-60	Myeloid	43 ± 64
KG-1	Myeloid	14 ± 35
ML-2	Myeloid	28 ± 57

Specific binding of ^{125}I-D-factor was observed with both sensitive (T-22, B-24) and resistant (R-1, R-4 and DR-3) clones, although the latter showed significantly less binding(22). The ^{125}I-D-factor did not bind to human myeloid leukemia cell lines (HL-60,

KG-1 and ML-2) which are not induced to differentiate
by treatment with mouse D-factor(22). Mm-1, a
macrophage-like cell line derived from spontaneously
differentiated M1 cells, and cell lines of unrelated
origin (FM3A, SV-3T3 and YAC-1), had no binding sites
for ^{125}I-D-factor(22).

Nicola and Metcalf(14) identified G-CSF as a protein
factor inducing differentiation of WEHI-3B cells.
Then, they demonstrated the absence of specific binding
of ^{125}I-G-CSF to the subline WEHI-3B(D⁻), which could
not be induced to differentiate by G-CSF.

Production of Inhibitory Factor for Cell Differentiation by Resistant Myeloid Leukemia Cell Lines and Sensitization of the Resistant Clones to Differentiation Inducers

The M1 cell clones that were resistant to D-factor
or dexamethasone, but not the sensitive clones, were
found to produce an inhibitory protein factor(I-factor)
for induction of differentiation of M1 cells(6,7,15).
Production of the I-factor by the resistant clones was
closely associated with their resistance to differentiation inducers, since inhibition of production of this
I-factor by a low concentration of actinomycin D
concomitantly restored the sensitivity of the resistnat
cells to the inducers(6,7). The resistant M1 cells
also became sensitive to differentiation inducers when
treated with low concentrations of other inhibitors of
RNA or protein synthesis (chromomycin A3, nogalamycin,
cordycepin, puromycin and cycloheximide), some anticancer agents (adriamycin, daunomycin, mitomycin C,
hydroxyurea, 5-fluorouracil and bleomycin), interferon
or DMSO, although none of these substances alone induced differentiation of the cells(6,7).

The I-factor was found not only in the CM of resistant M1 cells (R-1) but also in lysates of the cells
(16). The I-factor in a cell lysate of the R-1 cells
was mainly found in the membrane fraction, and this
I-factor in the membrane fraction was also associated
with resistance of R-1 cells to differentiation induc-
ers(16). We recently purified the I-factor in the
CM of R-1 cells to homogeneity(8). For this, the
I-factor in the CM was bound to Carboxymethyl-Sepharose
CL-6B and eluted with 0.27-0.4MNaCl. Although the
profile on gel filtration of the I-factor from Sephadex
G-200 showed considerable heterogeneity in molecular
size, the apparent molecular range of the main fraction
of I-factor was 60,000-80,000(8). This fraction was

purified to homogeneity by high performance liquid
chromatography and the apparent molecular weight of
the purified I-factor was estimated as 68,000 (8). The
purified I-factor also inhibited differentiation of
WEHI-3BD[+] cells induced by all-trans-retinoic acid, but
did not inhibit differentiation of normal bone marrow
hematopoietic stem cells (CFU-c) or human myeloid
leukemia cell lines (K562, HL-60 and ML-1 cells) (8).

IMPROVEMENT BY LOW DOSES OF ANTICANCER DRUGS OF DIFFER-
ENTIATION THERAPY OF EXPERIMENTAL ANIMALS INOCULATED
WITH MYELOID LEUKEMIA CELLS

In Vitro and In Vivo Studies

Based on the findings described above, we examined
the in vitro effects of differentiation inducers on
proliferation and differentiation of M1 cells and
human myeloid leukemia cells in "long-term cultures"
to develop a more effective strategy for differentiation therapy of myeloid leukemia, since little is known
about the therapeutically important, long-term effect
of differentiation inducers on growth and differentiation of myeloid leukemia cells (9).

We examined the effect of a typical differentiation
inducer, $1\alpha,25(OH)_2D_3$, on proliferation of M1 cells at
a constant product of time and concentration (480 nM
in 20 days). Results showed that continuous treatment
with 24 nM $1\alpha,25(OH)_2D_3$ was the most effective for
inhibition of cell proliferation (Table 2) (9). Similar
results were obtained when M1 cells were treated continuously with dexamethasone (9). This continuous
treatment of M1 cells with a low concentration of a
differentiation inducer resulted in complete arrest of
cell proliferation after several division cycles (9).
This treatment is cytostatic rather than cytotoxic to
M1 cells. Furthermore, the concentration required to
arrest cell proliferation completely was much less on
continuous treatment than on intermittent treatment (9).

Although proliferation of M1 cells in our long-term
culture system was markedly suppressed by continuous
treatment with a low concentration (24 nM) of $1\alpha,25(OH)_2D_3$,
resistant cells appeared 25 days after the start of
treatment (Fig.1) (9). In contrast, no resistant cells
appeared for at least 35 days when M1 cells were treated continuously with the inducer ($1\alpha,25(OH)_2D_3$ or dexamethasone) and a low concentration of an antileukemic
drug (daunomycin, Ara-C, or actinomycin D) (Fig.1) (9).

A similar long-term inhibitory effect of inducer plus
an antileukemic drug on proliferation in a human
monoblast-like cell line U937 cells was observed
previously(9).

TABLE 2.   Inhibition of growth of M1 cells by various
schedules of treatment with $1\alpha,25(OH)_2D_3$ (9)

Concentration (nM)	Time of treatment[a] (day)	Product of time and concentration (nM X day)	Cumulative mean cell no./ml on day 20 (X 10^8)
0	0	0	44,800
2.4	0-20	48	29.7
4.8	0-10	48	59.3
9.6	0-5	48	10,400
4.8	0-5,10-15	48	7,270
24	0-2	48	26,500
48	0-1	48	21,500
24	0-20	480	0.1
48	0-10	480	9.8
96	0-5	480	6,140
480	0-1	480	17,400
240	0-20	4,800	0.1
960	0-5	4,800	6,920
4,800	0-1	4,800	9,260

[a]The culture medium was renewed every 3 day. The cell density
was kept at 2-8 X 10^5/ml.

Most of the U937 cells treated with the inducer and
antileukemic drug differentiated into macrophages.
These results suggest that continuous treatment of
myeloid leukemia cells with a combination of a differentiation inducer and a low dose of an antileukemic
drug is effective for suppressing proliferation of leukemia cells by inducing terminal differentiation of the
cells.   The results also suggest that this combination
treatment may suppress the appearance of differentiation-resistant cells.
     Then, we examined whether simultaneous treatment
with $1\alpha(OH)D_3$ plus daunomycin could prolong the survival of syngeneic SL mice inoculated with M1 cells, since
we found previously that $1\alpha(OH)D_3$ was more effective
than $1\alpha,25(OH)_2D_3$ in increasing the survival of mice
inoculated with M1 cells(5).   SL mice inoculated with

3×10^5 M1 cells were treated with $1\alpha(OH)D_3$, daunomycin or $1\alpha(OH)D_3$ plus daunomycin 3 times a week. The mean survival time of untreated mice inoculated with M1 cells was about 19 days, while that of mice treated with 50 pmol $1\alpha(OH)D_3$ or 18 nmol daunomycin 3 times a week was 27 days; on the other hand, the survival of mice treated with $1\alpha(OH)D_3$ plus daunomycin was about 35 days (Fig.2)(9). Thus combination treatment with $1\alpha(OH)D_3$ and daunomycin was more effective therapeutically than treatment with either drug alone.

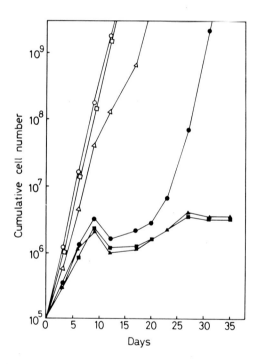

FIG. 1.   Inhibition of growth of M1 cells by continuous treatment with $1\alpha,25(OH)_2D_3$ and an anticancer drug(9). Cells were cultured with 24 nM $1\alpha,25(OH)_2D_3$ (●), 8.9 nM daunomycin (△), 36 nM cytosine arabinoside (□), 24 nM $1\alpha,25(OH)_2D_3$ plus 8.9 nM daunomycin (▲), or 24 nM $1\alpha,25(OH)_2D_3$ plus 36 nM cytosine arabinoside (■), or without $1\alpha,25(OH)_2D_3$ and anticancer drugs (○).

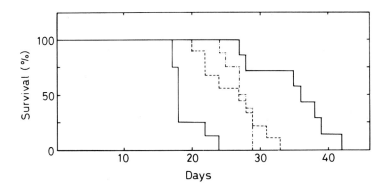

FIG. 2. Prolongation by 1α(OH)D_3 and daunomycin of
survival of SL mice inoculated with M1 cells(9). Mice
were inoculated intraperitoneally with 3×10^5 M1 cells
and treated with 50 pmol 1α(OH)D_3 (-----), 18 nmol
daunomycin (——·——), or 50 pmol 1α(OH)D_3 plus 18 nmol
daunomycin (▬▬) 3 times a week, or were not treated
(———).

Effects of Various Differentiation Inducers plus Anticancer Durgs in Differentiation Therapy of Myeloid
Leukemia

    The therapeutic effects of other differentiation
inducers on syngeneic SL mice inoculated with M1 cells
were also found to be markedly improved by simultaneous
treatment with low doses of several anticancer drugs
(Table 3)(2,5-7,9,10,19). Schlick and Ruscetti(19)
also reported recently that survival of Balb/c mice
inoculated with WEHI-3BD$^+$ cells, but not WEHI-3BD$^-$
cells, was markedly prolonged by treatment of the mice
with cyclophosphamide in combination with maleic
anhydride divinyl ether copolymer (MVE-2), which induces CSF secretion by macrophages and bone marrow
cells (Table 3). Serum from mice pretreated in vivo
with MVE-2, which contained CSF, induced terminal differentiation of WEHI-3BD$^+$ cells, but not WEHI-3BD$^-$
cells(19). These results suggest that the therapeutic
effect may be due to the induction of CSF or other differentiation factors.
    Fujii et al. (2) examined the therapeutic effect of
LPS, a differentiation inducer, in combination with
daunomycin on rat myelomonocytic leukemia (c-WRT-7).
The c-WRT-7 cells were initially confirmed to differen-

tiate both *in vitro* and *in vivo* into macrophage-like
cells and to lose their proliferative capacity when
treated with LPS(2). Although treatment of syngeneic
WKA rats with LPS alone did not markedly prolong the
survival of rats inoculated with the c-WRT-7 cells,
treatment of the rats with LPS in combination with
daunomycin completely inhibited the development of
leukemia, resulting in survival of all the animals
(Table 3)(2). These results clearly show that anticancer drugs enhance the therapeutic effects of differentiation inducers.

TABLE 3. Improvement by combination with anticancer
drugs in differentiation therapy in experimental
animals inoculated with various myeloid leukemia cell
lines (2,5-7,9,10,19)

Leukemia cell line	Animal	Differentiation inducer	Anticancer drug
M1	Mouse	LPS	Actinomycin D
M1	Mouse	Alkylethylene-glycophospholipid	Actinomycin D
M1	Mouse	$1\alpha,25(OH)_2D_3$	Actinomycin D
M1	Mouse	$1\alpha,25(OH)_2D_3$	Daunomycin
M1	Mouse	D-factor	Cyclophos-phamide
WEHI-3BD[+]	Mouse	Divinyl ether copolymer	Cyclophos-phamide
c-WRT-7	Rat	LPS	Daunomycin

SUMMARY

    The responsiveness of the myeloid leukemia cells
in *in vitro* culture to differentiation inducers was
found to be heterogeneous and unstable, resulting during long-term culture in the appearance of subpopulations of cells that were resistant to the inducers.
Several resistant clones isolated from mouse myeloid
leukemia M1 cells were found to produce an inhibitory
protein factor (I-factor) for induction of differentiation of sensitive M1 cells. The apparent molecular
weight of the purified I-factor was 68,000. Production
of the I-factor by the resistant M1 cells was associated with resistance of the cells to differentiation
inducers, since the sensitivity of the resistant cells
to the inducers was restored when the synthesis of

this I-factor was inhibited by treatment with low doses of some anticancer drugs.

Although proliferation of M1 cells in a long-term in vitro culture system was markedly suppressed by continuous treatment with a low concentration of a differentiation inducer, resistant cells appeared during long-term (3 weeks) culture. In contrast, no resistant cells appeared during long-term culture of M1 cells treated continuously with an inducer ($1\alpha,25(OH)_2D_3$ or dexamethasone) plus an anticancer drug (daunomycin, Ara-C, or actinomycin D). A similar effect of an inducer plus an anticancer drug on growth of human leukemia U937 cells was also observed. The survival of syngeneic SL mice inoculated with M1 cells was prolonged more by treatment with both $1\alpha(OH)D_3$ and daunomycin than by treatment with either drug alone.
The survival of experimental animals inoculated with M1 cells or other myeloid leukemia cells (WEHI-3BD$^+$ cells, c-WRT-7 cells) was also prolonged by treatment of the animals with a combination of a differentiation inducer and an anticancer drug.

These findings suggest that treatment of myeloid leukemia cells with a combination of a differentiation inducer and a low dose of an anticancer drug is effective for inducing terminal differentiation of the cells and that the appearance of differentiation-resistant cells is suppressed or retarded by this combination treatment. These findings also suggest the potential usefulness of combination therapy with a differentiation inducer and anticancer drug for maintenance therapy after induction of complete remission in leukemia, since this treatment might induce terminal differentiation and growth arrest of the small number of leukemic cells remaining after remission induction therapy.

REFERENCES

1. Cheson,B.D., Jasperse,D.M., Chun,H.G., and Friedman, M.A. (1986) : Cancer Treat. Rev., 13:129-145.
2. Fujii,Y., Yuki,N., Takeichi,N., Kobayashi,H., and Miyazaki,T. (1987) : Cancer Res., 47:1668-1673.
3. Hayashi,M., Gotoh,O., Kado,J., and Hozumi,M. (1981) : J. Cell. Physiol., 108:123-134.
4. Honma,Y., Kasukabe,T., Okabe,J., and Hozumi,M. (1977) : J. Cell. Physiol., 93:227-235.
5. Honma,Y., Hozumi,M., Abe,E., Konno,K., Fukushima, M., Hata,S., Nishii,Y., DeLuca,H., and Suda,T. (1983) : Proc. Natl. Acad. Sci. U.S.A., 80:201-204.

6. Hozumi,M. (1983) : Adv. Cancer Res., 38:121-169.
7. Hozumi,M. (1985) : CRC Crit. Rev. Oncol./Hematol. 3:235-277.
8. Kado,J., Kasuakbe,T., Honma,Y., Hayashi,M., and Hozumi,M. (1987) : Proc. Japn. Cancer Assoc., 45th Annu. Meet., p.236.
9. Kasukabe,T., Honma,Y., Hozumi,M., Suda,T., and Nishii,Y. (1987) : Cancer Res., 47:567-572.
10. Lotem,J., and Sachs,L. (1981) : Int. J. Cancer 28:375-386.
11. Metcalf,D. (1979) : Int. J. Cancer, 24:616-623.
12. Metcalf,D. (1980) : Int. J. Cancer, 25:225-233.
13. Metcalf,D. (1984) : The Hemopoietic Colony Stimulating Factors. Elsevier, Amsterdam.
14. Nicola,N.A., and Metcalf,D. (1984) : Proc. Natl. Acad. Sci. U.S.A., 81:3765-3769.
15. Okabe,J., Hayashi,M., Honma,Y., and Hozumi,M. (1978) : Int. J. Cancer 22:570-575.
16. Okabe-Kado,J., Hayashi,M., Honma,Y., and Hozumi,M. (1985) : Cancer Res., 45:4848-4852.
17. Reiss,M., Gamba-Vitalo,C., and Sartorelli,A.C. (1986) : Cancer Treat. Rep., 70:201-218.
18. Sachs,L. (1978) : Nature, 274:535-539.
19. Schlick,E., and Ruscetti,W. (1986) : Blood, 67:980-987.
20. Tomida,M., Yamamoto-Yamaguchi,Y., and Hozumi,M. (1984) : J. Biol. Chem. 259:10978-10982.
21. Tomida,M., Yamamoto-Yamaguchi,Y., Hozumi,M., Okabe,T., and Takaku,F. (1986) : FEBS Lett., 207:271-275.
22. Yamamoto-Yamaguchi,Y., Tomida,M., and Hozumi,M. (1986) : Exp. Cell Res., 164:97-102.

CLINICAL TRIALS OF DIFFERENTIATION THERAPY

Clinical Trials of Differentiation Therapy: Current Trials and Future Prospects

G.E. Francis and C.M. Pinsky*

*Department of Haematology, The Royal Free Hospital,
Pond Street, London NW3 2QG, UK;
*Biological Response Modifiers Program,
Division of Cancer Treatment, National Cancer Institute,
Frederick Cancer Research Facility, Frederick, Maryland 21701, USA*

Differentiation induction therapy is in its infancy. To be successful it is necessary to take over the controls of neoplastic or dysplastic cells rather than merely kill them. This requires detailed information about not only the molecular mechanisms of differentiation but also their malfunction in disease states. The group's aim has been to define the potential therapeutic roles of differentiation therapy, focussing on the underlying principles upon which they are based. These include views about the nature of the disease states being treated and the desired outcome, as well as the known or presumed mechanism of the inducer(s) used. We have also attempted to address some general questions: Does differentiation therapy have to be tailored for individual tissues, tumours, or even patients? How should our albeit limited knowledge of mechanisms of differentiation induction influence the design of clinical trials? In addition we have attempted to outline possible collaborative trials for the immediate future.

There are a number of potential clinical roles for differentiation therapy: differentiation extinction of tumours; improvement of differentiation in dysplasia; chemoprevention; modulation of the phenotype of tumour cells; adjuncts to chemo- or radiotherapy; extracorporeal purging of tumour cells. Since they are based to some extent on different principles, these roles and the clinical trials relating to them, will be dealt with separately. Much of this information has been provided prior to publication by members of the sub-group on "Clinical Trials of Differentiation Therapy" as personal communications to the co-chairmen and we are grateful for their contributions.

POTENTIAL CLINICAL ROLES OF DIFFERENTIATION THERAPY
AND STATUS OF CLINICAL TRIALS.

Differentiation Extinction of Tumours.

The principle here is that a tumour will be extinguished if any of the following take place:-
1) Tumour stem cells become committed to differentiate to non-dividing end cells; 2) Differentiation exceeds proliferation for sufficient time for the stem cell pool to become gradually exhausted; 3) The cells differentiate to a stage where the responsiveness to regulators is changed in a favourable way (e.g. loss of responsiveness to a growth factor or increased responsiveness to a physiological differentiation factor). Note that 1) would require an agent inducing an irreversible step whereas 2) could theoretically be achieved by protracted administration of any type of inducer so long as the ultimate cell product was a non-dividing cell.

Clinical trials of this approach include the use of alpha-interferon in hairy cell leukaemia, where complete or partial remissions have been achieved in 87% of patients (38). Although there is still debate about the relative contributions of cytotoxicity and the differentiation inducing effects of low dose cytosine arabinoside (ARA-C), complete and partial remissions are achieved with this regimen in acute myeloid leukaemia (AML). A recent review of 22 studies (a total of 238 patients with AML treated with low dose ARA-C) showed an overall rate of 31% complete remissions and 21% partial remissions (40). These results have to be viewed in light of the fact that this therapy has tended to be used for patients unresponsive to conventional treatment. New less toxic analogues of ARA-C with superior differentiation inducing capacity have been developed (see below) and will be worth evaluating.
The regression of cervical intraepithelial neoplasia with topical retinoic acid, has also been observed (22). Phase I trials of hexamethylene bisacetamide (HMBA) and N-methylformamide (N-MF) have taken place (6, 33) and phase II trials of HMBA in patients with melanoma and bladder cancer are in progress (PA Marks sub-group report, unpublished).

Improvement of Differentiation in Dysplasia.

Dysplastic tissues often show differentiation defects and these may make a significant contribution to morbidity, quite apart from any influence on the transformation to malignancy (which will be dealt with below). For example, in myelodysplasia the patients' major clinical problems derive from cytopenias of one or more haemopoietic lineages (16). Quantitative and qualitative improvement of differentiation reverses cytopenias and may improve lesions such as leukoplakia.

Myelodysplasia: single agent trials.
This subject has been extensively reviewed (24,30), so emphasis here will be placed on the more recent developments.
i) Low dose ARA-C. This is the most frequently used regimen. Comparison between trials has been difficult because of the variety of schedules used. Recent reviews demonstrate that responses vary widely (24,4).
ii) 13-cis-retinoic acid. Clark et al (7) have recently reported an increased survival with this agent versus suportive care. Several other groups have documented responses (23,37).
iii) Vitamin D3. This agent's clinical use has been complicated by symptomatic hypercalcaemia and Koeffler et al (29) recorded 8 minor but no complete responses in 18 patients.
iv) Interferons. Recombinant alpha interferon is also undergoing trials but initial results are disappointing (11). Human gamma interferon is undergoing phase II trials at present, undertaken by the South German Haemoblastosis Study Group (A D Ho, sub-group report, unpublished).
v) 5-azacytidine. A preliminary trial of this agent was reported at the first conference on differentiation therapy and is continuing. Using a continuous infusion of 75 mg/m2/day in 1 week courses, responses have been observed, but it is premature to evaluate response rate (LR Silverman and JF Holland, sub-group report, on behalf of Cancer and Leukaemia Group B, upublished).
vi) Recombinant colony stimulating factors. Although these factors have differentiation inducing effects one must not neglect their substantial growth stimulus (43). In addition bone marrow GM-CSF production increases prior to leukaemic transformation (13) and although not necessarily causally related, caution about the use of these agents in MDS seems warranted. These factors may only achieve their potential in differentiation therapy if the proliferation stimulus can be abrogated (see below).
Of nine patients treated with human recombinant GM-CSF (21) 7 showed increased leukocyte counts, one an increase in platelets and none an increase in reticulocytes. Significantly, increase in the percentage of circulating blasts was observed in 3 patients. Trials with recombinant G-CSF are in progress.

Myelodysplasia: combination agent trials.
The principle here is to exploit the synergistic interactions between agents which act on differentiation via different mechanisms (see below). The following combinations were highly synergistic in vitro (15,14,17) and are now being evaluated in vivo:-

i) 13-cis-retinoic acid and 6-thioguanine. Preliminary results (19) show responses where single agent therapy with either 13-cis-retinoic acid alone or low dose ARA-c alone have failed. The regimen used was 13-cis-retinoic acid 60-100 mg/m2/day orally with 6-thioguanine 20-40 mg/day orally in 14 day courses with a 3-4 week interval.

ii) 13-cis-retinoic acid and vincristine. Only a few cases have been studied, using 13-cis-retinoic acid 60-100 mg/m2/day orally for 4 days with 2mg vincristine on day 2 or 3, courses repeated every 2-3 weeks (19). Responses have occurred after failure of the 6-thioguanine regimen above and vice versa.

iii) 13-cis-retinoic acid with ARA-c. Despite good synergy in vitro on MDS, AML and normal cells (15,14,17) and also with cell lines (5), so far this looks the least promising of the 13-cis retinoic acid combinations with very few responses. Ho A. et al (26) used 13-cis-retinoic acid 60 mg/m2/day orally with cytosine arabinoside 5mg/m2/12h s.c. for 14 days repeated every 4-8 weeks. Clark et al (8) used ARA-c 10 mg/day sub cutaneously on 6 day/week, to which 20mg/day 13-cis-retinoic acid was added after 12 weeks. Both groups observed very low response rates. Chomienne et al (sub-group report, unpublished) found an increase in the number of responsive patients with retinoic acid plus ARA-C, but as in the studies above found responses surprisingly weak given the in vitro synergy between the agents. She has suggested that scheduling may be important since ARA-C in her in vitro experiments is most effective if added prior to retinoic acid (sub-group report, unpublished).

iv) ARA-C with fluoxymesterone. This trial (using 3mg/m2/day X 2 SC ARA-C and 1mg/kg/day fluoxymesterone) is still in progress (C Chomienne and L Degos sub-group report, unpublished). The treatment is well tolerated and half the patients have improved but there are very few complete remissions.

Other dysplastic conditions.
Leukoplakia. The current treatment for dysplastic oral leukoplakia is surgical excision, electrodessication or cryosurgery, but these approaches are not always feasible when the lesions are extensive. Encouraging results have been obtained in a trial of 13-cis-retinoic acid (1-2mg/kg/day for three months) in oral leukoplakia (27) in which the dysplasia was reversed in 54% of patients (13/24) compared with 10% (2/20) reversal in the placebo group. Since the lesions recur after cessation of therapy, this group is now comparing low dose 13-cis-retinoic acid (0.5mg/kg/day) versus beta-carotene (30mg/day) for maintenance therapy (W K Hong sub-group report, unpublished).

Chemoprevention

i) Prevention of de-novo tumours.

Epidemiological evidence and animal experiments (reviewed in 9) have provided the theoretical basis for this approach (e.g. the association of vitamin A deficiency and epithelial tumours). Retinol palmitate (300,000 I.U./day P.O.) is being evaluated by Pastorino et al (35) in a randomized clinical trial after complete resection of intrapulmonary non small-cell lung cancer (stage 1a). Two aspects of chemoprevention are being tested in this study, the occurrence of new primary tumours (usually beyond 3 years) and of cancer relapse (within 3 years). The latter aspect essentially tests effects on micrometastases (see below). Current trials also include evaluation of retinol palmitate in prevention of tumours in the second breast after mastectomy and trials of carotene or retinol palmitate in prevention of lung cancer in high risk groups (e.g. heavy smokers or patients with asbestosis). A chemoprevention trial in squamous cell carcinoma of the head and neck with 13-cis retinoic acid is also in progress (W K Hong sub-group report, unpublished). A breast cancer trial with the synthetic retinoid fenretinide 200mg/day with a 3 day drug holiday per month was initiated in March 87 (243 randomized subjects). Toxicity has yet to be evaluated (Pastorino et al sub-group report unpublished).

ii) Prevention of the dysplasia to malignancy transition.

This is based on the suspected contribution of defective differentiation to oncogenesis. Most attention to date has been given to myelodysplasia (where there are additional reasons for using differentiation therapy, mentioned above). However, since transformation rates are slow and analysis is complicated by the heterogeneity of the patient group there are no clear indications yet on this aspect. Regressions of bronchial metaplasia have been observed in heavy smokers given retinoids (25).

iii) Prevention of metastases.

There is some overlap with the differentiation extinction notion here, particularly for micrometastases, but differentiation status may also influence cells' ability to metastasize. In the trial mentioned above on evaluation of early relapse after resection of intrapulmonary non small-cell lung cancer using retinol palmitate (35), preliminary analysis of 170 patients (84 treated and 86 control group), presented at the ECCO 4 conference and kindly supplied by U Pastorino for the sub-group report, shows recurrence in 8 treated and 16 control subjects. When analysis is restricted to extrapulmonary relapses, these occurred in only 2 treated and 13 control subjects. Given the limited follow up (median approaching 12 months) one must interpret these results very cautiously .

Modulation of the Phenotype of Tumour Cells.

There are a number of inducible phenotypic changes which may be beneficial. It has, for example, been shown that malignant murine embryonal carcinomas can be converted to benign teratomas using differentiation induction in vivo with a combination of retinoic acid and dimethylacetamide (41).

In vitro studies show that some differentiation inducers change the expression of surface antigens. An increase in the expression of MHC class II antigens might be useful in vivo because it might render cells susceptible to host immune cytotoxic cells. Baldini et al (3) have suggested that an increase in HLA class II expression might contribute to the antileukaemic effect of interferon in hairy cell leukaemia.

One potentially important and apparently persistent phenotypic change is the observed reversion of transformation in ras-transformed cells by interferon (39). The mechanism apparently involves a DNA methylation event because the cells can be retransformed by 5-azacytidine (an inhibitor of DNA methyltransferase). The revertant cells still have an activated ras but are not tumorigenic. Since ras activation appears to have a contributory role in a high proportion of human malignancies (1), this may have wide applications.

The effects of cholesterol on cancer cell growth and differentiation are also currently being studied (G. Esposito sub-group report, unpublished) because of the possibility that the observed inverse relationship between serum cholesterol and cancer incidence (36) relates to hypocholesterolaemia-induced increased membrane fluidity. Increased membrane fluidity is a feature of metastasizing cells (34)

Adjuncts to Chemo- or Radiotherapy.

Several preliminary studies have demonstrated that agents known to have differentiation inducing effects (e.g. sodium butyrate and dimethylformamide) may alter the response of cells to radiation and cytotoxic drugs (2,10). Although it is not known whether this effect is actually due to the induction of differentiation, circumstantial evidence suggests that this may be the case. In AML, for example, there is a strong correlation between the phenotypic properties reflecting differentiation stage of the AML clonogenic cells and the ease with which remission can be induced with conventional cytotoxic regimens (45). The earliest stage is related to the worst response. This area is perhaps the logical one for the use of differentiation agents which are inducing reversible differentiation steps, or which are poorly tolerated by the patient, since the effect only need be maintained while the cells are exposed to the second agent.

Purging for Autologous Bone Marrow Transplantation.

Since in some systems it appears that brief exposure to differentiation inducers can alter the behaviour of tumour stem cells (inducing loss of stem cell capacity or a transition from malignant to benign phenotype), this raises the possibility of using differentiation inducing agents to eradicate (or render benign) tumour stem cells within bone marrow preparations prior to autologous transplantation. Animal models such as that of Speers et al (41) mentioned above, will allow this possibility to be investigated. Problems to be overcome will be the effect of the selected inducer on the normal haemopoietic stem cells. Relevant to this may be the use of bone marrow cultures for transplantation since stromal cells appear to protect haemopoietic stem cells from the influence of differentiation inducing compounds.

THE INFLUENCE OF KNOWN MECHANISMS OF DIFFERENTIATION INDUCTION ON THE DESIGN OF CLINICAL TRIALS.

The Complex Nature of Differentiation Machines

The sheer variety of pharmacological agents able to induce or inhibit differentiation in any individual cell system, reflects the number of molecular components involved in the differentiation event under study. Even single processes like changes in expression of one gene, can involve a number of molecular components (DNA-binding regulatory proteins and their binding sites, DNA methylation enzymes which may be influenced by the former, enzymes regulating chromatin structure, DNA topoisomerases which by regulating supercoiling influence DNA-protein binding, etc). Signal transduction systems are also complex. The differentiation "machinery" thus provides a series of targets for the action of the inducers/inhibitors.

There are three important implications for the clinician here. The first is that if differentiation machines are complex they will break down in a variety of different ways in different tumours of the same tissue. We must therefore anticipate heterogeneity of disease states at the molecular level. Second, if the differentiation inducers have different routes of action there is the possibility of utilizing synergistic and additive interactions between compounds active via different mechanisms. The caveat here is that there are also antagonistic interactions to be avoided. Third that where an experimental therapeutic approach fails in an individual patient, ensure that a functionally different "family " (see below) of differentiation inducer is tried next, since this will be impinging on the differentiation machinery in a different way.

Machine Components

Identification of the components of these differentiation "machines" is in progress. This is an area of rapid expansion which will ultimately fuel combination therapy design. One approach is to start with a particular gene (e.g. the globin genes in erythroid differentiation) and to dissect the molecular events associated with induced changes in its expression (32). Where key differentiation-specific genes have yet to be identified as, for example, in myeloid differentiation this approach cannot be used. Here, the first step is to identify different families of differentiation inducers (i.e. compounds with different mechanisms of action) since extensive studies of chemically unrelated compounds allow one to attribute the differentiation action to the biochemical properties shared by the family and to exclude other properties. Drug interaction studies are a powerful tool here because first order synergistic and antagonistic interactions usually preclude the possibility of two compounds having the same mechanism of action. Panels of interactions of many compounds produce a taxonomy useful because it discriminates broad categories (e.g. cytotoxic drugs) into distinct homogeneous "families" (cf. DNA methyltransferase inhibitors versus DNA synthesis inhibitors). The shared family property gives clues as to their underlying mechanism of action.

Studies on neutrophil-granulocyte differentiation illustrate this approach and show how it can be exploited in trial design. Studies of the interaction patterns of differentiation inducing agents identify at least eight families of differentiation inducing compounds, for neutrophil-granulocyte differentiation (17):-

1) Polar planar compounds (dimethylsulphoxide - DMSO and N-methylformamide - NMF).
2) Retinoids (13-cis and all trans retinoic acid).
3) DNA methyltransferase inhibitors (5-azacytidine, 5-aza-2'-deoxycytidine, L-ethionine).
4) DNA synthesis inhibitors (ARA-c, 6-mercaptopurine, 6-thioguanine, aphidicolin); exceptions are inhibitors of DNA topoisomerase II which inhibit neutrophil differentiation.
5) Bromodeoxyuridine.
6) Microtubule disrupting agents (vincristine).
7) Granulocytic colony stimulating factor (G-CSF)
8) Differentiation Inducing Factor (recently identified as tumour necrosis factor (42).

Sodium butyrate and hexamethylene bisacetamide - HMBA have not been fully analysed but are provisionally not assigned to group one. Alpha-interferon may also be in a distinct category (Francis G.E. unpublished).

The first information of clinical relevance provided by this work is to identify which families of compounds interact favourably (synergistically or additively) and which combinations are to be avoided because they are antagonistic. The interactions are reported in full elsewhere (17,18).

Although, as mentioned above, such a list suggests several mechanisms of action, many of these interactions fit a surprisingly simple unifying hypothesis concerning how these agents perturb components of a simple "differentiation machine" regulating transcription of a key gene or genes needed for granulocytic differentiation (17,20). The postulated components are: two DNA-binding proteins one a positive and the other a negative modulator of differentiation, a DNA methylation event or events (possibly regulated by these proteins) and DNA supercoiling changes mediated by DNA topoisomerase II (18). The decision-event of this putative machine occurs in S-phase of the cell cycle and is more likely when S-phase is lengthened.

Simple clinical implications of this hypothetical machine's structure include ideas like using 6-thioguanine to extend the S-phase responsive window for 13-cis-retinoic acid or treating patients who fail to respond to polar-planar compounds with 5-azacytidine because the DNA methylation component of the machine is a) separate and b) downstream of the one affected by the polar planar compounds. Also, only agents which lengthen S-phase without inhibiting DNA topoisomerase II, are suitable to enhance the actions of retinoids and polar planar compounds. Although the structure of this putative machine cannot be ascertained until we have identified the gene or genes regulated, this type of data set is so complex that it excludes many existing hypotheses and provides a rigorous constraint for any surviving hypothesis, since it requires that numerous interactions fit the model. It is therefore probably a robust way of generating tentative models of a wide variety of differentiation machines.

Different Tissues and Lineages

When the same agents are analysed in different systems many of the agents are active, but the details of the interactions vary. Monocytic differentiation clearly employs some molecular mechanisms not operating in granulocytic differentiation (28). One member of the group has performed an interaction analysis on erythroid differentiation (P Rowley, sub-group report, unpublished) which demonstrates that interaction patterns are different from those seen in neutrophil differentiation. Such results imply that although the components are similar they are built into different "machines" in different cells.

Because of the above view of a "repertoire" of similar components built into a very wide variety of machines, a good strategy for future screening programmes might be to adopt both a reductionist approach and examine individual components (in cell free systems perhaps) as well as exploiting available cell systems representative of individual tissues. Since the individual components are relevant to many tissues this seems an economical approach. Examination of the effects of agents (like polar-planar compounds) on the binding of specific proteins to differentiation specific enhancers is one example of this approach. Another would be analysis of activators of signal transduction components (e.g. protein kinase C).

Agents in Combination.

Because the interactions of these agents are dependent on the precise components of the differentiation mechanism operating in the tissue, cell-stage or individual tumour in question, it is particularly important to test interactions directly in vitro. Compounds which interact synergistically in one situation may easily interact antagonistically in another. Also, more is not necessarily better. One cannot assume that because drugs A + B and B + C are synergistic in these combinations that A + B + C will also be synergistic. All three together may well be an antagonistic combination.

The Proliferation Differentiation Balance.

One of the concepts central to differentiation therapy which seems likely to pose most problems for clinicians used to thinking in terms of conventional chemotherapy, is that of the proliferation/differentiation balance. Symptomatic of this confusion are statements like "this agent produces only a one log reduction in tumour cells, therefore it will not be useful". Such a differentiation inducing agent is however producing a dramatic shift in the proliferation/differentiation balance (the probability of a cell undergoing a differentiation step versus its probability of dividing). This, if operating for a long period in a system with a commitment step, could well extinguish the tumour stem cell pool. The ability of a self-renewing and differentiating tissue to achieve steady state is also dependent on this balance. If the ratio of probabilities (proliferation/differentiation) becomes too high, cell birth cannot be balanced by cell death and relentless expansion must ensue. Improvement in differentiation can restore the balance and allow the system to stabilize or even decline in size. This dynamic view of these two processes is central to the design of differentiation therapies. Calculated tumour growth rates give a measure of this imbalance and can be used to determine the extent to which differentiation must be increased to prevent tumour growth. Mathematical modelling could serve a useful purpose in this area.

Reversible and Irreversible (Commitment) Differentiation Steps.

Another source of confusion is the frequent assumption of the irreversibility of differentiation steps (usually indicated by

the use of the term commitment). It is now emerging that many
more differentiation steps than previously suspected are
reversible but the reversal is not fully tested in the cell
systems used (one needs to remove the differentiation stimulus
and, usually, to provoke cell division thus "diluting out" the
cell's differentiated properties - cf. the experiments on
haemopoietic cells of von Melchner et al (44)). As indicated
above this is crucial information vis à vis the type of
therapeutic strategy being considered for each agent/cell system
combination.

DOES DIFFERENTIATION THERAPY HAVE TO BE TAILORED
FOR INDIVIDUAL TISSUES, TUMOURS, OR EVEN INDIVIDUAL PATIENTS ?

In vitro studies of differentiation, probably for the reasons
outlined above, reveal enormous heterogeneity of response. How
much of a problem will this pose clinically ?
Variation in response between different cell types requires a
good working knowledge of the mechanisms of differentiation for
each type of tissue before therapies can be designed for tumours
derived from that tissue. In many cell systems this may include
the added complexity of a variety of different molecular events
occurring at different developmental stages. One of the major
sources of delay here seems the lack of good in vitro systems for
analysing differentiation in non-haemopoietic tissues. The data
on haemopoietic tissues should however help with the other
studies because they are uncovering a repertoire of components of
the differentiation mechanism which are likely to be involved in
differentiation machines of many tissues.
Although there is considerable intra-patient variation in
response even for an individual type of tumour, this may however
be less of a problem than it at first appears from in vitro
studies of freshly explanted neoplastic cells. It may well be
possible to devise combination differentiation therapies which
impinge on the differentiation mechanisms of the tissue in
question at several points. This will cater for the existence of
a variety of different defective components of the
differentiation machinery in the patient group. Thus we may be
able to have a strategy per tissue rather than one per patient.

PLANS FOR THE FUTURE

The need for Differentiation Markers as Tools
For Evaluation of Response in Differentiation Trials.

One of the most obvious deficiencies in trial design has been
lack of attention to this area, either because the clinical team
does not have access to the technology or simply because, for the
system in question, these tools do not yet exist. While it is
difficult to generalize one new approach seems well worth
implementing rapidly. That is the combined use of

immunofluorescence and a rapid and sensitive RNA in situ hybridisation technique permitting the detection of as few as 5 copies of mRNA per cell (12). Using this approach individual cells can be analysed for oncogene expression and at the same time be identified by antibodies to a lineage or stage-specific antigen. The aberrant expression of the oncogenes myc and sis in individual AML cells has already been analysed by this technique (expression is much higher than in all individual normal bone marrow cells so far examined). Individual cell analysis is crucial because in many tissues normal and neoplastic tissue is sampled together, complicating conclusions concerning levels of oncogene expression in unfractionated samples. Cell fractionation is at best time consuming and costly and at worst simply not feasible.

Current Myelodysplasia Trials Needing Collaborative Efforts.

Low dose ARA-C has been used by so many groups that it can serve as a good "yard stick" for the new trials. Randomization between low dose ARA-C and the current or new pilot trials could alleviate some of the problems of comparing results between different centers.

Although it is important to establish each agent in single agent trials, for the reasons outlined above, it is worth focussing the most effort on combination agent trials. The pilot trials of 13-cis-retinoic acid in combination with either 6-thioguanine or vincristine need to be extended. As mentioned above 13-cis-retinoic acid plus ARA-C has been assessed rather more than the former combinations and looks less promising, so it perhaps deserves less attention. There is also a national (UK) multi-centre trial of the 13-cis retinoic acid and ARA-C combination in progress (G J Mufti Personal communication) so that this will evaluate this combination in detail.

Single agent trials needing to be extended are those on 5-azacytidine and N-MF. For reasons outlined above single agent trials of recombinant G and GM-CSF warrant caution and should perhaps be limited and viewed mainly as a prerequisite to combination therapies involving these two agents (see below).

In Vitro Studies Relevant to Future Myelodysplasia Trials.

We have been looking at possible combinations for G-CSF in vitro (Irvine A E and Francis G E unpublished). The object of these studies was to design a drug combination to reduce/abolish the proliferative stimulus of G-CSF whilst retaining the differentiation stimulus (G-CSF has a substantial proliferation stimulus under some in vitro conditions which, if operative in vivo, would make the agent undesirable in myelodysplasias and myeloid leukaemias). The results are somewhat unexpected. Unlike the common pharmacological inducers of granulocytic differentiation (retinoic acid, DMSO, N-MF) which interact synergistically with most agents which slow proliferation, the differentiation induction action of G-CSF is antagonised by 6-thioguanine and vincristine. G-CSF also interacts somewhat antagonistically with retinoic acid and with recombinant interferon alpha-2b and these agents do not effectively remove the proliferative stimulus. So far the agent found which best restrains the proliferative effects of G-CSF and spares the differentiation inducing action is recombinant interferon .gamma.

Combinations not yet tried in myelodysplasia that are synergistic or additive in vitro are as follows:-
13-cis-retinoic acid plus 5-azacytidine (17)
N-methylformamide plus 5-azacytidine (17)
recombinant interferon alpha-2b plus ARA-C (Francis G. E. & Irvine A E unpublished).

New Differentiation Inducing Agents.

New Vitamin D3 analogues.
Structure function analyses have been performed by both M R Uskokovic (Roche Research Center, Nutley, New Jersey, USA) and by Chugai Pharmaceutical's Japan. Compounds with superior differentiation inducing capacity to 1,25-dihydroxyvitamin D3 and also with a reduced calcium mobilizing action have been demonstrated.

New ARA-C analogues.
Kong et al (3) have analysed a group of 2'-fluro and 5-substituted arabinosyl pyrimidines .and base-substituted pseudocytidine analogues using HL60 cells. Three compounds were found with superior differentiation inducing capacity and reduced cytotoxicity relative to ARA-C. Quite apart from the obvious potential of this observation, this series of compounds provides an important tool for analysing the relative contributions of cytotoxicity and differentiation induction to the effectiveness of ARA-C.

New retinoids.
There are a large range of these and again interesting structure-function relationships are emerging as well as more potent compounds. Different parts of the molecule may convey the induction of growth arrest and the differentiated phenotype (46).

Establishing an International Registry of Induction Trials

We plan to form a registry to serve several roles, not only acting as a general registry of completed trials (documenting agents used, conditions treated and responses obtained), but also serving as a standardized means for participating groups to handle patients' data entry and record keeping. We have arranged for collaborating groups to have direct access via a microcomputer based network.

REFERENCES

1. Aaronson, S.A., and Tronick, S.R. (1985): In: Carcinogenesis vol 10, edited by E. Huberman, and S.H. Barr, pp35-49. Raven Press, New York.

2. Arundel, C.M., Kenney, S.M., Leith, J.T., and Glicksman, A.S. (1986) Int. J. Radiat. Oncol. Biol. Phys., 12:959-968.

3. Baldini, L., Cortelezzi, A., Polli, N., Neri, A., Nobili, L., Maiolo, A.T., Lambertenghi-Deliliers, G., and Polli,E.E. (1986):Blood,67:458-464.

4. Buzaid, A.C., Garewal, H.S., and Greenberg, B.R. (1986): Am. J. Med., 80:1149-1157.

5. Chomienne, C., Balitrand, N., Degos, L., and Abita, J.P. (1986): Leuk. Res.,10:631-636.

6. Chun, H.G., Leyland-Jones, B., Hoth, D., Shoemaker, D., Wolpert-DeFilippes, M., Greishaber, C., Cradock, J., Davignon, P., Moon, R., Rifkind, R., and Wittes, R.E. (1986): Cancer Treat. Rep., 70:991-996.

7. Clark, R.E., Jacobs, A., Lush, C.J., and Smith, S.A. (1987): Lancet, i:763-765.

8. Clark, R.E., Ismail, S.A.D., Jacobs, A., Payne, H., and Smith S.A. (1987): Brit. J. Haematol.,66:77-83.

9. Costa, A., Pastorino, U., Andreoli, C., Barbieri, A., Marubini, E., and Veronesi, U. (1984): Int. Adv. Surg. Oncol., 7:271-295.

10. Dexter, D.L., DeFusco, D.J., McCarthy, K., and Calabresi, P. (1983): Proc. Amer. Assoc. Cancer Res. 24:267.(Abstract)

11. Elias, L., Hoffman, R., Boswell, S., Tensen, L., and Bonnem, E. (1987): Leukemia, 1:105-110.

12. Evinger-Hodges, M.J., Bresser, J., Cox, I., Beran, M., and Dicke K. (1987): Exp. Hematol.,15:500. (Abstract)

13. Francis, G.E., Wing, M.A., Miller, E.J., Berney, J.J., Wonke, B., and Hoffbrand, A.V. (1983): Lancet,i:1409-1412.

14. Francis, G.E., Guimaraes, J.E.T., Berney, J.J., and Wing, M.A. (1985): In: Haematology and Blood Transfusion Vol. 29. Modern Trends in Human Leukaemia VI, edited by R. Neth, R.C. Gallo, M.F. Greaves, and J. Janka, pp. 402-408. Springer Verlag, Berlin.

15. Francis, G.E., Guimaraes, J.E.T., Berney J.J., and Wing, M.A. (1985): Leuk. Res.,9:573-581.

16. Francis, G.E., and Hoffbrand, A.V. (1985): In: Recent Advances in Haematology -4, edited by A.V. Hoffbrand, pp. 239-267. Churchill Livingstone, Edinburgh, London, Melbourne,New York.

17. Francis, G.E., and Berney, J.J. (1986): In: Experimental Hematology Today - 1985, edited by S.J. Baum, D.H. Pluznik, and L.A. Rozenszajn,pp. 82-89. Springer Verlag, New York, Berlin, Heidelberg, Tokyo.

18. Francis, G.E., Berney, J.J., North, P.S., Khan, Z., Wilson, E.L., Jacobs, P., and Ali, M. (1987): Leukemia, 1:653-659.

19. Francis, G.E., Mufti, G.J., Knowles, S.M., Berney, J.J., Guimaraes, J.E.T., Secker-Walker, L.M., and Hamblin, T.J. (1987): Leuk. Res. (in press).

20. Francis, G.E., and Pinsky, C. (1987): In: Cancer Chemotherapy and Biological Response Modifiers Annual 9, edited by H.M. Pinedo, B.A. Chabner and D.L. Longo,. Elsevier Science Publishers B.V.

21. Ganser, A., Volkers, B., Greher, J., Walther, F., and Hoelzer, D. (1987): Onkologie, (in press). Published in connenction with a presentation and the German-Austrian Congress of Haematology.

22. Graham, V., Surwit, E.S., Weiner, S., and Meyskens, F.L. (1986): West. J. Med.,145:192-195.

23. Greenberg, B.R., Durie, B.G.M., Barwett, T.C., and Meyskens, F.L. (1985): Cancer Treat. Rep.,69:1369-1374.

24. Griffin, J., editor (1986): Myelodysplastic syndromes. Clin Haematol.,15:4.

25. Gouveia,J., Mathe, G., Hercend, T., Gross, F., Lemaigre, G., and Santelli, G. (1982): Lancet, i:710-712.

26. Ho, A.D., Martin, H., Knauf, W., Reichardt, P., Trumper, L., and Hunstein, W. (1987): Leuk. Res.(in press).

27. Hong, K.H., Endictott, J., Itri, L.M., Doos, M., Batsakis, J.G., Bell, R., Fofonoff, S., Byers, R., Atkinson, E.N., Vaughan, C., Toth, B., Kramer, A., Dimery, I.W., Skipper, P., and Strong, S. (1986): N. Engl. J. Med.,315:1501-1505.

28. Khan, Z., and Francis, G.E. (1987): Blood, 69:1114-1119.

29. Koeffler,H.P., Kirji, K., and Itra, L. (1985): Cancer Treat. Rep.,69:1399-1407.

30. Koeffler, H.P. (1986): Semin. Haematol.,23:284-299.

31. Kong, X-B., Andreeff, M., Fanucchi, M.P., Fox, J.J., Watanabe, K.A., Vidal, P., Chou, T-C. (1987): Leuk. Res.,(in press).

32. Marks, P.A., Sheffery, M., and Rifkind, R.A. (1987): Cancer Res., 47:659-666.

33. McVie, J.G., ten Bokkel Huinink, W.W., Simonetti, G., and Dubbleman, R. (1984): Cancer Treat. Rep. 68:607-610.

34. Nakazawa, I., and Iwaizumi, M. (1982): Tohoku J. Exp. Med., 137:325-328.

35. Pastorino, U., Soresi, E., Belloni, A., Clereci, M., Costa, A., Ongari, M., Valente, M., and Ravasi, G. (1986): Proceedings of the UICC - 14th International Cancer Congress, Aug 21-27 1986, Budapest.

36. Peterson, B., Trell, E., and Sternby, N.H. (1981): JAMA, 245:2056-2057.

37. Piccozzi, V.J., Swanson, G.F., Morgan, R., Hecht, F., and Greenberg, PL. (1986): J. Clin. Oncol. 4:589-95.

38. Queseda, J., Hersh, E.M., Manning, J., Revben, J., Keating, M., Scnipper, E., and Itri, L. (1986): Blood, 68:493-497.

39. Samid, D., Flessate, D.M., and Friedman, R.M. (1987): Mol. Cell Biol., 7:2196-2200.

40. Shatairid, M., Lotem, J., Sachs, L., and Berrebi, A. (1987): Eur. J. Haematol., 38:3-11.

41. Speers, W.C. (1982): Cancer Res.,42:1843-1849.

42. Takada, K., Iwamoto, S., Sugimoto, H., Takuma, T., Kawatani, N., Noda, M., Masaki, A., Mirise, H., Arimura, H., and Konno, K. (1986): Nature,323:338-340.

43. Vallenga, E., Young, D.C., Wagner, K., Wiper, D., Ostapovicz, D., and Griffin, J.D. (1987): Blood, 69:1771-1776.

44. Von Melchner, H., and Hoffken, K. (1985): Blood, 66:1469-1472.

45. Wilson, E.L., and Francis, G.E. (1987): J. Exp. Med., 165:1609-1623.

46. Yen, A., Powers, V., and Fishbaugh, J. (1986): Leuk. Res., 10:619-629.

Clinical Trials of Retinoids as Differentiation Inducers

F.L. Meyskens, Jr.

*Department of Internal Medicine and Arizona Cancer Center,
University of Arizona, Tucson, Az, USA 85724*

SCIENTIFIC BACKGROUND

Retinoid is the generic term for vitamin A and its natural
and synthetic derivatives The role of this essential natural
compound and its requirements for the normal differentiation of
epithelial tissues has been recognized for over half a century.
A limited number of studies conducted before World War II also
suggested that vitamin A could modulate the growth of malignant
tumors, but high doses with substantial attendant hepatic and
moderate central nervous system toxicity was evident. From the
early 1960's to the present a marked amount of effort has been
dedicated to developing vitamin A derivatives with decreased
toxicity and increased efficacy on target tissues.[3]

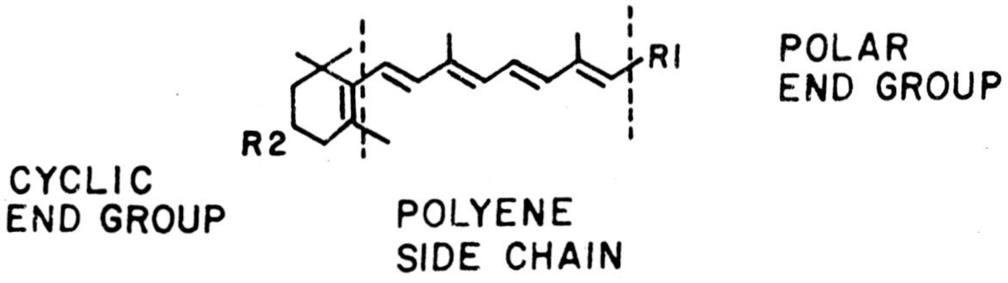

R_1	R_2	
-COH	-H	Retinol (Vitamin A)
-COOH	-H	β-Trans Retinoic Acid (Tretinoin)
-COOH	-H	13-cis-retinoic acid (Isotretinoin, Accutane)
-OOC$_2$H$_5$	-OCH$_3$	Aromatic (Etretinate)

FIG. 1. General structure of retinoids.

Vitamin A has three distinct domains: a cyclic end group, polyene side chain, and polar end group (Figure 1). Over 2000 derivatives have been synthesized; those listed represent compounds which are readily available for experimental or clinical use. Although a number of useful in vitro models have been developed to delineate the structure-function relationships for retinoids[30,31] more experience with in vivo and clinical systems suggests that the specificity seen in vitro is only general and not specific.[17-20]

TABLE 1. Effects of retinoids on cells is pleiotropic.

Biochemical
    Interaction with cellular membranes
    Binding to intracytoplasmic receptors
    Modulation of key enzymes
    Repression of oncogene expression
Cellular
    Blocks stage II promotion in carcinogenesis
    Inhibits proliferation
    Induces differentiation or maturation
    Enhances cellular immunity
    Enhances cell adhesions

Retinoids produce pleiotropic biological effects and use several biochemical strategies to effect the endpoint of controlled cellular growth (Table 1)[33]. The major biochemical mechanisms include direct interaction with the cellular membrane and its components, specific binding to intracytoplasmic receptors, modulation of intracellular enzymes, and repression of oncogene expression. Interaction of retinoids with the cell membrane indicates three major strategies: a) direct chemical covalent integration into the membrane via mannose phosphate linkages,[9] and b) indirect (via receptors) or direct interaction with growth factors and c) synthesis of new glycoproteins important in membrane function. Two major and highly specific intracytoplasmic receptors have been identified, including one which is specific for retinol (native vitamin A) and the other which is specific for retinoids with a free carboxyl group.[6,7] The interaction of retinoids with these receptors has been studied extensively, but the mechanisms involved remain only generally understood. The current hypothesis is that the holo-receptor interacts with the nuclear membrane to alter transcriptional regulation of genes with differential protein expression and subsequent phenotypic manifestations. A recent and intriguing idea put forth by Cope is that the apo-receptor functions as a substrate for protein kinase C while the holo-receptor inhibits this enzyme activity. Modulation of gene expression via regulation of nuclear events may then occur.[8] The third major mechanism may be through regulation of a number of enzymes including ornithine decarboxylase, although the selectivity of this process remains a puzzle.[29]

At the cellular level retinoids, in general, block stage II promotion of carcinogenesis, inhibit proliferation, induce differentiation or maturation and enhance cellular immunity and cell adhesion. A striking aspect about retinoids and their interactions with cells is the multiple biochemical pathways they affect and the diversity of phenotypic effects which they produce. These wide range of activities are to a large extent cell, tissue and species specific (Table 2) and hence therapeutic usage requires translation from the laboratory to the clinic in the forms of specific intervention trials.[2]

TABLE 2. Activity of retinoids as anticancer agents.[a]

	ANIMAL		HUMAN	
	in vitro	in vivo	in vitro	in vivo
Cutaneous Melanoma	+	+	−	±
Embryomal Cell Carcinoma	+	+	−	+[b]
Neuroblastoma	+	+	+	NT
Squamous Cell Cancers	+	+	+	+
Adeno Cell Cancers	−	−	−	−
Hematopoietic				
Myelodysplasia	NT	NT	±[c]	±[c]
ANNL	−	−	∓	∓
AML	−	−	−	−
APL	NT	NT	+[d]	+

[a]This chart is limited to antiproliferative and anticancer studies and does not include carcinogenesis. Symbols: +, positive; −, negative; NT, not tested.

[b]Positive in minimal disease choriocarcinoma and negative in testicular cell cancer.

[c]Active in vitro against erythrocyte lineage.

[d]Produces terminal differentiation of cells from HL-60 and fresh cultured APL from patients.

CLINICAL EFFECTS

The clinical effects of retinoids have been studied in a number of preventive and therapeutic settings and we have recently detailed these results in a number of long reviews. The important positive and negative therapeutic clinical results

are summarized below for established cancers (Table 3) and
premalignancies or hyperproliferative conditions. (Table 4).

TABLE 3.   Activity of retinoids in established human
           malignancies*.

Definite	Specific Reference
Mycosis fungoides (Cutaneous helper T-cell lymphoma)	15, 16
Squamous cell cancer of the skin	20
Probable	
Squamous cell cancer of head and neck	16
Acute promyelocytic leukemi	See 17, pt. II
Possible, More Testing Needed	
Malignant eccrine poroma	
Melanoma	
Choriocarcinoma	
Not Tested or Inadequate Numbers, More Testing	
Neuroblastoma	
Non-colon G.I.	
Bladder	
Negative	
Lung Lymphoma	24
Breast Ovarian	
Cervix Sarcoma	
Colon	

*The majority of the positive results are with the derivative
Accutane except for mycosis fungoides for which Etretinate is
also active.

   The activity of both Accutane and Etretinate against the
cutaneous T-cell lymphoma mycosis fungoides and squamous cell
cancer of the skin has been unequivocally demonstrated and this
therapeutic agent is now used widely. Two types of studies are
now needed to expand on these observations: a) in vitro
investigations of combinations using human mycosis fungoides and
squamous cell skin cancer lines and (2) phase III studies of
retinoids with electron beam and/or chemotherapy for mycosis
fungoides and clinical studies of the combination of retinoid
and interferon (α) for cutaneous squamous cell cancer.
   The in vitro differentiation response of cells from acute
promyelocytic leukemia has been impressive. Six clinical case
reports document that patients with acute promyeloctytic
leukemia can respond to Accutane. Substantiation of these
findings in larger defined clinical trials will be important.
   Two studies suggest that some (15-20%) squamous cell cancers
of the head and neck can respond to Accutane. These results,
and the high activity of retinoids against oral leukoplakia,

indicate that further trials should be performed including the use of retinoids as an adjuvant agent to prevent secondary malignancies in patients with stage I disease and in phase III studies of retinoid plus chemotherapy in the advanced setting.

To date 3 of 20 patients with metastatic melanoma have responded to Accutane with short term partial responses. Further exploration of this potential activity should probably be limited to in vitro testing of new retinoids and promising combination approaches. The responses seen in three women with choriocarcinoma were impressive (unpublished data) but a much larger trial is needed, which would be difficult since many effective chemotherapies are available for this cancer. A plethora of successful (although toxic) therapies for neuroblastoma also limits the chance for a clinical trial of retinoids. Based on in vitro studies a phase II trial would certainly seem warranted. These positive clinical results in a number of different malignancies indicates that further testing in patients with malignant eccrine poroma, bladder cancer, and non-colon gastrointestional cancer should be performed as well.

TABLE 4. Activity of retinoids in human preneoplastic and hyperproliferative states.

Definite	Specific Reference
Dermatologic	10
Actinic keratoses	
Keratoacanthoma	
Epidermal dysplasia verruciformis	
Oral leukoplakia	12
Laryngeal papillomatosis	1
Probable	
Cervical dysplasia	11
Bladder preneoplasias	
Possible, More Testing Needed	
Bronchial metaplasia	25
Myelodysplasia	
Not Tested or Inadequate Numbers, More Testing Needed	
Colon adenomas	
Negative	
Barrett's esophagus	
Dysplastic melanocytic nevi	

Considerable activity of both Accutane and Etretinate against dermatologic preneoplasias has been seen and this therapy has been widely adopted. Additionally these observations have been used as one rationale to move Accutane into the preventive mode. A number of chemopreventive trials are now being performed to

determine whether retinoids can block the development of
malignancy in patients at risk for cutaneous cancer. These
studies also suggest that the establishment of cell lines from
preneoplastic skin lesions would be a worthwhile endeavor. Many
phase II and a definitive randomized placebo-controlled phase
III trial with Accutane indicates that retinoids can cause
regression (perhaps permanent in some cases) of oral
leukoplakia. Additional studies should include identification
of a retinoid (or ? β-carotene) with fewer side effects and in
vitro investigations of leukoplakia cells. Laryngeal
papillomatosis has been unusually responsive to Accutane and
Etretinate and this therapy has been adopted by many groups.
This agent should be used more widely for this condition and
detailed investigations of the effect of retinoids on human
papilloma subtypes should be performed as well.

A series of detailed studies suggest that cervical dysplasia
can be reversed or suppressed by topically applied retinoic
acid. We are now conducting a placebo-controlled randomized
phase III trial to definitively document the validity of these
assertions. The studies of retinoids in bladder preneoplasias
(or proliferative states) suggest activity of both Accutane and
Etretinate. Definitive trials are needed as the natural history
of these lesions is complex. A phase III short term trial of
Etretinate in patients with bronchial metaplasia suggests that
this lesion can be suppressed. Longer follow-up with expanded
numbers and additional phase III studies are needed to document
this important observation.

In vitro studies on hematopoietic cells and clinical
responses in some patients with myelodysplasias suggests that
future study is needed. In particular, identification of the
biological features of responsive cells may identify a subset of
patients with a unique form of myelodysplasia.

Studies with Barrett's esophagus, a metaplastic condition
predisposing to adenocarcinoma (rather than the usual squamous
cell cancer), of the esophagus and dysplastic melanocytic
nevishow that these diseases are unaffected by retinoids.

These clinical results with a limited number of retinoids
(mainly Accutane and Etretinate) in a large number of patients
indicate overall that these differentiation agents have
significant activity against a considerable number of
premalignancies and malignancies and suggest a plan for further
clinical development.

For established malignancies:

1. More extensive and/or definitive trials are needed to
    confirm the activity of Accutane against a number of cancers
    in which probable or possible effects has been seen or in
    which testing has been inadequate.
2. Testing of newer retinoids should probably be initially done
    in malignancies that have shown retinoid sensitivity unless

there is compelling evidence for a particular tissue proclivity.
3. Screening of retinoids for anticancer activity should use human cell lines which are sensitive and insensitive to known retinoids.
4. Combination therapy with other differentiation or immunological-inducing agents or chemotherapy should be modeled in vitro using retinoid-sensitive lines (see below).

For premalignancies:

1. For diseases which are definitively sensitive to retinoids the emphasis should be to identify the minimally effective dose of a retinoid that is efficacious and other retinoids with intrinsically less side effects.
2. For preneoplasias with probable or possible sensitivity to retinoids definitive placebo-controlled randomized phase III studies need to be done. Currently only cervical dysplasia is undergoing definitive phase III testing.
3. Additional investigations of bladder precancers needs to be more carefully done to delineate the clinical and histologic subtypes and their responses. For myelodysplasia, the heterogeneity of the disease and its responses to retinoids indicates that careful clinical-biological correlations would be instructive.
4. There is a real need to study the biology of human preneoplasia in vitro. Even the most basic characterization of the majority preneoplasias has yet to be done.

Although the focus of this presentation is on therapeutic effectiveness of retinoids, mention should be made of the demonstrated activity of retinoids as antipromoters in in vitro and animal carcinogenesis models. Potential preventive activity of β-carotene and the retinoids for humans is being tested in phase III trials including skin and lung cancers.

MODELING OF COMBINATION THERAPY WITH RETINOIDS

Retinoid-responsive cells demonstrate changes in membrane glycoproteins, slowing of DNA synthesis, changes in differentiation markers, and excursions of key enzymes. These alterations suggest that the addition of retinoids to agents which affect or are affected by the state of the membrane, DNA, macromolecular synthesis, or key enzymes might produce unexpected and perhaps favorable effects in terms of controlled cellular regulation. Very few studies have addressed the effect of retinoids on the effectiveness of other biological modulators or cytotoxic agents (Table 5).

TABLE 5. Effect of retinoids on the ability of other agents to regulate tumor growth.

Retinoid	Other Agent	Tumor Cells	Effect[a,b]
Retinoic acid	4-hydroxytamoxifen	Human breast cancer	+ in vitro
Retinoic acid	1,25 (OH)$_2$ O$_3$	Murine B16 melanoma	- in vitro
Retinoic acid	Hydrocortisone	Human SV-40 transformed embyronic lung	++in vitro
Retinoic acid	Dex	Human melanoma	+
	DFMO		+
Retinyl palmitate	Vincristine	Murine P388 Leukemia in vivo	++in vitro and

			In Vivo
Retinyl palmitate	5FU	Murine ascites sarcoma 180	+
	MTX		+
	ACNU		+
	Adr		NE
	6MP		NE
	CDDP		NT
Retinyl palmitate	5FU	Murine P388	-
	MTX		+
	ACNU		++
	Adr		+
	6MP		+
	CDDP		++

[a]Effect: -, Inhibitory; NE, no effect; +, additive; ++, synergistic or potentiate; NT, not tested.
[b]References: 22, 12, 31, 4, 5, 26, 27.

The results summarized in Table 5, although meager, suggest that retinoids can have either positive or negative effects on the expression of other biologic regulators or cytotoxic agents. Exploration of the interaction of a number of compounds and retinoids may well provide interesting information about the mechanisms involved in cellular control and perhaps identify potentially important therapeutic combinations as well (Table 6).

TABLE 6. Potential therapeutic combination therapy involving retinoids.

Agents	Mechanism
Difluoromethylornithine	Ornithine decarboxylase
HMBA	Protein kinase C
Interferon	Clinically active in many of the same diseases
Cytokines	Effect on differentiation program
Cytotoxic	
Vinca Alkaloids	Membrane resistance
Others	Unknown

SUMMARY

Retinoids are powerful molecules which can affect and modulate many biochemical and biological properties of normal and abnormal cells. These agents produce clinical responses in a surprising number of human precancers and cancers. Further understanding of the mechanisms by which retinoids achieve a differentiation response or inhibit proliferation should assure continued logical development of new retinoids and combination therapy with other biological modulators and cytotoxic agents. My own assessment is that the range of activities of retinoids has not been fully appreciated in the experimental and clinical oncologic community. Despite the enormous amount of information generated about retinoids, we are just beginning to understand their potential experimental and clinical usefulness in oncology.

References

1. Alberts, D.S., Coulthard, S.W., and Meyskens, F.L., Jr. (1986): J. Biol. Resp. Mod., 5:124-128.

2. Bertram, J.S., Kolonel, L.N. and Meyskens, F.L., Jr. (1987): Cancer Res., 47:3012-3031.

3. Bollag, W. (1983): Lancet, 1:860-863.

4. Bregman, M.D., Buckmeier, J., Funk, C., and Meyskens, F.L., Jr. (1987): Pigment Cell Res., (in press).

5. Bregman, M.D., Peters, E., Sander, E., and Meyskens, F.L., Jr. (1983): J. Natl. Cancer Institute 71:927-932.

6. Chytil, F. (1986): J. Am. Acad. Dermatol., 15:741-747.

7. Chytil, F., and Ong, D.E. (1976): Nature, 260:49-51.

8. Cope, F.O., Howard, B.D., and Boutwell, R.K. (1986): Experientia, 42:1023-1027.

9. DeLuca, L.M. (1982): J. Am. Acad. Dermatol., 6:611-619.

10. Gensler, H.L.,and Meyskens, F.L., Jr., (1987) CRC Reviews - Special Issue, (in press).

11. Graham, V., Surwit, E.S., Weiner, S., and Meyskens, F.L.,Jr. (1986): West J. Med., 145:192-195.

12. Hong, W.K., Endicott, J., Itri, L.M., Doos, W., Batsakis, J.G., Bell, R., Fofonoff, S., Byers, S., Atkinson, N., Vaughn, C., Toth, B., Kramer, A., Dimery, I.W., Strong, S. (1986): New Engl. J. Med., 315:1501-1505.

13. Hosoi J., Abe E., Suda T., and Kuroki, T. (1985): Cancer Research, 45:1474-1478.

14. Kessler, J.F., Jones, S.E., Levine, N.E., Lynch, P.J., Booth, A.R., and Meyskens, F.L., Jr. (1987): Arch. Dermatol., 123:201-204.

15. Kessler, J.F., Levine, N., Meyskens, F.L., Jr., Lynch, P.J., and Jones, S.E. (1983): The Lancet, pp. 1345-1348.

16. Lippman, S.L., Kessler, J.F., Al-Sarraf, M., Alberts, D.S., Itri, L., Von Hoff, D., and Meyskens, F.L., Jr., (1987): Investigational New Drugs (in press).

17. Lippman, S., Kessler, J., Meyskens, F.L., Jr. (1987): Cancer Treat. Rep., Part I, 71(4):391-405, Part II, 71(5):493-515.

18. Lippman, S.M., and Meyskens, F.L., Jr., (1987): Am. J. Nutrition, (in press).

19. Lippman, S.M., and Meyskens, F.L., Jr. (in press, 1987): In: Nutrition and Cancer Prevention: The Role of Micronutrients, edited by T.E. Moon, M. Micozzi.

20. Lippman, S.M. and Meyskens, F.L., Jr. (1987): Ann. Int. Med., 107:499-601.

21. Lotan, R. (1980): Biochem. Biophys. Acta., 605:33-91.

22. Lotan, R. (1986): J. Nutr. Growth Cancer, 3:57-65.

23. Marth C., Mayer I., and Daxenbichler G. (1984): Biochem. Pharmacology, 33:2217-2221.

24. Meyskens F.L., Jr., Gilmartin, E., Alberts, D.S., Levine, N.S., Brooks, R., Salmon, S.E., and Surwit, E.A. (1982): Cancer Treat. Rep., 66:1315-1319.

25. Misset, J.L., Mathe, G., Santelli, G., Gouveia, J., Homasson, J.P., Suore, M.C., and Gaget, H. (1986): Cancer Detect. Prev., 9:167:170.

26. Moon, R.C., McCormick, D.L., and Mehta, R.G. (1983): Cancer Res., 43:2469-2475.

27. Nogae, I., Kikuchi, J., Yamaguchi, T., Nakagawa, M., Shiraishi,N., and Kuwano,M. (1987): Br. J. Cancer, 15:267-272.

28. Nakagawa, M., Yamaguchi, T., Ueda, H., Shiraishi, N., Komiyama, S., Akiyama, Shin-ichi, Ogata, J., Kuwano, M. (1985): Jpn. J. Cancer Res. (Gann), 76:887-894.

29. Russel, D.H. (1985): Drug Metab. Rev., 16:1-88.

30. Sporn, M.B., and Roberts, A.B. (1984): J. Natl. Cancer Institute, 73,1381-1387.

31. Sporn, M.B., Roberts, A.B. (1984): In: The Retinoids, edited by M.B. Sporn, A.B. Roberts, and D.S. Goodman, etc., pp. 235-279. Academic Press, Orlando.

32. Stanulis-Praeger, B.M., Jacobus, C.H., and Nuttall, A.E. (1986): Nutr. and Cancer, 8:171-184.

33. Wolf, G. (1984): Physiol. Rev., 64:873-937.

Therapeutic Trials of Acute Myeloid Leukemia and of Myelodysplastic Syndromes by LD-ARA C and Treatment of Promyelocytic Leukemia by Retinoic Acid

L. Degos[1], S. Castaigne[1], C. Chomienne[1], M.E. Huang[2],
H. Tilly[3], D. Bordessoule[4], J.M. Miclea[1], G. Thomas[1],
Y. Najean[1], J.P. Abita[1] and Z.Y. Wang[2]

[1]*Institut de Recherche sur les Maladies du Sang, Hopital Saint-Louis;
2 rue Claude Vellefaux 75010 Paris, France;*
[2]*Medical University of Shangaï, Chine;*
[3]*Department of Haematology, Centre Henri Becquerel,
Rue d'Amiens 76000 Rouen, France;*
[4]*Department of Haematology - Hopital Universitaire Dupuytren,
2, Avenue Alexis Carrel - 87031 Limoges Cedex, France*

In order to evaluate the therapeutic ability of differenciating agents, we have conducted two trials : one, in acute non lymphoblastic leukemia of elderly patients comparing LD-ARA C alone versus a combination of anthracycline plus ARA-C at conventional doses, and the second one in myelodysplastic syndrome comparing very low dose of ARA-C with or without androgens.

Furthermore we report chinese data (Shangai, Medical University n°2) on the treatment by all-trans retinoic acid in a series of 23 patients with promyelocytic leukemia, showing 95% of complete remission with all the cirteria of a differentiating effect.

In vitro studies were simultaneously performed in order to delineate the adequation of a type of a malignancy and the efficacy of a differentiating agent.

I – LD –ARA C VERSUS COMBINATION OF ANTHRACYCLIN PLUS ARA-C IN ELDERLY PATIENTS WITH ACUTE MYELOID LEUKEMIA
(H. Tilly, S. Castaigne, D. Bordessoule and L. Degos)

In order to compare the effectiveness and the toxicity of Low dose Aracytine (LD-ARA C) and conventional intensive chemotherapy in acute non lymphoblastic leukemia (ANLL) of elderly patients, a multicenter randomized study was begun in January 1984. Whatever the mechanism of low dose ARA-C is (differentiation and/or cytotoxic effect), we and other have demonstrated that this treatment may induce remissions in acute non lymphoblastic leukemia (ANLL) (1) (11). The overall toxicity of this regimen seems to be rather low, which is particularly appreciable in the elderly patients.

Patients

Only patients over 65 years of age with de novo ANLL were registered. Patients with severe heart, renal or hepatic disease or whose performance was above 3 (WHO nomenclature) three months before diagnosis were not eligible for randomization and were treated with LD ARA C (GROUP C).

Protocole

Patients were randomized to receive either (GROUP A) intensive induction therapy (Zorubicin 100 mg/m2 day 1 to day 4 ; Ara-C 200 mg/m2 continuous infusion day 1 to day 7) or (GROUP B) LD-ARA C (Ara-C 10 mg/m2) subcutaneously every 12 hours day 1 to day 21, 1 or 2 cycles at 14 days interval.

Patients who entered complete or partial remission received either alternate maintenance courses of conventional dose chemotherapy (GROUP A) or LD-ARA C (same dose 14 days every 4 weeks) (GROUP B).

Results

124 patients entered in the trial (45 Group A, 39 Group B and 40 Group C). The mean age was 72 years old.

No difference in the survival curve was found. More cases with complete remission were obtained by intensive chemotherapy (55% Group A versus 33% Group B). Additioning the complete and partial remissions, similar results were found in the two groups. More early deaths occurred with the intensive therapy (30 % Group A, versus 5 % Group B).

Patients with low dose ARA-C received less transfusions than those with intensive therapy (70 % amount of RBC transfusion and 50 % of platelets transfusions) for the same obtention of CR.

Four patients among 39 (Group B) treated by low dose ARA-C were never transfused, nor hospitalized and achieved CR, while all the patients treated with intensive chemotherapy had profond aplastic anemia.

In conclusion, one drug at low dose gives the same results than two drugs at conventional doses, as judged by the survival curve. Some cases were treated as outpatients (even without any transfusions) in the group treated by low dose ARA-C and the general consumption of transfusions was lesser in this group.

II – VERY LOW DOSE OF ARA-C WITH OR WITHOUT ANDROGEN THERAPY IN MYELODYSPLASTIC SYNDROMS (MDS)
(C. Chomienne, Y. Najean, G.Thomas and L. Degos)

Myelodysplastic syndroms probably represent an heterogeneous group of hematopoietic disorders characterized by an impaired maturation resulting in pancytopenia with a risk of ending in acute leukemia. No treatment really improve the disorders. The hypothesis of a treatment for malignancy based on inducing cellular differentiation has opened new possibilities of treatment for MDS. We have previously observed that low dose ARA-C (10 mg/m2 twice daily SC) has shown to be toxic in such patients due to a true aplastic phase.

Based on these clinical reports (8) (12) and on our in vitro differentiating (2) and pharmacokinetic data of ARA-C (10) we launched a trial with very low doses (VLD-ARA C) in order to test the efficacy and the toxicity of this dose. In one case out of two, by randomization, an androgen, fluoxymesterone, was added.

Patients

At the time of writing, 73 patients have entered the study and 32 have completed the first part of the treatment : 20 in the ARA-C group and 12 in the ARA-C + androgen group. Only 14 cases have started a maintenance therapy. All these patients fulfilled the criteria of the FAB MDS groups III and V. There is no difference in the clinical and biological data of the two groups before treatment. All patients are more than 50 years of age, with a median of 70 years.

The bone marrow blast infiltration was always more that 5% but never exceeded 30%.

Protocole

Patients received 2 courses of 21 days of VLD-ARA C per month (3 mg/m2 twice daily, in subcutaneous injections) followed ,when in complete or partial remission, by a maintenance therapy of 15 days per months at the same dose.

The patients with fluoxymesterone (1 mg/kg/day orally) were treated continuously for at least 6 months.

The evaluation was done at the end of 2 courses of 21 days treatment on blood and bone marrow data and then every two months.

Complete remission was judged on normal morphology and count of blood and bone marrow ; partial remission required two of the following criteria : an increase of the level of hemoglobin of ≥ 2 g/dl, of polymorphonuclear leucocytes (PMN) of $\geq 1.10^9$/l and platelets of $\geq 50.10^9$/l.

Results : (table I)

Table 1 : COMPARISON OF HEMATOLOGICAL DATA BEFORE AND AFTER
TREATMENT IN BOTH GROUPS.

VLD–ARA C ALONE	BEFORE TREATMENT	AFTER TREATMENT
Hemoglobin (g/dl)	9.1 ± 1.89	8.89 ± 1.65
Polymorphonuclears (10^9/L)	1 ± 0.9	1.23 ± 1.06
Platelets (10^9/l)	117 ± 69.36	127.9 ± 69.38
Bone marrow blasts (%)	11.89 ± 5.63	8.39 ± 6.16

VLD – ARA C + ANDROGENS		
Hemoglobin (g/dl)	8 ± 1.85	10.3 ± 2.26
Polymorphonuclears (10^9/L)	1.3 ± 1.4	1.6 ± 0.9
Platelets (10^9/L)	112 ± 88	149 ± 84
Bone marrow blasts (%)	12 ± 5	9 ± 6

Both groups have an increase in most parameters of the peripheral blood. In at least 15 patients out of 32 (50%) there was a response to the treatment. There are 2 complete remissions, one in each group, with a present follow up of 6 and 12 months. 4 patients have died during the first two months of treatment, all in the ARA-C alone group, one from an infection that was already present before entry in the study, and 3 from overt leukemia.

The treatment was well tolerated. The PMN and platelet count falls of about 50% in most cases at the begining of the treatment , with maybe a protective effect of androgens. Only 3 cases were hospitalized in each group and for a period inferior to 15 days.

The results of the trial are still preliminary considering the short length of treatment and follow up and no statistical analysis is yet possible.

In conclusion, the present results demonstrate that : 1) the hematological tolerance of 3 mg/m2 ARA-C is good and that the treatment can, be managed at home ; 2) an improvement of the Hb PMN and platelet count is seen in the majority of the patients and complete remission possible ; 3) this improvement is in some cases progressive and more that 2 regimens is sometimes necessary ; 4) however little modification of the bone marrow blast infiltration is noted.

III – TREATMENT OF ACUTE PROMYELOCYTIC LEUKEMIA WITH ALL–TRANS RETINOIC ACID (M.E. Huang and ZY Wang).

Acute promyelocytic leukemia (ALP) is considered as a distinct entity among acute myeloid leukemia (M3 in FAB classification). Hemorragic diathesis attributed to severe disseminated intravascular coagulation (DIC) often occurs. Anthracyclin greatly raised the rate of complete remission but incidence of death during the induction of therapy due to consequences of DIC is a major complication.

ALP cells are also distinguishable by their sensitivity of in vitro differenciation by retinoic acid derivatives. Few cases treated by retinoic acid were reported (5) (6) (7) (9) generally with success-full results. We have treated 23 ALD patients with all trans retinoic acid (RA)

Patients

23 patients (10 females, 12 males, mean age 33,7 years, all chinese) were treated.

Protocole

Treatment of patients

2 cases (case 1 and case 2) of APL received therapy consisting of RA (20-45 mg/m2/d and chemotherapeutic regimen including HOAP and HOCP [H=Harringtonin (0.02-0.07 mg/kg/d), O=Oncovin (0.02-0.03 mg/kg/d), A=Ara-C (1.7 mg/kg/d), P=Prednisone (0.5-0.7 mg/d), C=Cyclophosphamide (3.3d-6.7 mg/kg/d)].

5 cases (case 3-7) were treated by RA 20-80 mg/m2/d in combination with low dose ARA-C 10 mg/m2/d or harringtonin 0.03 mg/kg/d. 7 cases (case 8-14), resistant to chemotherapy, were treated by all-trans RA alone and other 9 previously untreated cases were also treated by RA as sole agent.

All the patients had whole blood transfusions (200 ml 1-2 times a week) during the induction of remission, but no platelet or white blood cell transfusion as general treatment. They received antibiotic therapy if necessary.

Maintenance Therapy

22 cases were followed up from 1-12 months after obtaining CR (N=20) or bone marrow remission (N=2). The maintenance therapy was as followed : (1) with RA alone in 9 cases, (2) RA, low dose Ara-C or other chemotherapy alternatively in 8 cases, (3) with low dose Ara-C alone in 4 cases, (4) with HOCP regimen in 1 case.

Results

Table 2 summarizes the treatment outcome of 23 patients with APL.

TABLE II : OUTCOME OF 23 APL PATIENTS

Treatment	Cases	Medullar remission (days)	CR (days)
RA + HOAP or HOCP	2	52 ± 29.6 (n=2)	54.2 ± 26 (n=2)
RA + LD-H or LD Ara-C	5	61.4 ± 15.8 (n=5)	78.8 ± 13.2 (n=5)
RA*	7	22.3 ± 5.6 (n=7)	35.8 ± 17.8 (n=7)
RA**	9	26.7 ± 5.7 (n=9)	41 ± 5.7 (n=7)***

LD=low dose,   H=Harringtonin,   O=Oncovin,   A=Aracytine,
P= Prednisone, C=Cyclophosphamide
  * Patients who were resistant to previous chemotherapy.
** Previously untreated patients.
*** Two cases with persistant anemia, but CR on myelogram.

In 21 cases, responding to the induction of differentiation effect of RA, L-CFU growth was predominant (231.9 ± 297.3 colonies) and GM-CFU suppressed (0.42 ± 1.16 colonies) before RA treatment, while GM-CFU reached normal level (116.6 ± 87.4 colonies) with little or no growth in L-CFU (1.1 ± 1.6 colonies) after obtaining CR.

Systetamic observation of peripheral blood counts during RA treatment in these previously untreated patients revealed a specific pattern. There was a rise in total white blood cells after starting the RA treatment and it reached a peak after 7-14 days. The cell count then fell, with a progressive maturation of granulocytes. The rise of platelet count was most prominant after three weeks. The elevation of hemoglobin concentration appeared reluctant and slow. Bone marrow aspirates revealed that the cells between day 10 and day 14 had more condensed chromatin and fewer azurophilic granules. Medullar remission could usually be expected in one month.

Coagulation parameters were measured simultaneously at the initiation of RA and during the treatment in 16 cases (7 previously treated and 9 untreated). 14 cases who were normal in coagulation parameters before RA therapy had no significant changes during treatment. The other two previously treated cases who had DIC positif tests before became negative in 7-10 days during RA therapy.

9 cases treated with RA alone as maintenance therapy are still in remission for a duration of 1-8 months. 4 cases maintained by low-dose Ara-C and 1 case maintained by HOCP regimen are also in CR. Among 8 cases maintained by RA, low dose Ara-C or other chemotherapy alternatively, 6 cases are still in remission with the longest more than 12 months, 2 cases (case 7, case 11) relapsed in 4 and 5 months respectively. Case 7 (non responder to RA alone) was reinduced with HOAP regimen and CR was again obtained. In case 11, the leukemic cells isolated at relapse were resistant to RA-induced differentiation in vitro.

Therapy with oral all-trans RA was accompanied by mild toxicity that consisted of dryness of lips and skin (100%), headache (21.7%), nausea (17.4%), moderate bone and joint pain (13%) and mild exfoliation (8.7%). One case had an increased SGPT. All of these side effects were well tolerated or alleviated when the dosage of oral RA was decreased.

IV - IN VITRO STUDIES
(C. Chomienne, J.P. Abita, and L. Degos)

The establishment of human myeloid leukemic cells lines consisting of a homogeneous population of leukemic cells, has provided a valuable tool for the study of differentiating effects of drugs. Various agents have now been screened on these cell lines : physiologic (such as vitamin A and D3 derivatives) or low dose antimetabolic agents (namely, Ara-C, Methotrexate (MTX), and VP16). With this in vitro model, we have shown that Ara-C at low concentration (10^{-7}M) induces monocytic differentiation of two human myeloid leukemic cell lines, the promyelocytic HL-60 and the monoblastic U-937 cell line, with a concomittant negative effect on cell proliferation (2). Retinoic acid (RA) at 10^{-6} M triggers HL-60 cells to mature into polymorphonuclear cells and U-937 cells into monocytes, with, on the contrary, a very weak effect on cell proliferation. These effects were also confirmed on a rapid modification of RNA transcript levels of c-myc and c-fos (3). The exact mechanisms which induce cells to differentiate is not fully understood. An arrest of proliferation may be essential to restore the normal equilibrium between proliferation and differentiation and allow the cell to continue its differentiation. This could be one possible mechanism for low dose antimetabolic drugs that diminish cell proliferation but not for drugs such as RA or 1-25 (OH) 2 D3 which barely modify cell growth. This is corroborated by the synergic or at least additive effect observed when the drugs of these two groups, such as we have found with RA and Ara-C, are associated (4). It remains however difficult to explain why a certain lineage pathway of differentiation is chosen or determined (granulocytic or monocytic).

Methods

Faced with the heterogeneity of response and multiple possibilities of mechanisms for the induction of differentiation in the leukemic cell lines, as with the incomplete efficacy of the clinical trials based on these differentiating drugs, we launched an in vitro study of the differentiation of fresh human myeloid blasts with drugs known to induce HL-60 and U-937 cell lines. Since investigations reported in the litterature have shown a lack of correlation between the data obtained with the leukemic cell lines and fresh human blasts, our aim was to determine if initial parameters of proliferation and differentiation status of the myeloid blast could predict its response to a certain category of differentiating drug. Blasts from 31 patients with acute myeloid leukemia (AML) were isolated fy Ficoll-Hypaque gradient from heparinized blood and/or bone marow specimens. To maintain culture conditions as close as possible to that of leukemic cell lines, only specimens with more that 90% blast invasion were studied and cultured in RPMI 1640 with 15% fetal calf serum at 10^6 cells/ml. Initial cellular proliferation was assessed using incorporation of radioactive (3HDT) thymidine into DNA, RNA transcript levels of c-myc expression and in vitro multiplication after 5 days in culture. The differentiation status of the blasts was determined by morphological and cytochemistry data (FAB classification by the Hematology Laboratory) and the Nitro-blue tetrazolium (NBT) test. The effect of low dose antimetabolic drugs (Ara-C 10^{-7}M, MTX 2.10^{-8}M, VP16 2.10^{-8}M) and physiologic drugs (RA 10^{-6}M and 1-25 (OH)2 D3 2.10^{-8}M) on blast prolifera- tion and differentiation was monitored after 5 or 6 days incubation with the drugs, on morphological and NBT criteria and after 3 days incubation, with sither Ara-C or RA, on RNA transcript levels of the oncogenes c-myc and c-fos.

Results

All proliferation criteria were correlated in all patients. The blast cells were able to proliferate in vitro, to a degree related to the initial proliferation status but variable from one case to another. Low concentration antimetabolic drugs reduced cell proliferation in all cases. However, only 58 % differentiated with Ara-C ; VP16 induced much the same degree of cell arrest and differentiating effect (absolute number of NBT positive cells) of each drug was well correlated. MTX was totally ineffective. RA and even more 1-25 (OH)2 D3 induced little cell growth arrest. Their differentiating capacity was here again not linked to the degree of initial proliferation status nor to their effect on cell growth. Therefore in this study no correlation between a differentiating effect of a drug and a blast initial proliferation status was found.

Concerning the predictive characteristic of a blast differentiation status and its response to induction of differentiation, a correlation was found with only RA and the FAB M3 promyelocytic subtype, confirming previously reported data. Nevertheless, as the differentiating effect of agents from the two groups were not correlated, it implied that an increased differentiating effect could be obtained by their association. Alone RA and Ara-C induced some differentiation in respectively 55 and 58% of the cases, whereas 73% were responsive to the association.

However, in the 26 cases studied, the association was additive in only 8 cases.

The differentiating effect observed in this study was weak. The different parameters usually used to assay the level of induced cell differentiation (NBT reduction, latex bead phagocytosis, FMLP receptors) are characteristic of a terminally differentiated granulocyte or monocyte-macrophage. Morphological assessment though very subjective gives often more signs of a triggered differentiation. With short term cultures, such as those presently used to study blast induction of differentiation, it is clear that markers of early differentiation would be more useful. This had been our aim while assessing the modification of c-myc and c-fos oncogenes. However little variation in the transcript levels were observed after three days treatment with Ara-C and RA.

Further studies to determine what specific intrinsic feature of a blast makes it responsive to differentiation (like RA and the M3 promyelocytic leukemia) and what parameters are best to study the different stages of differentiation, are future projects in this field.

REFERENCES

1. Castaigne, S., Daniel, M.T., Tilly, H., Herait, P., Degos, L. (1983): *Blood*, 62, 1: 85-86

2. Chomienne, C., Balitrand, N., Degos, L., Abita, J.P. (1986) : *Leuk. Res.*, 10, 6 : 631-636

3. Chomienne, C., Emanoil-Ravier, R., Balitrand, N., Garcette, M., Degos, L., Abita J.P. (1987) : *Journal of Biol. Reg. and Homeos. Agents*, 1, 2 : 69-72

4. Chomienne, C., Najean, Y., Degos, L., Thomas G. (1987) : *Acta Haemat.* (in press)

5. Daenen, S., Vellenga, E., Van Dobbenburgh ,O.A, Halie, M.R. (1986): *Blood* 67 : 559-561

6. Flynn, P.J., Miller, W.J., Weisdorf, D.J., Arthur, D.C., Brunning, R., Branda, R.F. (1983) : *Blood* , 62 : 1211-1217

7. Fontana, J.A., Roger, J.S., Durham, J.P. (1986) : *Cancer,* 57 : 209-217

8. Mufti, G.J., Oscier, D.G., Hamblin, T.J., Bell, A.J. (1983) : *N. Engl. J. Med,* 309, 26 : 1654

9. Nilsson, B. (1984) : *Br. J. Haematol.* 57 : 365-371

10. Poirier, O., Chomienne, C., Castaigne, C., Degos, L., Abita J.P., Najean, Y. (1986) : *Lancet ii :* 1436-1437

11. Tilly, H., Castaigne, S., Bordessoule, D., Sigaux, F., Daniel, M.T., Monconduit, M., Degos, L. (1985) : *Cancer* 55, 8 : 1633-1636

12. Wisch, J.S., Griffin, J.D., Kufe, D.W. (1983) : *N. Engl. J. Med.* 309, 26 : 1599-12603

Treatment with Interferon Gamma in Myelodisplastic Syndromes: A Pilot Study

F. Gavosto[2], A.T. Maiolo[1], M. Aglietta[2], G. Alimena[6],
C. Bernasconi[3], G. Castoldi[4], M. Cazzola[5], A. Cortelezzi[1],
F. Mandelli[6], L. Resegotti[7] and E. Polli

(Gruppo cooperativo italiano per lo studio delle mielodisplasie)

[1]*Clinica Medica I, Univ. di Milano, 20122 Milan;*
[2]*Clinica Medica I, Dip. Scienze Biom. Oncol. Umana,*
Univ. di Torino, 10126 Turin;
[3]*Divisione di Ematologia, Policlinico S. Matteo, 27100 Pavia;*
[4]*Cattedra di Ematologia, Univ. di Ferrara, 44100 Ferrara;*
[5]*Clinica Medica II, Univ. di Pavia, 27100 Pavia;*
[6]*Cattedra di Ematologia, Univ. di Roma, 00161 Rome;*
[7]*Divisione Med. Gen. E, Serv. Ematologia Osp. S. Giovanni, 10126 Turin*

INTRODUCTION

Myelodisplastic syndromes (MDS) consist of a rather heterogeneous group of diseases, involving the myeloid system. Different terminologies have been used to define diseases belonging to MDS (Table 1). Although the clinical course may be rather variable, several clinical and biological characteristics unify these disorders. MDS are neoplasias due to the clonal proliferation of myeloid progenitor cells. It is believed that the transformation event involves an immature progenitor cell (multipotent or totipotent) (2,7). On peripheral blood examination variable cytopenias, involving one or more cell lineages is the main feature. In contrast to these cytopenias, the bone marrow is generally normo or hypercellular

TABLE 1. Different terminologies used to define diseases belonging to myelodysplastic syndromes.

Refractory anemia
Preleukemic anemia
Sideroblastic anemia
Sideroacrestic anemia
Hemopoietic dysplasia
Preleukemic leukemia
Early leukemia
Smouldering leukemia
Refractory sideroblastic leukemia
Acquired idiopathic diserythropoietic anemia
Refractory anemia with excess of BM blasts
Atypical leukemia
Chronic myelomonoc. leukemia
Oligoblastic leukemia
Subacute myeloid leukemia
Panmyelopathy
Preleukemia
Dismyelopoietic syndrome

as a consequence of the accumulation of myeloid cells which show marked maturation abnormalities. This results in a maturation block which is, however, less evident than in patients with acute leukemia. The heterogeneity of the clinical presentation as well as of the clinical course of the different MDS is a reflection of the degree of maturation arrest. The FAB classification of MDS (Table 2) considers 5 classes: the first two are classical refractory anemias with or without ringed sideroblasts, one the myelomonocytic leukemia; the other two implie the presence of an excess of blasts. These last two classes (FAB 3 and 5) deserve further consideration: in some situations, infact, the leukemic clone is already established, although not invasive and could, therefore, be considered smouldering leukemias. Despite many attempts, treatment remains unsatisfactory (2, 7). Aggressive cytostatic therapy is poorly tolerated, as most MDS patients are old and the pancytopenia is generally very prolonged. Moreover the neoplastic cells appear intrinsecally rather resistent: only a small percentage of subjects who recover from the aplasia enter a complete remission which is generally short lasting (2, 7). Allogeneic bone marrow transplantation may be a potentially effective form of treatment; however, only few MDS patients may benefit from this therapeutic approach in view of the age of presentation and the availability of hystocompatible donors (9).

Supportive treatment is also rather unsatisfactory: it does not influence the progression to a frank leukemic picture and leaves the patient susceptible to bleeding and infection. Moreover, iron overlood is a frequent complication in polytransfused individuals (2, 7).

The knowledge that the maturation arrest of the neoplastic cell population in MDS is only partial, has led to the development of alternative therapeutic approaches aiming to act on the automaintenance of the pathological clone by inducing MDS cells to terminal differentiation. Low dose cytosine arabinoside (ara-c) appears effective only in a minority of patients and its bone marrow toxicity is not irrelevant (1, 13, 14, 15). Whether low dose ara-c acts by inducing terminal differentiation or an antiproliferative effect still remains uncertain. Retinoic acid, a potent in vitro inducer of differentiation of myeloid

TABLE 2. <u>Main clinico-hematological parameters used for the</u>
<u>FAB classification of MDS.</u>

Disease	Periph.blood	Bone marrow
1) Refractory anemia (RA)	Blasts < 1%	Blasts < 5%
2) Refractory anemia with ringed side= robl. (RAS)	Blasts < 1%	Blasts < 5%; ringed siderobl. >15% nucleated cells
3) Refractory anemia with excess blasts (RAEB)	Blasts < 5%	Blasts 5-20%
4) Chronic myelo= monoc. Leuk. (CMML)	>1,000 monoc./μl + neutrofilia	As above + promonocytes
5) RAEB in tran= sformation RAEB-T	As RAEB or blasts >5% or Auer rods	Blasts 20-30% or Auer rods

leukemic cells, may play a therapeutic role in a selected group of patients (4, 6). In vitro data suggest that interferon-gamma (IFN-gamma), may influence the proliferation as well as the differentiation of myeloid cells. In addition to its direct antiproliferative effect, particularly evident at high concentrations, IFN-gamma may induce terminal differentiation and Hb syntesis of myeloid leukemic cells (5, 8,12). Moreover at low concentrations it is capable of inducing CSF and IL-3 release by cells belonging to bone marrow micro-environment (monocytes, T-lymphocytes) (10, 11).

In a few cases of myeloproliferative disorders an in vivo effect of IFN-gamma has been demonstrated. Preliminary evidences indicate that this lymphokine may be active in chronic myelogenous leukemia. Moreover, four patients with acute myeloid leukemia have been treated with IFN-gamma (5). One partial and one complete response were observed. IFN-gamma action on myeloid cells may, therefore, be multiple. It might have a direct antiproliferative effect. Moreover its action may result in an enhancement of the differentiation of myeloid cells which is often blocked at different levels. This differentiative effect can be obtained either through a direct action on the neoplastic cell either indirectly by an activation of the immune system. One these basis, a multicenter trial was initiated in Italy, in patients with MDS, using two different doses to evaluate the toxicity of IFN-gamma and to establish whether it could have a role in the treatment of these disorders.

METHODS

Patient selection

Eligibility criteria.
They were: diagnosis of MDS, FAB types 3, 4, 5 or types 1-2 if clonal cytogenetic abnormalities (beside 5q-) were present. Age 18-75 years. Normal hepatic and renal function, karnofsky performance status > 50%, lack of previous cytostatic therapy; written informed consent according to the Helsinki declaration.

Treatment schedule.

Patients were randomized in two groups (14 patients/group) of treatment with recombinant IFN-gamma (Boehringer Ingelheim), 2x10^7 u/mg protein. Group 1 (higher dose) received IFN-gamma 0.1 mg/m^2 /3 week s.c.; group 2 (lower dose) received IFN-gamma 0.01 mg/m^2 /3 week. The duration of treatment was 6 months. All patients who reached 4 weeks of treatment were considered evaluable.

Evaluation of response.

Complete remission corresponds to disappearance of all signs of disease and normalization (if abnormal at diagnosis) of the caryotype. Partial or minor response: Increase of Hb > 2gr/dl; increase of platelets > 20,000/ul; increase of GN > 1,000 ul; reticulocytosis. Stable disease corresponds to any significant changes. Progressive disease: Increased percentage of blasts or appearance of Auer rods; progression to a higher FAB type.

Withdrawal criteria.

They were: evidence of progression to overt leukemia; intercurrent illness; unacceptable side effects; lack of patient compliance.

RESULTS

Thirty one patients entered the study. Three are evaluable for toxicity only, (1 for a misdiagnosis; one for withdrawal of the informed consent; one for an hemorrhagic complication during the second week of treatment). Of the remaining patients 14 received the lower dose and 14 the higher dose of IFN-gamma.

Tables 3 and 4 show the main clinical-hematology features, at diagnosis, of MDS patients treated respectively with the lower and the higher dose of IFN-gamma.

Table 5 shows the clinical results obtained with the 2 treatment schedules. It is clear that about half of patient obtained some benefit by treatment with IFN-gamma.

Tables 6 and 7 show the variation of some hematological parameters in the responding patients during treatment.

In addition to the clinical evaluation, some biological parameters were studied during

TABLE 3. <u>Clinical parameters, at diagnosis, of MDS</u>
<u>patients treated with the lower dose IFN-gamma</u>.

Diagnosis	RAEB	RAEB-t	RAS
Number	5	8	1
M/F	5/0	7/1	1/0
Age	52 (32-62	53 (27-73)	55
Time from diagnosis	4,2 (1-10)	16,4 (1-89)	37
Hb (gr/dl)	8 (5.5-11.5)	9.3 (7.6-11.4)	9.1
Leukocytes (10^9/l)	6.1 (2.8-10.0)	3.3 (1.3-7.4)	6.2
Granulocytes (10^9/l)	2.3 (0.08-7.25)	1.26 (0.07-4.29)	3.4
P.B Blasts (10^9/l)	0-0.6	0-0.4	0
Platelets	111 (14-163)	107 (17-340)	386
Reticulocytes (10^9/l)	26.6 (3.6-45.5)	20 (2.5-42.3)	8.8
BM blasts (%)	13 (8-19)	26 (21-30)	3.5
Spenomegaly	3/5	0/8	0
Hepatomegaly	3/5	4/8	0

TABLE 4. Clinical parameters, at diagnosis, of MDS
patients treated with the higher dose IFN-gamma.

Diagnosis	RAEB	RAEB-T	LMMC
Number	12	1	1
Sex (M/F)	(9/3)	1/0	1/0
Age	64	66	74
Time from diagnosis to treatment (months)	6 (1-27)	18	6
Hb (g /dl)	9.0 (7.1-10.8)	13	11.2
Leukocytes (10^9/l)	4.5 (1-11.9)	4.1	48.9
Granulocytes (10^9/l)	1.8 (0.01-5)	0.16	34.2
PB blasts (10^9/l)	0.03	0.2	7.8 (monoc.)
Platelets (10^9/l)	143 (54-334)	67	174
Reticulocytes (10^9/l)	27.6 (0-65)	25.3	61.5
BM blasts (%)	12 (6-19)	23	15
Splenomegaly	0/12	0	1
Hepatomegaly	0/12	1	1

TABLE 5. Responsiveness of MDS to treatment with IFN-gamma (lower and higher dose).

	HIGHER DOSE	LOWER DOSE
Enrolled Patients	16	15
Evaluable Patients	14	14
Complete Response	0%	0%
Partial Response	14%	7%
Minor Response	43%	29%
Stable Disease	14%	21%
Progressive Disease	29%	43%

(Partial Response 14% + Minor Response 43% = 57%; Partial Response 7% + Minor Response 29% = 36%)

TABLE 6. Variation of some hematological parameters in patients treated with higher IFN-gamma dose (0.1 mg/sqm) and considered responsive to treatment.

RESPONDING PATIENTS - HIGHER DOSE

	BEFORE TREATMENT	1 MTHS	3 MTHS	6 MTHS
BM Blasts (%)	13	7	6.5	6.2
Retic./μl	29,000	77.000	70,000	70,000
Transfusions (U./month)	3	1	0	0

TABLE 7. Variation of some hematological parameters in patients treated with lower IFN-gamma dose (0.01 mg/sqm) and considered responsive to treatment.

RESPONDING PATIENTS - LOWER DOSE

	BEFORE TREATMENT	1 MONTH	3 MONTHS
BM Blasts (%)	17	12	11
RETIC./μl	17,000	34,600	55,000
TRANSFUSIONS (U./month)	7	2	3

TABLE 8. Toxicity and complications during treatment with IFN-gamma at two different treatment schedules.

Toxicity and Complications	Higher dose	Lower dose
Fever	100%	73%
Myalgias	46%	27%
Hepatic	7%	33%
Renal	7%	7%
Cardiac	7%**	0%
Nervous system	20%	7%
Infections	20%	33%
Thrombosis/hemorrages	0%	20%

** 1 case of sudden death

treatment. In the majority of patients leukocyte alkaline phosphatase (variable at diagnosis) did not show significant changes. In 3 cases, only, a consistent increase was documented.

The majority of patients had caryotype abnormalities at diagnosis. In only one the caryotype reverted to normal during treatment. It should, however, be noted that most of the cytogenetic data presently available are those carried out after 1 month of treatment only.

The in vitro growth of granulo-monocyte progenitor was, in most patients, markedly reduced, with a cluster/colony ratio generally normal. A certain degree of fluctuation of the in vitro growth, unrelated, however, to the percentage of BM blasts, was observed during the treatment.

The treatment with IFN-gamma was not devoid of toxicity. Except from one patient who suffered from severe peripheral neuropathy, (partially reversibile), the toxicity was, however, generally mild and mainly consisting of flu-like symptoms (Table 8). Most of the other complications (thrombosis or hemorrhages, infections) were not clearly related to treatment.

DISCUSSION

The aim of the present study was to investigate whether IFN-gamma could play a role in the treatment of MDS and to assess in such patients the toxic effects of a prolonged treatment. Although our patients were rather old and in most cases leuko-thrombocytopenic, we did not observe a marked hematological toxicity during treatment. The majority of patients complained of flu-like symptoms particularly in the higher dose group, which only partially regressed during treatment. In one case, only, the side effects induced to refuse further continuation of treatment. Except for one case of severe peripheral neurotoxicity, IFN-gamma did not give rise to major toxic complications. These findings suggest that IFN-gamma, at both doses, is well tolerated by patients with MDS.

With regard to the possibile therapeutic effect of this compound it must be noted that, despite a prolonged treatment, no patient entered a complete remission. It appears, however, that the molecule

shows some degree of activity since 36% of the
patients treated with the lower dose and 57% of the
patients in the higher dose group display some
clinico-hematological improvement. It is of
interest that while the leukocyte and platelet
counts did not change significantly during
treatment, a reticulocytosis and a decreased blood
transfusion requirement were frequently observed,
pointing to a possible selective effect of the
molecule on the erythroid cell compartment. Bone
marrow blasts decreased in about 50% of patients;
the effect, however, was most often transient. A
complete analysis of biological parameters is not
available as yet. However, the lack of
normalization of the neutrophil alkaline
phosphatase in the patients with a low score before
treatment, the persistence of a reduced in vitro
growth of myeloid progenitors following treatment
and the lack, except for one case, of a
normalization of the caryotype, are in keeping with
the clinical evidence of only a partial response of
MDS patients to IFN-gamma treatment. The presently
available data do not allow to determine whether
IFN-gamma deferred the evolution to overt acute
leukemia. The quite large proportion of patients in
whom the disease progressed seems to indicate a
rather low activity in this context. It should,
however, be considered that most patients (RAEB-T)
were at high risk of evolution. Only a larger
trial, randomized with patients receiving
supportive treatment only, will help to answer this
question.

In vitro data indicate that IFN-gamma may
suppress myeloid leukemia proliferation either via
an antiproliferative effect or by acting as a
differentiation inducer. Our in vivo observations
do not allow to clarify the mode of action. The
lack of bone marrow aplasia during treatment may be
in favour of a differentiative effect, mainly on
the erythroid lineage; this effect, however, was
often limited.

In conclusion our data show that IFN-gamma is
well tolerated by patients with MDS and that both
doses we tested can induce a partial remission of
the disease. The percentage of responding patients
seems somewhat greater with the higher dosage,
which, however, produced more marked secondary
effects, namely the persistent flu-like syndrome.

In consideration of these results, a larger

trial on the effect of IFN-gamma in MDS comprehensive of an arm with an higher dose oh the drug alone or combination with other differentiation agents, as for instance retinoic acid, seems warranted.

REFERENCES

1. Baccarani, M., Zaccaria, A., Bandini, G., Cavazzini, G., Fanin, R., Tura, S. (1983): Low dose arabinosyl-cytosine for treatment of myelodysplastic syndromes and subacute myeloid leukemia. Leuk. Res., 7:539-545.

2. Bagby, G.C. Jv. (1985): The preleukemic syndrome. CRC press, Boca Raton, U.S.A.

3. Beran, M., Andersson, B., Keating, M., Rios, A., McCredie, K. B., Freireich, E.J., Gutterman, J. (1987): Hematological response of four patients with smouldering acute myelogenous leukemia to partially pure gamma interferon. Leukemia, 1:52-57.

4. Clark, R.E., Ismail, S.A.D., Jacobs, A., Payne, H., Smith, S.A. (1987): A randomized trial of 13-cis retinoic acid with or without cytosine arabinoside in patients with the myelodysplastic syndrome. Br.J. Haematol., 66:77-83.

5. Dayton, E.T., Matsumoto-Kobayashi, M., Perussia, B., Trincheri, G. (1985): Role of immune interferon in the monocytic differentiation of human promyelocytic cell lines induced by leukocyte conditioned medium. Blood, 66:583-594.

6. Gold, E.J., Mertelsmann, R.H.,Itri, L.M., Gee, T., Arlin, Z., Kempin, S., Clarkson, B.D., Moore, M.A.S. (1983): Phase I Clinical trial of 13-cis retinoic acid myelodysplastic syndromes. Cancer Treat. Rept., 67:981-986.

7. Koeffler, H.P. (1986): Myelodysplastic syndromes (Preleukemia). Seminars Hematol., 23:284-299.

8. Koeffler, H.P., Ranyard, J., Yelton, L., Billing, R., Bohman, R., (1984): Gamma interferon induces expression of the HLA-D antigens on normal

and leukemic human myeloid cells. Proc. Natl. Aca. Sci. (USA): 81:4080-4084.

9. O'Reilly, R.J. (1983): Allogeneic bone marrow transplantation: current status and future directions. Blood 62:941-964.

10. Piacibello, W., Lu, L., Aglietta, M., Rubin, B.Y., Cooper, S., Wachter, M., Gavosto, F., Broxmeyer, H.E. (1986): Human gamma interferon enhances release from phytohemoagglutinin stimulated T4 lymphocytes of activities that stimulate colony formation by granulocyte-macrophage, erythroid, and multipotential progenitor cells. Blood, 68:1339-1347.

11. Piacibello, W., Lu, L., Wachter, M., Rubin, B.Y., Broxmeyer, H.E. (1985): Release of granulocyte-macrophage colony stimulating factors from major histocompatibility complex class II antigen-positive monocytes is enhanced by human gamma interferon. Blood, 66:1343-1351.

12. Ralph, P., Harris, P.E., Punjabi, C.J., Welte, K., Litcofshy, P.B., Ho, M.K., Rubin, B.Y., Moore, M.A.S., Springer, T.A (1983): Lymphokine inducing terminal differentiation of the human monoblast leukemia cell line U937: a role for gamma interferon. Blood, 62:1169-1175

13. Roberts, J.D., Ershler, W.B., Tindle, B.H., Stewart, J.A. (1984): Low dose cytosine arabinoside in myelodysplastic syndromes and acute myelogenous leukemia. Cancer, 56:1001-1005.

14. Tricot, G., De Bock, R., Dekker, A.W., Boogaerts, M.A., Peetermans, M., Punt, K., Verwilghen, R.L. (1984): Low dose cytosine arabinoside (Ara-c) in myelodysplastic syndromes. Br. J. Haematol., 58:231-240.

15. Wisch, J.S., Griffin, J.D., Kufe, D.W. (1983): Response of preleukemic syndromes to continuous infusion of low dose cytarabine. N. Engl. J. Med., 309:1599-1602.

Clinical Trials of Polar Differentiation Agents

M.J. Egorin

Division of Developmental Therapeutics
University of Maryland Cancer Center, 655 West Baltimore Street
Baltimore, Maryland 21201, USA

Low molecular weight, polar-planar compounds constitute a major class of agents that induce differentiation of malignant cells (2,17,29,31,33). Tumor cells that have been induced to differentiate by these agents lose their ability to proliferate, to clone in vitro, and to propagate when transplanted into animals (2,17,30,32,33). Hexamethylene bisacetamide (HMBA, NSC 95580) is the most potent inducer of differentiation yet defined in this group of compounds (11,24–27,34) and has a number of characteristics which render it among the most interesting and of greatest potential clinical use. HMBA was selected for introduction into clinical trials after analysis of the structure-activity relationships of a series of bisacetamides indicated it had maximum differentiating activity (25,27,34). Importantly, HMBA differs from differentiating agents, such as DMSO and NMF, which have been disappointing in clinical evaluation (1,10,19–21,35,37,38), in that animal toxicologic and pharmacokinetic studies (5) indicated the ability to achieve HMBA concentrations in plasma equal to those required for induction of differentiation in vitro. HMBA induces in vitro morphological and functional differentiation of a variety of murine and human leukemic and solid tumor cell lines, and this induction has been carefully characterized with regard to the temporal and concentration requirements for HMBA exposure (6,11,14-16, 22-276,31,34).

Five phase I clinical trials of HMBA have been reported in the literature (8,12,13,18,28,36) and a larger number have been initiated based on data accrued in those initial trials. This manuscript describes the clinical and pharmacologic data from the initial 5 clinical trials. It also will attempt to identify the ongoing clinical trials and will describe some unique concepts of the use of HMBA which have been rationally based on the agent's pharmacokinetics and pharmacology.

INITIAL PHASE I TRIALS

The first five clinical trials of HMBA have all been phase I trials, each using a continuous infusion schedule (8,12,13,18,28,36). The choice of continuous infusion therapy was based on the extensive preclinical data indicating that prolonged contact of HMBA with tumor cells was required for induction of differentiation. The first two trials, at the University of Maryland Cancer Center (UMCC) (8) and Johns Hopkins

Oncology Center (28), were initiated with 5-day continuous infusion schedules and involved dosage escalations of 4.8, 9.6, 16, 24, 33.6, and 43.2 $gm/m^2/d$. The results of these two trials were remarkably consistent both with regard to their clinical and pharmacologic observations.

Clinical Toxicities

Both studies identified three important clinical toxicities associated with the 5-day continuous infusion schedule. In each study thrombocytopenia was noted, but the dose-limiting toxicities consisted of an anion gap, metabolic acidosis and neurotoxicity (including agitation obtundation, confusion and hallucinations).

Metabolic Acidosis

The acidosis associated with HMBA therapy was hypochloremic and metabolic in character and was associated with an anion gap of 5-8 meq/l. This toxicity was reversible and clearly dose-related, not being observed at doses less than 24 $g/m^2/d$ in the Hopkins study (28) or less than 33.6 $g/m^2/d$ in the UMCC study. More importantly, and, as described in more detail later, this toxicity has not been noted in any patient with HMBA steady-state concentrations (C_{ss}) less than 2 mM. The exact etiology of this toxicity remains unknown, but the list of possible causes is relatively short. One possible etiology, renal insufficiency has been noted in several of the acidotic patients, but not all of the patients developing acidosis have had reduced creatinine clearances or elevated serum concentrations of creatinine or urea nitrogen. Ketoacidosis has not been documented in any patient with HMBA-induced metabolic acidosis. At the UMCC, patient plasma was checked for acetone and no positive reactions were found. However, the question of B-hydroxybutyrate production, which would not have been detected with the test employed, remains undefined. As discussed later, the biotransformation of HMBA and its metabolites involves two documented deacetylation reactions and the potential for liberation of at least two additional acetate moieties (Fig. 1) (4). As a result, the question of a contribution from ketoacidosis remains of interest. The documentation of 6-acetamidohexanoic acid (AcHA) and 6-aminohexanoic acid (AmHA) as metabolites of HMBA (4) made attractive the possibility that HMBA-associated acidosis reflected generation of significant concentrations of acidic metabolites. As described later, quantification of the plasma concentrations of AcHA and AmHA has ruled this out as a sole source of HMBA-induced acidosis. The final possible cause for an anion gap, metabolic acidosis could be lactic acidosis. It is currently unknown whether HMBA or any of its metabolites could, for example, poison oxidative phosphorylation and, as a result, induce this type of acidosis.

It is clear that the etiology of HMBA-induced metabolic acidosis is multifactorial. This has implications in terms of developing strategies

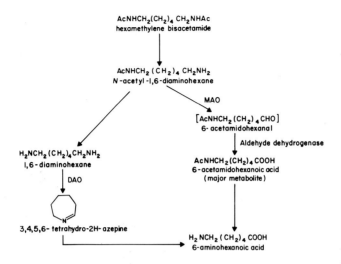

FIG. 1. Proposed metabolic pathways leading to the metabolites of HMBA in humans, a. deacetylase; b. monoamine oxidase; c. aldehyde dehydrogenase or aldehyde oxidase; d. diamine oxidase and aldehyde oxidase. Ac. acetyl.

to mitigate this toxicity. The current phase I trial at the UMCC is evaluating the utility of sodium bicarbonate, administered concomitantly with HMBA, as a means to overcome the acidosis or to allow higher HMBA doses or plasma C_{ss} to be achieved before the acidosis would become dose-limiting. As discussed later, monoamine oxidase has been shown to be the enzyme that converts N-acetyl-1,6-diaminohexane (NADAH), the initial deacetylated metabolite of HMBA, to AcHA (7). This has raised the potential for using monoamine oxidase inhibitors, such as tranylcypromine or pargyline, to block generation of AcHA as another means to reduce the acid load generated from HMBA and thereby allow higher doses or C_{ss} be achieved. We are currently conducting preclinical studies in this regard and, should they prove promising, hope to initiate clinical trials to investigate this issue.

Neurotoxicity

The neurotoxicity associated with HMBA, although reversible and dose-related, is otherwise poorly characterized. As with acidosis, neurotoxicity has not been observed at doses less than 24 g/m^2/d and, in all cases but one, required doses greater than 24 g/m^2/d. It is unknown what, if any, role acidosis plays in the neurologic changes noted in patients receiving HMBA. Electroencephalographic evaluation of patients receiving HMBA has not proven useful in following patients or in defining the cause of the observed central nervous system abnormalities (28). The pathways for catabolism of HMBA and its various metabolites (Fig. 1), described later in this article, provide several intriguing possibilities for neurotoxic materials being generated, but to date, this issue remains undefined.

Thrombocytopenia

Although preclinical toxicology studies of HMBA provided no evidence of this agent being myelosuppressive, each of the initial 5-day continuous infusion trials of HMBA identified reductions in platelet counts as a dose-related, adverse effect associated with HMBA therapy (8,28). The dose relationship involved both the frequency and severity of this problem. Although a major toxicity, in neither the UMCC nor Hopkins trials with 5-day continuous infusion schedules did thrombocytopenia prove to be a dose-limiting toxicity. The data from the UMCC trial has been analyzed further, recognizing the significant variation in C_{ss} associated with the same dose of HMBA in different patients and the fact that, for most drugs, a better relationship exists between plasma concentration and drug effect than between dose and drug effect. When examined in this fashion, a clear relationship was defined between drug exposure as measured by area under the curve (AUC) and the percentage change platelet count observed in each patient (Fig. 2).

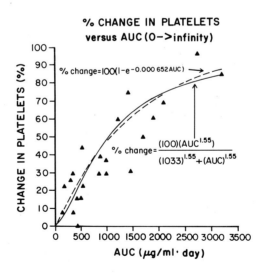

% CHANGE IN PLATELETS versus AUC (0—>infinity)

$$\% \text{ change} = 100(1 - e^{-0.000\,652\,AUC})$$

$$\% \text{ change} = \frac{(100)(AUC^{1.55})}{(1033)^{1.55} + (AUC)^{1.55}}$$

FIG. 2. Relationship of th HMBA AUC of individual patients to the percentage of decrease in platelet count observed in that same course.

While modeled as AUC, the possibility that the effect was actually related to plasma C_{ss} could not be ruled out because the AUC associated with continuous infusion therapy is proportional to the C_{ss}. Nevertheless, the data implies that dose-limiting thrombocytopenia would prevent a 10-day continuous infusion schedule of HMBA maintaining 2 mM C_{ss} HMBA. In fact, this has been the case in both of the two 10-day continuous infusion studies (18,35). The exact etiology of HMBA-induced platelet suppression remains unknown. However, blood smears of patients receiving HMBA do not reveal platelet clumping, and the time course of platelet suppression, with nadirs at 15-22 days and recovery by days 20 to 29, suggests a myelosuppressive effect rather than peripheral destruction.

Other Toxicities

Nausea and vomiting associated with HMBA therapy have been mild to moderate, dose-related and have ended when the drug infusion ceased (8,28). Several patients in the UMCC phase I trial had reactivation of herpes simplex or herpes zoster, although this problem was not dose-related (8). A number of patients treated at the Johns Hopkins Oncology Center with 24 or 33.6 $g/m^2/d$ were described as having mucositis with soreness, erythema, and ulcers on their lips, gums, palate, and pharynx (28). Whether these lesions represented herpetic reactivation is unknown since the results of viral cultures were not reported.

Subsequent Phase I Trials

Two phase I trials, each employing a 10-day continuous infusion schedule repeated every 28 days, have been reported (18,36). The first of these was performed at the Johns Hopkins Oncology Center, and not surprisingly, found dose-or exposure-related thrombocytopenia to be the dose-limiting toxicity at a maximum tolerated dose (MTD) of 20 $g/m^2/d$ (18). In this study, central nervous system, renal and metabolic toxicities were rare; however, the HMBA concentrations achieved were much lower than those associated with these toxicities in the trials which employed 5-day continuous infusion schedules. An unusual toxicity associated with HMBA was noted in this trial. A 65 year old female with metastatic leiomyosarcoma, who was receiving HMBA at 15.8 $g/m^2/d$, developed a leukocytoclastic vasculitis (29). The second trial employing a 10-day continuous infusion schedule has been performed at the Memorial Sloan Kettering Cancer Center (36). As in the study at Hopkins, thrombocytopenia was identified as the dose-limiting toxicity, but this second trial felt that an MTD of 24 $g/m^2/d$ was possible. As in the Hopkins 10-day infusion trial, this 10-day infusion trial at Memorial Sloan Kettering produced no instances of central nervous system, renal or metabolic toxicity.

PHARMACOKINETIC AND CLINICAL PHARMACOLOGY STUDIES

The initial trials of HMBA have been marked by an intensive investigation of the metabolism and disposition of this agent (4,7,8,12,13,18,28,36). This pharmacologic information is important because it has either been incorporated into or, in certain cases, has actually stimulated subsequent clinical trials.

Pharmacokinetics

Plasma Pharmacokinetics (Table 1)

Plasma C_{ss} of HMBA are achieved between 12 and 24 hr after initiation of an HMBA continuous infusion, and in individual patients, the C_{ss} of HMBA remains quite constant, with day to day variation usually less than 10% of the mean C_{ss}. After cessation of the HMBA infusion, plasma concentrations of HMBA decline in monoexponential fashion with a half-life of 2 to 4 hr. Plasma C_{ss} of HMBA increase with increasing dosage, however, at every dosage there is variation in the plasma HMBA C_{ss} noted among the patients studied so that the standard deviation represents an average of 30% of the mean C_{ss} determined at that dosage (Table 1). The two 5-day continuous infusion trials described earlier (8,28) both documented the ability to achieve C_{ss} HMBA of 1.5 to 2 mM with HMBA dosages of 24 to 33.6 $g/m^2/d$.

Despite an initial impression that the pharmacokinetics of HMBA were linear with dosage, this has not proven to be the case. More detailed studies have shown the clearance of HMBA to have two components (4,13). The first of these components is linear and proportional to creatinine clearance, being described by the equations: HMBA renal clearance = (0.56 ± 0.28) creatinine clearance. The other component of HMBA clearance is saturable and exhibits Michaelis-Menten characteristics with Km = 251 ± 73 mg/l and Vmax = 1991 ± 409 mg/hr.

Individualized and Optimized Dosing

These plasma pharmacokinetic data have had a major impact on several ongoing and recently initiated clinical trials. Based on the initial data from the two 5-day continuous infusion trials (8,28), the MTD for a 5-day continuous infusion of HMBA would be 33.6 $g/m^2/d$ and the recommended dose for phase II trials would be 24 $g/m^2/d$. However, the significant variability in the plasma of HMBA C_{ss} achieved at any dosage of HMBA implies that a number of patients treated with HMBA at 24 $g/m^2/d$ would not achieve an HMBA C_{ss} of 2 mM. In that 2 mM concentrations of HMBA were not associated with serious toxicities, we have argued against empiric dosing of HMBA. As an alternate, we have proposed the concept of pharmacokinetic monitoring of patients receiving HMBA with the plan of defining a maximum tolerated plasma concentration or a recommended plasma concentration for phase II trials. To this end, we have developed an adaptive control dosing

TABLE 1

Summary of HMBA Pharmacokinetics

Dosage (g/m^2/d)	C_{ss} ug/ml	C_{ss} mM	AUC (ug/ml h)	t 1/2B (h)	CL_{TB} (ml/min)	%Dose Excreted in urine/24 h
4.8 (7/3)[a]	43.5 + 15[b]	0.22	52 + 1801	3.81 + 1.81	150 + 63	28.5 + 18.9
9.6 (6/4)	89.8 + 17.3	0.45	10774 + 2081	2.44 + 0.63	120 + 24	19.8 + 4.3
16 (3/3)	176.2 + 79.8	0.88	21143 + 9573	2.83 + 0.69	109.7 + 36.2	33.8 + 12.8
24 (7/6)	253.8 + 82.9	1.27	30458 + 9959	2.27 + 0.80	116.8 + 35.0	43.8 + 12.5
33.6 (4/3)	405.3 + 108.4	2.03	48633 + 13005	2.02	89.8 + 26.6	39.2 + 16.3
43.2 (1/1)	636	3.18	6152	5.65	86.7	43.0

a Numbers in parentheses, number of course per number of patients

b Mean $\pm$ S.D.

strategy which uses a MAP-Bayesian parameter estimator and daily measurement of HMBA plasma concentrations, and we have shown this type of dosing strategy suitable to produce HMBA C_{ss} of 1.5 to 2 mM without central nervous system, renal or metabolic consequences (12,13). This dosing strategy is serving as a means for determining HMBA dosage in a number of the ongoing clinical trials.

We have carried our proposal of maximum drug therapy beyond the concept of a maximum tolerated concentration. As described earlier, the thrombocytopenia associated with HMBA therapy is related to drug exposure, and we and other workers have published mathematical models to describe this relationship (8,33). With such a model and a patient's pretreatment platelet count, it is possible to predict the maximum duration of an infusion that maintains a given C_{ss}, e.g. 1.5 or 2 mM and which will produce the maximum tolerable reduction in platelet count. In this regard we have utilized our adaptive control dosing algorithm and our model relating drug exposure and platelet reduction to describe a further refined dosing scheme which allows the maintenance of a maximum tolerated plasma concentration for a maximum tolerated duration giving thereby maximum tolerable exposure. We will employ this dosing strategy in our soon-to-be initiated trials of HMBA therapy for uterine cervical dysplasia and oral leukoplakia.

Saliva

As an adjunct to the idea of therapeutic drug monitoring and the idea of treating neoplasia in the oral cavity, we have studied the salivary concentrations of HMBA in patients receiving 5-day continuous infusions of the drug. These studies, which have recently been submitted for publication, show that salivary concentrations of HMBA increase rapidly and, after approximately 2 hr, are essentially equal to concomitant plasma concentrations of HMBA. These results sampling and document the excellent delivery of HMBA to the oral cavity and may help monitor HMBA therapy in patients with venous access too poor for frequent plasma.

Urine

The third aspect of HMBA pharmacokinetics that has been defined in published trials and which has implications in terms of ongoing or planned clinical trials is the drug's urinary excretion (8,18,28,36). Urinary excretion of HMBA accounts for 20 to 45% of the daily administered dose (Table 1). When considered in terms of urinary concentrations of HMBA instead of absolute excretion, i.e., concentration x volume, it is apparent that even the lowest dose of HMBA used in clinical trials produces urinary concentrations of HMBA between 3 and 15 mM (Table 2). This result is not surprising when one considers that grams per day of a material with a molecular weight of 200 are administered and that a large percentage of that dose is excreted in a daily urinary volume of 1 to 2 liters. The fact that concentrations which are active in vitro can easily be achieved in urine with HMBA doses that produce low plasma concentrations of HMBA means that therapeutic concentrations can be achieved in the bladder without the risk of central nervous system, renal or metabolic toxicity.

TABLE 2

URINARY CONCENTRATIONS OF HMBA AND METABOLITES

Dosage	HMBA (mM)	AcHA (mM)	NADAH (mM)	DAH (mM)
4.8	3.3 ± 0.8[a]	3.8 ± 0.6	3.3 ± 0.6	0
	7.9 ± 0.3	5.5 ± 0.8	1.6 ± 1.9	0
	10.8 ± 3.6	3.6 ± 1.6	2.8 ± 0.7	0
9.6	22.0 ± 11.6	20.7 ± 10.8	15.9 ± 8.5	1.5 ± 0.6
	5.8 ± 2.7	15.2 ± 6.2	8.5 ± 4.4	0.7 ± 0.7
	8.8 ± 0.9	5.5 ± 0.5	6.9 ± 0.7	0.6 ± 0.2
16	11.8 ± 8.5	10.2 ± 1.6	12.7 ± 0.4	1.0 ± 0.9
	38.0 ± 9.3	28.8 ± 3.5	7.4 ± 1.4	0
	65.5 ± 36.4	16.2 ± 4.3	14.5 ± 3.8	0.4 ± 0.0
24	74.4 ± 48.6	16.8 ± 1.1	12.0 ± 0.4	0
	20.0 ± 0.9	11.5 ± 5.6	8.7 ± 3.6	0.5 ± 0.6
	90.6 ± 22.9	26.8 ± 11.5	27.8 ± 11.0	1.0 ± 0.2
33.6	16.9 ± 13.2	15.3 ± 4.5	6.6 ± 2.7	0
	62.5 ± 11.1	21.5 ± 1.9	11.2 ± 1.2	0
	57.5 ± 16.8	21.6 ± 7.5	7.2 ± 2.9	0
43.2	12.1 ± 1.6	24.1[b]	14.4[b]	0[b]

[a] Mean $\pm$ S.D. of concentration of HMBA and metabolites in 24 h urine collections obtained from individual patients on days 2, 3, 4, and 5 of their 5 d continous infusions of HMBA.

[b] Urinary concentrations of HMBA and metabolites in the one patient treated with $43.2 g/m^2/d$. Values represent urinary concentrations on day 1 of treatment only because insufficient material remained from urine voided on days 2,3,4, & 5.

Moreover with the knowledge of plasma concentrations achieved with $5 \, g/m^2/d$ of HMBA and the model relating drug exposure to platelet suppression, it is possible to estimate that a 30-day infusion should be feasible without dose-limiting thrombocytopenia. These facts have been utilized by investigators at the Memorial Sloan Kettering Cancer Center who have formulated a trial of HMBA in superficial carcinoma of the bladder.

Metabolism of HMBA

Clinical and pharmacologic studies of HMBA have not been restricted to defining the pharmacokinetics of the drug. Rather, the metabolism of this compound has been defined in depth (4,7,9) and the results of these studies may have implications in terms of the toxicities seen. Initial studies with gas chromatography/mass spectrometry (4) documented the presence of 5 HMBA metabolites in the urine of patients receiving HMBA (Fig. 1). These metabolites included the monodeacetylated, monoamine compound, NADAH; its oxidation product, AcHA; its deaminated product, 1,6-diaminohexane (DAH); and the product of DAH oxidation, 6-aminohexanoic acid (AmHA) with its lactam, caprolactam. Subsequent studies have documented the concentrations of each of these compounds in the plasma (Fig. 3) and urine (Table 3) of patients treated with varying doses of HMBA (9). At all HMBA dosages, AcHA was the major metabolite present in both plasma and urine. Plasma concentrations of AcHA were at steady-state by 24 hr after the start of the HMBA infusion, and, within any patient, there was little day-to-day variation in plasma C_{ss} of AcHA (Fig. 3). For individual patients the daily variation about the mean C_{ss} of AcHA in plasma obtained at 24, 47, 71, 95, and 120 hr was usually less than 25% (Fig. 3). As observed with HMBA (8,28) there was variation among the AcHA C_{ss} achieved in the individual patients treated at each dosage (Fig. 3). Plasma AcHA C_{ss} increased with increased HMBA dosage, but this rate of increase was less than that of the increase in C_{ss} HMBA. As a result, the ratio of plasma C_{ss} AcHA to plasma C_{ss} HMBA decreased with increasing HMBA dosage (Fig. 4).

Plasma concentrations of NADAH were less than plasma concentrations of either HMBA or AcHA. At HMBA dosages of 4.8, 9.6, and $16 \, g/m^2/d$, NADAH was not measurable in plasma. In three patients treated with $24 \, g/m^2/d$, plasma NADAH C_{ss} were 0.05 ± 0.02, 0.19 ± 0.08, and 0.23 ± 0.01 mM. In 2 patients treated with $33.6 \, g/m^2/d$ and 1 patient treated with $43.2 \, g/m^2/d$, NADAH C_{ss} were 0.08 ± 0.01 mM, 0.21 ± 0.04 mM and 0.19 ± 0.04 mM, respectively. These concentrations represented between 33% and 80% of concomitant plasma concentrations of AcHA and between 6% and 38% of concomitant plasma concentrations of HMBA. DAH and AmHA were not detected in the plasma of any patient.

Upon completion of the 120 hr infusion of HMBA, plasma concentrations of NADAH declined monoexponentially with a half-life of

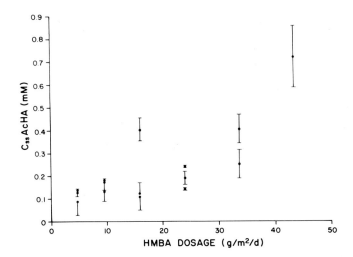

FIG. 3. Relationship of steady-state concentration of 6-acetamido-hexanoic acid in plasma and HMBA dosage. Points, means for individual patients, bars, SD. Concentrations of 6-acetamidohexanoic acid in plasma samples obtained at 24,47, 71, 95, and 120 h in the 120-h infusion of HMBA were used to calculate means of SD.

approximately 2-4 hr. Plasma concentrations of NADAH declined in parallel with the decline in plasma concentrations of HMBA. In contrast, plasma concentrations of AcHA declined little, if at all, during the 6 to 8 hr after the infusion from which samples have been available.

Within each patient, the daily urinary excretion of AcHA, NADAH, and DAH was consistent from day to day (Table 3). Urinary excretion of AcHA accounted for 12.7 + 3.9% of the daily dose of HMBA. The percentage of the daily HMBA dose that was excreted as NADAH decreased with increased HMBA dosage, from 10.8 + 6.0% at 4.8 g/m^2/d to 4.2 + 1.2% at 33.6 g/m^2/d (Table 3). Urinary excretion of DAH was not dose-related, and never accounted for more than 3% of the daily dose of HMBA and in most cases, accounted for less than 1% of the daily HMBA dose (Table 3). The data also define the range of concentrations of HMBA and each metabolite achieved in urine when various dosages of HMBA are administered by continuous infusion (Table 2).

As mentioned earlier, these results indicate that the acidosis associated with toxic doses of HMBA is not entirely due to production of acidic metabolites since the plasma concentrations of AcHA measured in patients treated with 33.6 and 43.2 g/m^2/d are insufficient by

TABLE 3
URINARY EXCRETION OF HMBA AND METABOLITES
% Daily Dose Excreted As:

Dosage (g/m^2/d)	HMBA	AcHA	NADAH	DAH	Total
4.8	36.9 $\pm$ 18.4[a]	10.1 $\pm$ 2.4	10.6 $\pm$ 6.0	0.2 $\pm$ 0.3	74.4 $\pm$ 27.0
9.6	18.3 $\pm$ 7.9	18.7 $\pm$ 10.7	14.2 $\pm$ 6.9	1.4 $\pm$ 0.6	68.4 $\pm$ 21.7
16	30.7 $\pm$ 9.7	14.5 $\pm$ 6.2	9.7 $\pm$ 4.1	0.4 $\pm$ 0.6	84.2 $\pm$ 21.2
24	41.6 $\pm$ 20.7	9.6 $\pm$ 3.8	8.3 $\pm$ 4.9	0.3 $\pm$ 0.3	84.8 $\pm$ 17.2
33.6	44.3 $\pm$ 18.7	10.4 $\pm$ 5.1	4.2 $\pm$ 1.2	0	79.9 $\pm$ 19.8
43.2	46.7[b]	12.7	5.5	0	64.9

[a] Mean $\pm$ S.D. of mean daily excretion by 3 patients at each dosage except 43.2 g/m^2/d. Mean daily excretion for each patient was based on the 24 hour excretion of HMBA and each metabolite on days 2, 3, 4, and 5 of the 5 day continous infusion.

[b] Daily excretion by the one patient treated with 43.2 g/m^2/d. Values represent the excretion from day 1 of treatment only because insufficient material remained from urine voided on days 2, 3, 4, and 5.

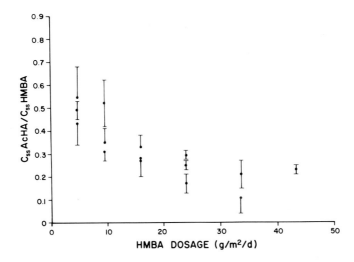

FIG. 4. Relationship of steady-state concentrations of 6-acetamido-hexanoic acid to those of HMBA at different HMBA dosages. Points, means for individual patients; bars, SD. Ratios of plasma concentrations of 6-acetamidohexanoic acid to those of HMBA in plasma samples obtained at 24, 47, 71, 95, and 120 h in the 120-h infusion of HMBA were used to calculate means $\pm$ SD

themselves to account for the anion gap encountered in those patients. In addition, documentation of the metabolic pathways for the interconversion of HMBA and its metabolites has implications with regard to the drug's associated neurotoxicity. Consideration of the potential metabolites produced by sequential beta oxidation of AmHA yields gamma aminobutyric acid and glycine, each a known neurotransmitter. Ongoing in vivo work in our laboratories is attempting to define and quantify the degree of such metabolism.

A final aspect of the clinical pharmacology and metabolism of HMBA involves documentation of the enzymes responsible for each metabolic step. Our laboratory has shown that monoamine oxidase is the sole enzyme responsible for conversion of NADAH to AcHA and that diamine oxidase is the enzyme responsible for converting DAH to AmHA (Fig. 1) (7). As described earlier, this information may prove clinically exploitable through trials combining monoamine oxidase inhibitors with HMBA in attempts to increase the dosage of HMBA that can be delivered.

At this time, a number of clinical trials of HMBA are ongoing or are planned. Some of these are phase I trials aimed at evaluating various pharmacologic aspects of HMBA or evaluating various maneuvers that might mitigate the drug's known toxicities and thereby allow higher doses of drug to be delivered. Included in this group of trials are the UMCC's evaluation of sodium bicarbonate as a means to ameliorate HMBA-associated acidosis. Also in this class of studies is an ongoing collaborative trial of the Walter Reed Army Medical Center and the NIH which is using enterally administered solutions of HMBA. This trial is delivering HMBA by nasogastric tube due to the unpalatable nature of the drug and is trying to assess a number of pharmacokinetic issues such as: 1) the bioavailability of HMBA when delivered in this fashion; 2) the rate of absorption of an enterally administered dose; 3) the peak concentrations achieved with various enterally administered doses; and 4) whether suitable plasma concentrations can be maintained with a reasonable schedule of enterally given drugs. In a complementary activity, efforts are being directed at producing a suitable capsule or tablet formulation of HMBA. These pharmaceutical efforts are being undertaken with the realization that it may be unrealistic to deliver an efficacious dose of approximately 50 g/d as 1 g tablets. On the other hand, such a formulation may be a very useful alternative to a 30-day continuous infusion of low-dose HMBA if the Memorial Sloan Kettering trial in bladder cancer provides encouraging results.

A second group of ongoing or planned clinical trials are being pursued in selected tumor types in an effort to document some therapeutic efficacy of HMBA. Included in this group of studies are 3 trials of HMBA in myelodysplastic syndromes, the Memorial Sloan Kettering Cancer Center's trial in bladder cancer, a trial in oral leukoplakia, and a trial in uterine cervical dysplasia. Each of these disease entities has been considered one in which tissue accessibility and the availability of objective measures of cellular differentiation will allow careful investigation of possible therapeutic pharmacodynamic responses to HMBA. Each of these studies is relatively early in its course and data with regard to their results has not been published. It is these trials that will provide important clinical data with regard to HMBA during the next year.

REFERENCES

1. American Cancer Society. (1983): Unproven methods of cancer management: Dimethylsulfoxide (DMSO). CA, 33:122-125.
2. Block, A.: (1984): **Cancer Treat. Rep.**, 68:199-205.
3. Calabressi, P., Dexter, D.L. and Heppner, G.H. (1979): **Biochem. Pharmacol.**, 28:1933-1941.
4. Callery, P.S., Egorin, M.J., Geelhaar, L.A. and Nayar, M.S.B. (1986): **Cancer Res.**, 46:4900-4903.

5. Chun, H., Leyland-Jones, B. and Hoth, D. (1986): **Cancer Treat. Rep.,** 70:991-996.
6. Collins, S.J., Bodner, A., Ting, R. and Gallo, R.C. (1980): **Int. J. Cancer,** 25:213-218.
7. Conley, B.A., Callery, P.S., Egorin, M.J., Subramanyam, B., Geelhaar, L. and Pan, S. (1987): **Proc. Am. Assoc. Cancer Res.,** 28:311.
8. Egorin, M.J., Sigman, L.M., Van Echo, D.A., Forrest, A., Whitacre, M.Y. and Aisner, (1987): **J. Cancer Res.,** 47:617-623.
9. Egorin, M.J., Zuhowski, E.G., Cohen, A.E., Geelhaar, L.A., Callery, P.S. and Van Echo, D.A. (1987): **Cancer Res.** (in press).
10. Ettinger, D.S., Orr, D.W., Rice, A.P. and Donehowr, R.C. (1985): **Cancer Treat. Rep.,** 69:489-493.
11. Fibach, E., Reuben, R.C., Rifkind, R.A. and Marks, P.A. (1977): **Cancer Res.,** 37:440-444.
12. Forrest, A., Conley, B., Egorin, M., Zuhowski, E., Bachur, N.R. and Van Echo, D.A. (1987): **Proc. Am. Soc. Clin. Oncol.,** 6:39.
13. Forrest, A., Egorin, M.J., Zuhowski, E. and Van Echo, D.A. (1987): **Clin. Pharmacol. Therap.,** 41:178.
14. Gazitt, Y. and Friend, C. (1980): **Cancer Res.,** 40:1727-1732.
15. Hughes, E., Schut, H.A.J. and Thorgeirsson, S.S. (1982): **In Vitro,** 18:157-164.
16. Kloog, Y., Axelrod, J. and Spector, I. (1983): **J. Neurochem.,** 40:522-529.
17. Marks, P.A. and Rifkind, R.A. (1984): **Cancer,** 54:2766-2769.
18. McGuire, W.P., Rowinsky, E.K., Ettinger, D.S., Grochow, L.B., Luk, G.D. and Donehower, R.C. (1987): **Proc. Am. Assoc. Cancer Res.,** 28:193.
19. McVie, J.G., tenBokkel Huinink, W.W., Simonetti, G. and Dubbelman, R. (1984): **Cancer Treat. Rep.,** 68:607-610.
20. O'Dwyer, P.J., Donehower, M., Sigman, L.M., Fortner, R.C., Aisner, J. and Van Echo, D.A. (1985): **J. Clin. Oncol.,** 3:853-857.
21. Orr, D.W., Ettinger, D.S., Rice, A.P., Colvin, O.M., Grochow, L.B. and Donehower, R.C. (1983): **Proc. Am. Soc. Clin. Oncol.,** 2:24.
22. Palfrey, C., Kimhi, Y., and Littauer, U.Z. (1977): **Biochem. Biophys. Res. Comm.,** 76:937-942.
23. Rabson, A.S., Stern, R., Tralka, T.S., Costa, J. and Wilczek, J. (1977): **Proc. Natl. Acad. Sci. USA,** 74:5060-5064.
24. Reuben, R.C. (1979): **Biochim. Biophys. Acta,** 588:310-321.
25. Reuben, R.C., Khanna, P.L., Gazitt, Y., Breslow, R., Rifkind, R.A. and Marks, P.A. (1978): **J. Biol. Chem.,** 253:4214-4218.
26. Reuben, R.C., Rifkind, R.A. and Marks, P.A. (1980): **Biochim. Biophys. Acta,** 605:325-346.
27. Reuben, R.C., Wife, R.L., Breslow, R., Rifkind, R.A. and Marks, P.A. (1976): **Proc. Natl. Acad. Sci. USA,** 73:862-866.

28. Rowinsky, E.K., Ettinger, D.S., Grochow, L.S., Brundrett, R.B., Cates, A.E. and Donehower, R.C. (1986): **J. Clin. Oncol.,** 4:1835-1844.

29. Rowinsky, E.K., McGuire, W.P., Anhalt, .J., Ettinger, D.S. and Donehower, R.W. (1987): **Cancer Treat. Rep.,** 71:471-474.

30. Sartorelli, A.C. (1985): **Br. J. Cancer,** 52:293-302.

31. Speers, W.C., Birdwell, C.R. and Dixon, F.J. (1979): **Am. J. Pathol.,** 97:563-584.

32. Sporn, M.B., Roberts, A.B. and Driscoll, J.S. (1985): In: **Cancer Principles and Practice of Oncology,** edited by V.T. Devita, S. Hellman, and S.A. Rosenberg, S.A. Second edition, pp. 49-65, J.B. Lippincott Co., Philadelphia.

33. Spremulli, E.N. and Dexter, D.L. (1984): **J. Clin. Oncol.,** 2:227-241.

34. Tanaka, M., Levy, J., and Terada, M. (1975): **Proc. Natl. Acad. Sci.,** 72: 1003-1006.

35. Tauer, K., Kemeny, N. and Hollander, P. (1985): **Proc. Annu. Meet. Am. Assoc. Cancer Res.,** 26:169.

36. Walsh, T.D., Fanucchi, M.P., Williams, L., Lokos, G., Stevens, Y.-W., Cassidy, C. and Young, C.W. (1987): **Proc. Am. Assoc. Cancer Res.,** 28:188.

37. Wiemann, M.C., Cummings, F.J., Posner, M.R., Weens, J.H., Crabtree, G.W., Birmingham, B.K., Moore, A., and Calabresi, P. (1985): **Proc. Am. Soc. Clin. Oncol.,** 4:38.

38. Yagoda, K., Sternberg, C., Scher, H. and Hollander, P. (1985): **Proc. Am. Soc. Clin. Oncol.,** 4:105.

FUTURE STRATEGIES

The Incorporation of Differentiation Induction into the Design of Cancer Therapy

S. Waxman and F. Takaku*

*Division of Medical Oncology, Mt. Sinai School of Medicine,
1 Gustave L. Levy Place, New York, NY 10021;*
Third Departments of Internal Medicine, University of Tokyo, Tokyo, Japan

INTRODUCTION

The unstable phenotype of neoplasia, predicted by developmental biologists, well recognized by experimental pathologists and clinical oncologists for many years, and now being defined at the molecular level, is ready to be utilized therapeutically. Most current cancer therapies, based on maximal cytotoxicity, fail to exploit the unstable phenotype of the cancer cell, and in practice are neutralized by provoking the emergence of a more malignant phenotype and/or drug resistance. In contrast, several cytotoxic agents alter gene expression in tumor cells and induce differentiation and a commitment to terminal cell division (TCD) in vitro (Table 1) and in vivo (see reviews in this volume). This differentiation property may not be directly related to the cytotoxic mechanism of the drug, occurs at lower drug levels, and can be augmented by combination with other drugs and physiologic factors. Therefore, the gene alterations associated with cytotoxic based therapy may be more characteristic of the tumor cell than its normal component, and may contribute to the success or failure of the treatment (13). The rationale for the introduction of differentiation induction into the design of cancer therapy will be critically reviewed using leukemia as the best studied model. An attempt will then be made to develop a design for differentiation induction as part of cancer therapy based on information provided by the participants in the Conference on Differentiation Therapy.

LEUKEMIA AS A MODEL FOR DIFFERENTIATION THERAPY

Studies on the differentiation of myeloid leukemic blast cells started with mouse MI cells. These cells were shown by Ichikawa to differentiate into granulocytes and macrophages by a conditioned medium of mouse embryo cells in which there was a factor - later termed D-factor (4). Subsequent studies by others demonstrated that differentiation of Friend leukemia cells into erythroid cells could be induced by dimethyl sulfoxide (DMSO) (3), and several human leukemia cell lines were established which were susceptible to various differentiation inducers. The most frequently used human leukemia cell lines for the study of differentiation are HL-60 and K562. Many factors or compounds have been shown to differentiate leukemic blast cells into granulocytes, macrophages and erythroid cells in in vitro culture conditions. Various differentiation inducing agents and human leukemia cell lines susceptible to such agents are listed in Table 1.

It has also been demonstrated that fresh human leukemic cells can undergo differentiation after administration of retinoic acid and 1a,25-dihydroxycholecalciferol (Vitamin D_3). These vitamin derivatives have been used clinically in the treatment of skin diseases or osteoporosis, and their safety is well documented. In clinical trials they have been given to patients with acute myeloid leukemia (AML), as well as to patients with refractory anemia who have an excess of blast cells (RAEB). However, administration of these agents in increasing doses to patients was limited by their toxicity, and though there are several reports on the efficacy of these vitamin derivatives in the treatment of acute promyelocytic leukemia (APL) or RAEB, the results have not always been conclusive. More evidence is needed to demonstrate that human leukemic blast cells have actually been differentiated in vivo by these agents. Assuming that differentiation has occurred, does it necessarily mean that it is the contributing factor to the remission observed in patients treated with these vitamin derivatives?

Cytosine arabinoside (Ara-C), thioguanine and aclacinomycin are known to induce differentiation of human leukemic cell lines in vitro, as shown in Table 1. These findings have provided the rationale for using low doses of Ara-C for the treatment of

TABLE I. <u>Differentiation Inducing Agents and Cell Lines Responding to These Inducers.</u>

Differentiation Inducing Agents	Cell Line	Differentiated Cells
I. Proteins		
D-factor	HL-60	G
Arginase/Histone H/Proteinase	HL-60/K562	M
II. Lipids		
o-alkylphospholipid/ ganglioside GM3	HL-60/M1-1,2,3/U937	M
neolacto long chain ganglioside	HL-60	G
short chain fatty acid	K562	E
III. Vitamins		
Retinoic acid	HL-60/H1-92	G/M
1α25 dihydroxy D₃	HL-60	M
B₁₂	K562	E
IV. Polar compounds		
Dimethylsulfoxide	HL-60/ML-1/HL-92/PL-21	G
Hexamethylene-bis-acetamide	HL-60	G
V. Nucleic acids & BSA Derivatives		
Cytosine arabinoside	HL-60/ML-1	G/M
	K562/KMOE	E
6-thioguanine/5-fluorouracil	K562	E
VI. Carcinogenesis promotors		
TPA/Teleocitidine	HL-60/ML-1/KG-1/K562/ THp-1/RC-2A	M
	K562/CMK	Meg
VII. Antibiotics and Inhibitors of Nucleic acid synthesis		
Bleomycin/Mitomycin C/ Actinomycin D	K562	E
Acitnomycin D/Aclacinomycin	HL-60/K562	M
VIII. Polysaccharide and Inhibitors of Polysaccharide		
Latosillan/Tunicamycin	HL-60	M
IX. Others		
Hemin/δ-aminolevulinate/ Dithiothreitol/Cadeverine/ Ouabain	K562/KMOE/HEL	E

smoldering refractory acute leukemia or myelodysplastic syndrome. Treatment of these disorders by
low dose Ara-C induced complete or partial remissions. It is difficult to demonstrate that low dose
Ara-C did, in fact, induce differentiation of
leukemic cells. However, the report by Fearon et al.
(2) demonstrated the persistence of single dominant
hematopoietic clones in granulocytes of patients with
acute non-lymphocytic leukemia after complete
remission, which suggests in vivo differentiation of
leukemic cells. Further evidence for differentiation
induction of human leukemic blast cells in vivo
associated with the remission of leukemia is urgently
needed.

Future strategies for the development of
differentiation therapy involves the discovery or
development of new agents to treat human
hematopoietic malignancies. Among the recently
reported differentiating agents, granulocyte colony
stimulating factor (G-CSF) is considered the most
promising. Differentiation of mouse leukemic blasts
such as WEHI-3 or MI cells by mouse G-CSF and human
G-CSF is well documented (7,11). Fresh human
leukemic blast cells can also be induced to
differentiate to a more mature granulocytic series by
exposing them to G-CSF in vitro. Though the differentiating activity of G-CSF is less than that of
purified D-factor, and not all leukemic blast cells
have receptors for G-CSF, this hematopoietic factor,
which is now available as a pure recombinant product
(10), has the advantage of not causing any significant side effects. Phase I and II studies of human
recombinant G-CSF revealed almost no side effects
except for a marked increase of granulocyte counts,
which was associated with neither subjective nor
objective symptoms. It is expected that recombinant
G-CSF or other recombinant hematopoietic factors will
become readily available and be clinically tested for
differentiation therapy of human leukemias. Recent
reports by Yuo et al. (14) on in vitro G-CSF
activation of granulocyte functions in myelodysplastic syndrome suggest that G-CSF will be a
useful treatment in this syndrome.

Biological response modifiers (BRM) such as
interferons (IFN) can be used for differentiation
therapy. Gavosto et al. (see review in this volume)
reported the results of a multicenter trial on the
effectiveness of IFN- gamma in the treatment of
myelodysplastic syndrome. Degos and his co-workers
(see Sigaux et al. review in this volume), based on

the results of his group's experiments, hypothesized that IFN-alpha exerts its action on Hairy-Cell Leukemia through inhibition of an autocrine loop involving a B Cell Growth Factor (BCGF) -like molecule. It appears reasonable to speculate that an increasing number of BRM will be introduced into clinical trials in the near future for differentiation therapy of leukemias as single agents, or in combination with other BRM, or with anti-leukemic agents.

The combination of differentiation inducing agents and low doses of conventional anti-leukemic chemotherapeutic agents represents another possibility for clinical application of differentiation therapy. Efficacy of this combination has been demonstrated by animal experiments (5). Rationale for this combination is the suppression of the production of an inhibitor of differentiation by anti-leukemic chemotherapeutic agents (Hozumi et al., see review in this volume). Many trials are being carried out to determine the best combination.

Alterations of the expression of some oncogenes, especially c-myb and c-myc, in association with the differentiation of myeloid cells, has been reported. Though the significance of oncogene alterations has not yet been clarified, differentiation therapy in leukemia, by modifying these oncogenes or their expression, may become feasible in the future. If the gene(s) regulating the differentiation of myeloid cells can be cloned, it may be possible to clarify the molecular mechanism of the defect in differentiation in leukemia cells, and treat leukemia by manipulating the differentiation gene.

This Conference has presented data to demonstrate that the clinical responses of two unusual leukemias (Hairy Cell and APL) by two non-cytotoxic agents (interferon-alpha and trans-retinoic acid, respectively) is probably due to differentiation induction (Sigaux et al., Degos et al., see review). However, the remissions were not sustained with or without further treatment. The remission of AML following treatment with cytotoxic drug regimens in some patients is associated with evidence of in vivo differentiation (Raza et al., see review in this volume). The failure to cure these patients may be partially explained by the evolution of a proliferative clone not controlled or responsive to differentiation induction.

This result can be predicted from the work of Scott and others reviewed in this volume. Their models demonstrate that the outcome of the cancer cell placed in a G_o-G_1 growth arrest by nutrient restriction, and theoretically as a result of cytotoxic drugs, may be differentiation induction with or without TCD, proliferation without differentiation, or TCD without differentiation. These four different responses are cell-type specific, dependent on local exogenous factors, can be recognized in vitro by commitment assays and in vivo by morphology and markers for differentiation, and should be considered in the development of therapeutic design (Fig 1).

THE INCORPORATION OF DIFFERENTIATION INDUCTION INTO CANCER THERAPY

In order to initiate maximal tumor cell reduction, a schematic therapeutic cycle should begin with high dose conventional cytotoxic agents for lethal, anti-proliferative effects (Fig. 1). In addition to cell death, these agents should also cause non-lethal growth arrest in some cells (dependent on cell cycle) making them more responsive to differentiation induction. This can be followed by lower (non-cytotoxic) doses of the same or similar type agents with differentiation induction capability in combination with other differentiation inducers (see Table 1) for 7 days of continuous treatment based on optimal synergistic levels (8,12). This should commit a population of tumor cells to TCD. The combination of cytotoxic agents (i.e., mitomycin, irradiation) to disturb DNA synthesis with a chemical differentiation inducer (i.e. DMSO) is synergistic for the induction of differentiation and TCD of MEL cells. Oishi and co-workers have identified two differentiation factors which offer a biochemical basis for this observation (see review in this volume by Watanabe et al.). Evidence, both in vitro and in vivo, to support this combination is presented by the working group on Clinical Trials of Differentiation also reported in this volume. The pre-clinical and clinical studies of HMBA by Rifkind et al. and Egorin (see review) provide further bases for introducing polar solvents in trial with conventional cytotoxic chemotherapy.

The choice of anti-proliferative cytotoxic agent(s) will continue to be tumor cell type specific. However, these agents should be assessed

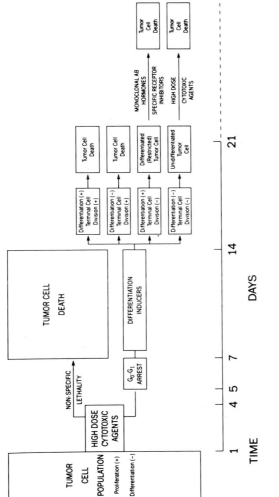

INCORPORATION OF DIFFERENTIATION INDUCTION INTO THE DESIGN OF CANCER THERAPY

Figure 1

for differentiation induction, particularly at various concentrations. In the three dimensional primary culture of human squamous cell carcinomas described by Chang et. al. (see review), agents such as IFN gamma and TNF alpha caused cell death in part through induction of differentiation. Cytotoxic agents known to affect squamous cell carcinoma cells such as radiation and bleomycin, should be studied for differentiation induction in this system. The mechanism responsible for the loss of proliferation following treatment with cytotoxic agents should be separated into non-specific toxicity and differentiation induction. Previous studies using analogues of purine nucleosides, anthracyclines and mitomycin to separate non-specific cytotoxicity from differentiation induced TCD suggest that drug structural design may allow for more selective anti-proliferative therapy. Pharmacologic structure correlation with the biologic mechanism of anti-proliferation may also be studied by evaluating the effect of various analogues of cytotoxic agents on specific oncogene expression in the tumor being studied. This may become more significant when the therapeutic strategy is developed for eradicating the differentiated-proliferating tumor cell if a malfunction or overabundance of one or more of these oncogenes is detected.

The scheduled combination of high-dose anti-proliferative cytotoxic agents with differentiation inducers (low dose cytotoxic, chemical, biologic and physiologic) could result in a markedly reduced tumor cell population with a restricted (differentiated) phenotype (6). The tumor cell with the restricted phenotype may be less divergent, more homogeneous and responsive to selective therapy such as hormones, monoclonal antibodies and biological modulation. Further studies are necessary to determine whether this differentiated but proliferative tumor cell population will exhibit a decrease in malignant phenotype and drug resistance. The undifferentiated tumor cell population remains the target for a new cycle of combination cytotoxic and differentiation therapy.

When considering gene expression in the design of differentiation therapy, the effect on normal tissue, pre-neoplastic cells and the fully transformed cell must be considered. The analysis of differentiation related proteins and mRNA localization in mouse normal skin, papillomas and squamous carcinomas is an excellent model for this purpose (see review by Yuspa and Roop). Identification of specific differentiation defects in the transformed cell may be helpful in evaluating differentiation inducers in vitro and in vivo. Similarly, it is possible to measure the selectivity of recombinant hematopoietic growth and differentiation factors, using long-term (Dexter) bone marrow cultures, in normal and leukemic cells (Moore and Dexter, see review).

The responsiveness of tumor cells (i.e., myeloid leukemia cell lines) to differentiation inducers is asynchronous, heterogeneous and unstable, and during long-term culture subpopulations of resistant cells appear. Resistance has been reported to be associated with the production of an inhibitory protein factor which could be reversed by treatment with low concentrations of RNA or protein inhibitors (Hozumi et al., see review). The emergence of differentiation resistant cells was prevented by the combined use of a differentiation inducer and a cytotoxic drug in long-term culture of luekemic cells. These findings support the concept that combination differentiation therapy is not only synergistic in promoting TCD but may also suppress the emergence of differentiation resistant cells.

The enhancement of the level of commitment to differentiation and TCD is an important area for further research. Leukemic cells obtain "commitment-memory" during brief exposure to differentiation agents which can be called upon for a rapid commitment to differentiation and TCD in the presence of other differentiation inducers (see review by Hickman and Friedman). Such interactions between HMBA and DMSO were recently demonstrated by DiMambro et al. (1). The use of "commitment memory" can simplify differentiation therapy and perhaps decrease the duration and toxicity. Although the biochemical mechansims involved in commitment remain to be determined there are several enzyme and oncogene alterations that have been associated with the process, which could be used to monitor therapeutic efficacy.

ADDITIONAL SITES FOR THE APPLICATION OF DIFFERENTIATION TO CANCER THERAPY

If, as suggested by Christman (see review in this volume), most tumors result from a combination of enhanced expression of altered oncogenes and inactivation of dominant suppressor genes, then a drug such as 5 azacytidine or its deoxy-derivative may be effective by activating a wide spectrum of genes. Preliminary studies in patients with myelodysplastic disease treated with 5-azacytidine show some benefit, but have not been studied for oncogene expression and differentiation in a manner similar to that reported in this meeting by Preisler et al. A major concern is the evidence that a variety of familial and sporadic human tumors are associated with the loss of both functional alleles of a gene whose role is presumably to produce protein(s) that act as suppressors of tumor development (9). As discussed by Ellen Solomon at this meeting, major progress has been made in cloning and analysis of several of these genes. Whether the irreversible loss of tumor suppression activity can be compensated by inducing differentiation genes remains to be determined.

The pivotal role that the cell surface membrane plays in the action of growth factors, differentiation inducers and cell-cell and cell-stromal actions has been demonstrated (see review by Lotan and Abita). The design of combination differentiation therapy can include exploiting membrane events by inhibiting receptors that make the tumor cell less responsive to growth factors, so that they accumulate in the G_1 phase of the cell cycle and become more responsive to differentiation induction. Signal transduction may be modulated as a result which may lead to alterations in gene expression. The tumor cell membrane can be induced to increase existing receptors so that its growth can be inhibited by physiologic factors or by immunological mechanisms. Retinoids, G-CSF, tumor necrosis factor, interleukin-2 and interferon(s) may be useful for this action.

In addition to treating the tumor at the cellular level, a scheme must be designed for dealing with the tumor as a multi-cellular tissue or organ. As the tumor cellular population changes spontaneously through multiple divisions, or as a result of therapeutic interventions, the tumor as an organ becomes unstable. Cell-cell and cell-stromal interactions play a significant role in normal fetal developmental processes, but is less well documented in neoplastic development (see review by Medina and Huberman). Differentiation and proliferation of tumor cells can be modulated by direct cell contact and by diffusable factors produced by stromal

cells. Conversely, the expression of stromal cell
functions can be modulated by specific inducers,
(e.g., Vitamin D_3, TGFbeta) that further influence
growth factors and also affect tumor cell adhesion.
The loss of cell-cell relations and local breakdown
of tissue boundaries are characteristic of malignant
epithelial neoplasms. Further malignant progression
requires neovascularization, and thus the tumor as an
organ becomes "angiogenesis dependent" (see review by
Ingber and Folkman). Hence, specific inhibitors of
capillary growth interfere with malignant histodifferentiation and provide another non-cytotoxic
focus into the design of cancer therapy (see review
by Ingber and Folkman). The development of pharmacologic methods for controlling extracellular matrix
metabolism could provide additional means of controlling tumor progression by inhibiting tumor cell
responsiveness to soluble angiogenic factors and
provoke capillary involution.

SUMMARY

Early recognition and prevention of cancer will
be based on the identification of clonal abnormalities by probes for specific DNA sequences. It is
possible that this will be associated with abnormalities in specific gene expressions that can be the
site of differentiation directed therapy. Biological
characteristics of the fully transformed cell, such
as invasiveness and metastatic ability, are due to
gene alterations and their protein products may be
redirected or blocked by differentiation inducers.
Experimental models utilizing the two stage carcinogenesis assay suggest a role for new oncogene
expression in pre-neoplasias and a subsequent co-
carcinogenic event in the progression to complete
neoplastic transformation. The identification of the
genes and gene products responsible for these biological phases of malignant transformation should
also allow for the development of more specific
differentiation therapy. In the complete expression
of malignancy with manifest disease, it is most
probable that non-specific, cytotoxic chemotherapy
together with combination differentiation therapy
will continue to be the basis of cytoreductive
therapy. However, more predictable tumor extinction
will require the design of cytotoxic agents which
have differentiation capability and can be synergis-

tic when combined with agents designed to alter specific gene expression for commitment to differentation and/or TCD.

ACKNOWLEDGEMENTS

The authors wish to acknowledge all of the Participants in the Conference on Differentiation Therapy for their co-operation in sending their progress reports to their co-chairmen. We also wish to acknowledge all of our corporate sponsors, as well as NIH grant G45381, which was awarded to the Conference. Finally, we wish to thank Serono Symposia for their continuing support of our efforts.

REFERENCES

1. DiMambro, E., Galanti, M., and Levy, S.B. (1987): Blood, 70:1565-1571.
2. Fearon, E.R., Burke, P.J., Schiffer, C.A., Zehnbauer, B.A., and Vogelstein, B. (1986): New Eng. J. Med., 315:15-24.
3. Friend, C., Scher, W., Holland, J.F., and Sato, T. (1971): Proc. Natl. Acad. Sci. USA, 18:378-382.
4. Ichikawa, Y. (1969): J. Cell Physiol., 74:223-234.
5. Kasukabe, T., Honma, Y., Hozumi, M., Suda, T., and Nishii, Y. (1987): Cancer Res., 47:567-572.
6. Lotan, R., and Nicholson, G.L. (1987): Biochem. Pharmacol. (in press).
7. Nicola, N.A., and Metcalf, D. (1984): Proc. Natl. Acad. Sci. USA, 81:3765-3769.
8. Scher, W., Scher, B.M., and Waxman, S. (1983): Exp. Hematol., 11:490-498.
9. Solomon, E., Voss, R., Hall, V., Bodmer, W.F., Jass, J.R., Jeffreys, A.J., Lucibello, F.C., Patel, I., and Rider, S.J. (1987): Nature, 328:616-618.
10. Souza, L.H., Boone, T.C., Gabrilove, J., Lai, P.H., Zsebo, K.M., Murdock, D.C., Chazin,V.R., Bruszweski, J., Lu, H., Chen, K.K., Barendt, J., Platzer, E., Moore, M.A.S., Mertelsmann, R., and Welte, K. (1986): Science, 232:61-65.
11. Tomida, M., Yamamoto-Yamaguchi, Y., Hozumi, M., Okabe, T., and Takaku, F. (1986): FEBS Letter, 207:271-275.
12. Waxman, S., Scher, W., and Scher, B.M. (1986): Cancer Det. and Preven. 9:395-407.

13. Waxman, S. (1987): Cancer Invest. (in press)
14. Yuo, A., Kitagawa, S., Okabe, T., and Takaku, F. (1986): FEBS Letter 207:271-275.

Subject Index